Cervical Cancer

Cervical Cancer
A Guide for Nurses

Ruth Dunleavey

Department of Haematology/Medical Oncology
St Vincents Hospital
Sydney, Australia

⟨W⟩WILEY-BLACKWELL

A John Wiley & Sons, Ltd., Publication

This edition first published 2009
© 2009 John Wiley & Sons

Wiley-Blackwell is an imprint of John Wiley & Sons, formed by the merger of Wiley's global Scientific, Technical and Medical business with Blackwell Publishing.

Registered office
John Wiley & Sons Ltd, The Atrium, Southern Gate, Chichester, West Sussex PO19 8SQ, United Kingdom

Editorial office
John Wiley & Sons Ltd, The Atrium, Southern Gate, Chichester, West Sussex PO19 8SQ, United Kingdom

For details of our global editorial offices, for customer services and for information about how to apply for permission to reuse the copyright material in this book please see our website at www.wiley.com/wiley-blackwell.

Library of Congress Cataloging-in-Publication Data

Dunleavey, Ruth.
    Cervical cancer : a guide for nurses / Ruth Dunleavey.
        p.   ;   cm.
    Includes bibliographical references.
    ISBN 978-0-470-06101-5 (pbk. : alk. paper)   1. Cervix uteri–Cancer–Nursing.   I. Title.
    [DNLM: 1. Uterine Cervical Neoplasms–Nurses' Instruction.   WP 480 D921c 2009]
    RC280.U8D86 2009
    616.99′466–dc22
                                                                    2008032238

A catalogue record for this book is available from the British Library.

Set in 9.5 on 10.5 pt Sabon by SNP Best-set Typesetter Ltd., Hong Kong
Printed in Singapore by Markono Print Media Pte Ltd

1   2009

Contents

Acknowledgements

I would like to thanks the following people for their suggestions, reviewing chapters or general help:

Rosie Millar, Aberdeen Royal Infirmary
Alison Griffiths, Medway NHS Trust
Martha Rabwoni, Palliative Care Association, Uganda
Rose Kiwanuka, Palliative Care Association, Uganda
Richard Hillman, Westmead Hospital, Sydney
St Vincent Hospital Sydney Library staff
Ellen Barlow, Royal Hospital for Women, Randwick, Sydney
Mary Ryan, Royal Hospital for Women, Randwick, Sydney
Alison Nightingale, Jo's Trust
Philip Beale, Sydney Cancer Centre
Johnathon Carter, Sydney Cancer Centre
Norelle Lickiss, Royal Hospital for Women, Sydney
Gerald Wain, Westmead Hospital, Sydney
Isabel White, Cancer Research UK Nursing Research Training Fellow
Gill Sanderson, Sue Ryder Care, Nettlebed
Carol Stott, Royal Hospital for Women, Sydney
Ian Frazer, Princess Alexandra Hospital, Brisbane
Susan Jolley, Nottingham University Hospitals Trust
Sheree Patterson, Royal Hospital for Women, Sydney
Anne Merriman, Palliative Care Association, Uganda
Sally Watts, Royal Hospital for Women, Sydney
Emma Chaplin, Southend Hospital
Lorna Maule, Ninewells Hospital
Rose Kiwanuka, Palliative Care Association, Uganda
Nicky Carter, Royal Surrey County Hospital
Karen Donnelly, St Mary's Hospital, Manchester
Karen Johnson, Christie Hospital, Manchester
Kay Welton, Addenbrooks Hospital, Camberidge
Dr N Hacker, Royal Hospital for Women, Randwick, Sydney
Viet Doh, Westmead Hospital, Sydney
Tish Lancaster, Westmead Hospital, Sydney
Kathryn Nattress, Sydney Cancer Centre
Professor Michael Quinn, Royal Women's Hospital, Melbourne

Chapter 1

Dysplasia, HPV and cervical cancer

'In theory, recognition that a pandemic infection is responsible for more than half a million cancer cases each year would attract huge media attention and infection control would become the subject of preventative efforts from the global health agencies. Media attention would likely be particularly acute if the majority of deaths was among women rearing families in the developing world and if the disease were sexually transmitted. A vaccine capable of preventing the disease would be diligently pursued and, once available, promptly distributed for the health and welfare of humankind. Human papilloma virus (HPV) infection fits this scenario; however, HPV has yet to make an impact on either the media or public thinking as outlined in the previous paragraph, even though the link between HPV infection and cervical cancer has been recognised for more than 20 years.'

(Frazer et al. 2006)

Introduction

Our understanding of cervical cancer has increased enormously in recent years, principally through a greater appreciation of the role of the human papilloma virus (HPV). Whilst HPV alone does not cause cervical cancer, it is certainly an extremely important factor. Infection with the virus can trigger a number of cellular changes to the cervix which if left unchecked have the potential to develop into cervical cancer.

This chapter begins with a review of the worldwide incidence of cervical cancer. This is followed by a discussion of the form and function of the normal, healthy cervix and the pathological processes which can occur to disrupt it. The role of HPV in the development of cervical neoplasia is assessed, together with other causative factors. The different stages of pre-cancerous cellular abnormality are outlined, with a description of their cytological and histological grading systems. The final section of the chapter looks at the progression of abnormal cervical cells into carcinoma and describes the main staging system for squamous cell carcinoma of the cervix.

The size of the problem

Cervical cancer is the second most common cancer amongst women worldwide, accounting for more than 273,000 deaths a year – 9% of all female cancer deaths. One in ten female cancers diagnosed worldwide are cancers of the cervix (Ferlay et al. 2004).

The distribution of the disease is not uniform – cervical cancer rates are estimated to vary eight-fold throughout the world, with a seventeen-fold variation in mortality rates

(Ferlay et al. 2004, Sankaranarayanan and Ferlay 2006). This disparity in incidence is principally between developed and developing nations. Globally, cervical cancer accounts for over 2.7 million years of life lost among women between the ages of 25 and 64. When this is broken down by country, 2.4 million years of life lost occur in developing areas, with only 0.3 million in developed countries (Yang et al. 2004).

Within the UK, cervical cancer is the second most common cancer after breast cancer in women under the age of 35, with 625 new cases diagnosed in 2003 (Cancer Research UK 2006). Within Australia 1 in 183 women will develop cervical cancer by the age of 75 (Cancer Council 2006). The incidence and mortality rates of cervical cancer in the UK, USA and Australia are shown in Table 1.1 and some other cervical cancer facts and figures can be found in Box 1.1.

Largely as a result of cervical screening, cervical cancer rates within the developed world are, for the most part, falling. For example, in the UK the mortality rate fell by 60% between 1975 and 2004 (from 7.5 to 2.8 per 100,000 females) (Cancer Research UK 2006). There are a few exceptions to this trend. For reasons which are not really understood the mortality rate for cervical cancer is rising in a number of developed countries such as Spain, Romania and Bulgaria (Cancer Research UK 2006, Office for National Statistics 1999). Where cervical cancer is declining, there has been a concomitant increase in the diagnosis of carcinoma in situ in women under the age of 30 (Quinn et al. 2001). This is also attributable to the success of cervical screening programmes.

Table 1.1 Incidence and mortality rates from cervical cancer in developed countries (per 100,000 women)

	Incidence	Mortality
UK	8.3	3.1
Australia	6.9	1.7
USA	7.7	2.3

Source: www.dep-iarc.fr/GLOBOCAN 2002
Taken from National Health and Medical Research Council (NHMRC) powerpoint presentation) http://www.cancerscreening. gov.au/internet/screening/publishing.nsf/Content/FCB2AB96D1 D5E15BCA2571D80078876F/$File/presentation-june06.pdf (accessed 17/6/07)

Box 1.1 Cervical cancer statistics

Cervical cancer statistics: Australia

Cervical cancer is the thirteenth most common cancer in women in Australia
740 women are diagnosed with cervical cancer each year
270 women die of cervical cancer each year in Australia
http://www.nswcc.org.au/editorial.asp?pageid=54 (accessed 5/7/07)

Cervical cancer statistics: UK

Cervical cancer is the twelfth most common cancer in women in the UK
2800 women are diagnosed with cervical cancer each year
1100 women die of cervical cancer each year in the UK, giving a European age-standardised death rate of 2.8 per 100,000 females and a crude rate of 3.6 per 100,000.
http://info.cancerresearchuk.org/cancerstats/types/cervix/ (accessed 5/7/07)

The healthy cervix

The role of the cervix in a healthy woman is principally concerned with reproduction – it helps to keep the developing foetus in the uterus and has a part to play in the initiation and progression of labour. The mucus produced by the cervix is considered important in female fertility (Moghissi 1972). The cervix is also thought to have a function in the female sexual response (Grimes 1999).

The cervix is cylindrical in shape and lies in the inferior, fibromuscular part of the uterus, accounting for approximately one third of the uterus. The remaining two thirds of the uterus are known as the body or corpus. It is located within the pelvic cavity, posterior to the bladder and anterior to the recto-sigmoid and rectum. It is attached to the bladder by the two vesicouterine ligaments. The tissue lateral to the cervix between the paravesical and pararectal spaces is known as the parametrium. The nerve supply to the cervix is derived from the hypogastric plexus and its blood supply from the internal iliac arteries. Its regional lymph nodes include: the parametrial, external iliac, obturator, hypogastric (internal iliac) and common iliac.

The cervix generally measures about 3–4 cm in length and 2.5 cm in diameter, although its size varies according to age. At its upper boundary, where it meets the corpus of the uterus, there is a narrowing known as the isthmus or internal os. The lower boundary of the cervix is known as the external os and opens into the vagina – indeed, the lower half of the cervix protrudes into the vagina.

Within the cervix itself, the anatomy is subdivided into the *endocervix* and the *exocervix* or *ectocervix*. The endocervix is the name for the upper two thirds of the cervix and the ectocervix the lower two thirds – this is the part that is more easily visualised on colposcopic examination (see Chapter 2).

The ecto and endocervix are lined with two different types of epithelium – the endocervix with *columnar glandular epithelium* and the ectocervix with *squamous epithelium*. The squamous and glandular epithelium meet at the *squamocolumnar junction (SCJ)*. The squamocolumnar junction appears as a sharp line with a step due to the difference in the height of the squamous and columnar epithelium.

The cervix undergoes significant changes over a lifetime. Puberty, pregnancy and menopause all serve to alter its structure and location. For example, when a woman reaches puberty the cervix grows and the squamocolumnar junction moves down, exposing the

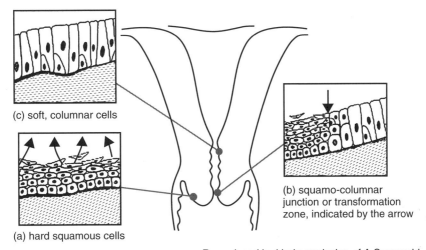

(c) soft, columnar cells

(a) hard squamous cells

(b) squamo-columnar junction or transformation zone, indicated by the arrow

Reproduced by kind permission of A Saraworld

Figure 1.1 Different types of epithelium within the cervix

thin, glandular epithelium of the endocervical canal to the acidic environment of the vagina. This leads to the destruction of the columnar epithelium which is replaced by newly formed *metaplastic squamous epithelium.*

The term *metaplasia* refers to the replacement of one type of epithelium with another. The region of the cervix where the columnar epithelium has been or is being replaced by the new metaplastic squamous epithelium is referred to as the *transformation zone*. It is at the transformation zone that most of the cellular abnormalities associated with cervical cancer arise.

After menopause the SCJ moves back up the endocervical canal and the cervix becomes smaller. Because the maturation of the squamous epithelium is dependent on oestrogen, after menopause the cells do not mature and the epithelium becomes thin and atrophic.

Types of cervical cancer

There are two main types of cervical cancer. The most common is squamous cell carcinoma (SCC) involving the squamous epithelium lining the ectocervix. However, a further 20% of cervical cancers are adenocarcinomas involving the glandular epithelial cells which are scattered along the endocervical canal (Scorge et al. 2004). A small percentage of cervical cancers are also composed of rare histological types such as lymphomas, sarcomas and neuroendocrine tumours.

This chapter will concentrate exclusively on squamous cell carcinoma because it is the most prevalent kind of cervical cancer. However, adenocarcinoma appears to be growing in incidence and is becoming an increasingly significant problem within the developed nations (Smith et al. 2000). Cervical adenocarcinoma, its pre-malignant phases and its management are discussed in Chapter 2.

Cervical cytology grading

One important factor which distinguishes cervical cancer from most other cancers is the fact that it is preceded by a long pre-cancerous phase. Changes to the cervix begin an average of 10 to 15 years before its progression into malignancy. A whole spectrum of events may occur before the development of cervical cancer, beginning with cellular atypia, then various grades of dysplasia and finally invasive disease. It is this feature of cervical cancer which allows the diagnosis and management of cervical abnormalities prior to the development of cancer.

The early detection of cervical abnormality relies – certainly within the developed world – on obtaining samples of the cervical epithelial cells for analysis. This is achieved by taking a Pap smear. Whilst in recent years a number of developments have been made in cervical cytology testing, the cervical smear remains the most important cervical screening test in the western world. Details of the Pap smear procedure are given in Chapter 2 and some of the terms used to describe cervical cellular abnormalities are explained in Box 1.2.

The Bethesda System (TBS)

Originally, all cervical smear test cytology samples were graded by the Papanicolaou Class System which was introduced in 1943 and used for about 40 years. Since then a number of grading systems have been developed in an effort to improve and standardise cervical cytology reporting. Perhaps the most important of these is the Bethesda System (TBS). 'The Bethesda System for Reporting Cervical/Vaginal Cytologic Diagnoses' was approved at a National Cancer Institute Workshop in the USA in 1988 (Anderson 2004). Development of the system had been prompted by much publicised media reports of women dying of cancer despite having cervical smears interpreted as normal (Cox 2005). Since then

---

Box 1.2 Some cytology terms seen on cervical smear reports (see also Table 1.3)

Dyskaryosis: an abnormality of nuclei seen in exfoliated cells, often cells from the uterine cervix, in which the cytoplasm remains unchanged but the nuclei exhibit hyperchromatism, irregularity or enlargement, or an increase in number. (It refers to the nuclear changes seen in cells derived from lesions histologically described as Cervical Intraepithelial Neoplasia or CIN). It is a term now rarely used outside the UK and has been replaced with Squamous Intraepithelial Lesion (SIL) (Johnson and Patnick 2000).
Dysplasia: abnormal development or growth of tissues, organs or cells.
Neoplasia: a pathological process that results in the formation and growth of a neoplasm.

Koilocytosis: a cavitation of cellular cytoplasm, usually as a result of viral infection. It is also sometimes called koilocytic atypia, and is seen as halo-like structures around the nuclei of the abnormal cells. Koilocytosis is not dysplasia but may be considered a 'pre-dysplastic' change in some cases.
http://medical-dictionary.thefreedictionary.com

---

there have been two revisions, one in 1991 and most recently in 2001. This system has subsequently been adopted in its original or a modified form in a number of countries around the world (see Table 1.2).

TBS grades cervical squamous cellular abnormalities from low to high severity. Low grade disease is referred to as low grade squamous intraepithelial lesions (LSIL), and high grade as high grade squamous intraepithelial lesions (HSIL). The next category of dysplasia refers to cancer cells.

The system also has two additional categories known as atypical squamous cells-unspecified (ASC-US) and atypical squamous cells-high grade (ASC-H). These terms were introduced in the 2001 amendments and replaced the previous category atypical squamous cells of undetermined significance (ASCUS – see Box 1.3). It is a classification applied to cells which are not normal but cannot easily be categorised into any of the other groups.

Most women with a diagnosis of ASC-US will on further investigation be found to have no serious pathology. Their cellular changes may have been caused by trauma from benign changes related to tampon use, intercourse, bacteria, yeast, viral infection with Human Papilloma Virus (HPV) or the cellular effects of aging (Cox 2005).

After extensive consultation by the Australian Society of Cytology, Australia also chose to adopt the Australian Modified Bethesda System in 2004. The National Health and Medical Research Council (NHMRC) approved Australian terminology is based on, but has some differences from, the Bethesda System 2001 (NHMRC 1994). The major differences relate to the classification of low-grade abnormalities.

The UK has different terminology for its categories of cervical abnormality, but these can to a greater extent be compared with the Bethesda System categories as illustrated in Table 1.2. The British altered their terminology and classification system in 2002 and brought it closer to TBS. Whilst there could be an argument for the British moving closer still to the Bethesda system, this would clearly have widespread ramifications for the current screening system, necessitating retraining of cytologists, clinicians, nurses and a whole range of ancillary staff including coders and data managers.

Within the developed world most cervical smears taken through screening programmes will turn out to be normal – nine out of ten in the UK. A small number will have pre-cancerous changes which can be treated. Less than 1 in 1000 will demonstrate invasive cancer (Cancer Research UK 2006) (See also Table 1.3).

Cervical histopathology grading

A histological diagnosis is considered to be the 'acid test' of a cancer and can provide information about the level of abnormality in the cervical tissue as a whole rather than

Table 1.2 Comparison of cervical cytology staging systems (Rana et al. 2004, NHMRC 2005)

BSCC Terminology (UK) 1986	The Bethesda System (USA) 2001	ECTP terminology (Europe)	Australian Modified Bethesda System (2004)
Negative	Negative for intraepithelial lesion or malignancy	Within normal limits	Negative
Inadequate	Unsatisfactory for evaluation	Unsatisfactory due to — (spec)	Unsatisfactory
Borderline nuclear change	(1) Atypical squamous cells of undetermined significance (ASC-US) (2) Atypical squamous cells possible high grade lesion (ASC-H)	(1) Koilocytes (without changes suggestive of intraepithelial neoplasia) (2) Squamous cell changes (not definitely neoplastic but merit early repeat)	(1) Possible low-grade squamous intraepithelial lesion (2) Possible high grade squamous lesion
Mild dyskaryosis	Low grade squamous intraepithelial lesion	Mild dysplasia (CIN 1)	Low grade squamous intraepithelial lesion
Moderate dyskaryosis	High grade squamous intraepithelial lesion	Moderate dysplasia	High grade squamous intraepithelial lesion
Severe dyskaryosis	High grade squamous intraepithelial lesion	(1) Severe dysplasia (CIN 3) (2) Carcinoma in situ (CIN 3)	High grade squamous intraepithelial lesion
Severe dyskaryosis/? Invasive	Squamous cell carcinoma	(1) Severe dysplasia ? invasive (2) Invasive squamous cell carcinoma	Squamous cell carcinoma

Box 1.3 Shades of grey

Cytology is subjective. With subjectivity comes great difference in interpretation, even among expert cytopathologists.

(Cox 2005)

Determination of the different levels of cytological abnormality in a cervical smear specimen is a task performed by a cytologist looking under a microscope. And it is not always easy.

The famous Californian photographer, Ansel Adams, always photographed in black and white and identified, for the purposes of his photography, nine different shades of grey. Parallels can be drawn with the reporting of cervical cytology. Whereas the highly normal and the highly abnormal cells are relatively simple to diagnose, it is the grey areas in the middle that are problematic. This category is the abnormal squamous cells of undetermined significance (ASCUS) classification.

It was proposed by some cytologists prior to the 2001 Bethesda update to abolish the ASCUS category but in doing this it was found that some high grade epithelial abnormalities would have been missed. Instead the 2001 review of TBS resulted in a break-down of the ASCUS category into two – ASC-US to include cytologic changes suggestive of a lesion but difficult to interpret fully, and ASC-H in which there are changes suggestive of a high grade lesion but once again inadequate criteria for a definite diagnosis (Smith 2001).

As Cox explains, the problem is that cytology is subjective, and with subjectivity comes difference in interpretation – even amongst cytologists. 'The ASCUS diagnosis is not reproducible. In fact, ASCUS is not a "diagnosis", but an interpretation that is very subjective' (Cox 2005).

The ALTS trial was a large study set up in the USA in order to look specifically at some of the issues associated with the management of low grade cervical lesions (ALTS 2003). Here it was found that only 43% of the Pap tests originally submitted as ASCUS by clinical centre pathologists were interpreted as ASCUS in a blinded review by pathologists involved in the trial (Stoler et al. 2001). It has been suggested that a large number of samples assigned to the ASC category in the USA is from concern over a 'missing lesion' and potential litigation that could result from this (Cox 2005).

Table 1.3 Abnormal cytology in NHS cervical screening programmes (as percentage of evaluable cervical smears)

	UK(Health and Social Care Information Centre Statistics 2005)
Year	2005–2006
Negative	93.8%
Borderline	3.2%
LSIL/mild dyskaryosis	1.8%
HSIL/moderate dyskaryosis	0.5%
HSIL/severe dyskaryosis	0.6%
Suspected invasive cancer or glandular neoplasia	0.1%

just amongst individual cells. Following the identification of an abnormality on cervical cytology, generally the next stage is to confirm the abnormality by performing a colposcopy. The colposcopy procedure is described in Chapter 2. The following section focuses on cervical histology grading and explains the commonly-used cervical intraepithelial neoplasia (CIN) system.

Whereas cytology grading systems have, to a certain extent, developed independently in different countries, histolopathologists tend to use the same system worldwide. Until the 1970s, cervical biopsies were graded as dysplastic, (mild, moderate or severe). The next category of dysplasia was referred to as squamous cell carcinoma in situ. This is known today as the World Health Organisation (WHO) grading system, but has now been replaced in many countries by the CIN system.

In 1973 Richart introduced the cervical intraepithelial neoplasia (CIN) system which has three levels. The CIN categories are:

- CIN 1: mild dysplasia in which the abnormal cells only occupy the basal half of the epithelium.
- CIN 2: moderate dysplasia whereby the cells occupy the basal two thirds of the epithelium.
- CIN 3: severe dysplasia with almost full thickness involvement of the epithelium by abnormal cells, leaving only a thin mantle of differentiated cells at the surface.

The next level of abnormality is carcinoma in situ (CIS) in which there is full thickness involvement of the epithelium by undifferentiated cells, but the basement membrane is still intact (Richart 1973, Chang 1990). Because both the cytologic and histologic differences between severe dysplasia and cervical carcinoma in situ are often subjective, CIN 3 encompasses both of these categories.

Correlating the cervical *cytology* result with cervical *histology* means translating a two-grade system (LSIL/HSIL) into a three grade system (CIN 1/2/3). This can sometimes be problematic for histologists and for this reason some prefer to apply the terms high and low grade lesions to histology samples as well as cytology samples. There is a call from some histologists to revise the whole histology grading system so that it reflects cytological grading more closely (Cooper et al. 1983).

Generally speaking, LSIL will be found to correspond to CIN1 on biopsy. Similarly, HSIL indicate at least CIN2. That said, even within low grade lesions there may be small areas of CIN2 or CIN3 which are not represented on the smear. Thus, the cytological degree of dyskaryosis should be taken to indicate the minimum degree of cellular abnormality that is likely to be present in the histology sample (Johnson and Patnick 2000).

As with cervical cytology, the CIN cervical histology grading system is reliant on humans and is therefore not perfect. The criteria are subjective, with significant levels of intra- and inter-observer variability (Schneider 2003).

Causative factors in cervical neoplasia

Cervical neoplasia is a disease for which the principle causative agent has been clearly identified. Whilst a number of other factors will influence the progression and development of the disease, the key to cervical neoplasia and cervical cancer is the human papilloma virus (HPV).

Cervical cancer thus joins the 15% of cancers which are attributable to infectious agents (Pisani et al. 1997). Other cancers within this category include Burkitts lymphoma (strongly associated with the Epstein Barr virus), hepatocellular carcinoma (associated with Hepatitis B and C viruses) and gastric cancer (associated with *Helicobacter pylori*).

HPV DNA is found in 99.7% of cervical cancers and the virus is found in up to 94% of women with CIN. It is currently being debated whether any HPV negative cervical carcinoma exists (Herrington 1999, Walboomers et al. 1999, Schiffman and Castle 2003). Evidence indicating a role for HPV in cervical cancer is now so strong that the International Agency for Research on Cancer (IARC), and part of the World Health Organisation (WHO) – the National Toxicology Program – has officially acknowledged high risk HPV as a known human carcinogen (IARC 1995, US Department of Health and Human Services 2004). HPV is also associated with a number of other cancers such as oral, vulval, vaginal, penile and anal (Kahn and Bernstein 2005).

However, infection with HPV does not inevitably mean that cervical cellular abnormality will develop – indeed, HPV can be detected in up to 46% of cytologically normal women (Scheurer et al. 2005). Why is it, then, that some women are infected with HPV and do not experience any cervical cellular change, whereas others develop CIN, and others still invasive cancer? The answer is that we do not really know. However, in recent decades our understanding of HPV and its mode of action has increased significantly and is discussed more fully below.

Human papilloma virus

Human papilloma viruses are small viruses. Their structure is different from many other viruses in that they are spherical in shape, a little like a golf ball. In order to fully understand the lifecycle of HPV it is necessary to review the normal pattern of cellular regeneration in the skin.

It will be recalled that the innermost layer of the cutaneous epidermis is the *basal layer*. The cells in this layer are continuously dividing, pushing the older cells up towards the surface. During the process of upward migration the cells lose their capacity to divide and become fully differentiated, mature epithelial cells. At the skin surface they eventually die and are shed in the normal process of skin shedding.

The human papilloma virus is a small virus of approximately 8000 base pairs. In order to become established within a host, HPV requires cells to be actively dividing and differentiating. For this reason the fully differentiated cells on the skin surface are of no use to the virus. The virus requires access to cells at a much earlier stage in their development, whilst they are still in the basal layer.

The HPV genome codes for only eight proteins (Jansen and Shaw 2004, Mahdavi and Bradley 2005). These are divided into 'early' (E) and 'late' (L), the 'early' proteins being expressed during the early stages of the viral infection and the late proteins in the later stages.

The current hypothesis suggests that HPV enters the body through areas of epidermis which are vulnerable and thin, such as the transformation zone of the cervix or anus, or through micro-abrasions in the epithelium produced during sexual activity (Frazer et al. 2006). Once the virus enters the actively-dividing cells of the basal membrane it 'hijacks' the cellular resources in order to replicate its own genetic material and express HPV proteins (Frazer et al. 2006). In the meantime it does not disrupt the cells' normal process of division. On the contrary, because it is so reliant on cellular division continuing for its own multiplication, the virus expresses certain proteins ('early' proteins) whose role it is to inhibit cellular differentiation and stimulate continued cellular proliferation (Frazer et al. 2006).

It is not difficult to extrapolate that interfering with cellular replication in this way might also be associated with oncogenesis. And this indeed appears to be the case. E6 and E7 seem to be particularly important in this process. In high risk HPV sub-types, these proteins bind to and inactivate the tumour suppressor gene products p53 and retinoblastoma protein (Kahn and Bernstein 2005), with the clear potential for uncontrolled cell division and ultimately carcinogenesis.

The 'late' proteins which are coded by the L1 and L2 part of the genome are the virus capsid proteins, that is, the structural part of the virus. These proteins are not expressed until the virus is much more advanced in its lifecycle and the invaded cell has migrated upwards, closer to the skin surface. Thus, by the time the virally invaded cells reach the surface of the epidermis the viral genome has been replicated by the E proteins and the only remaining step is to apply the viral capsid or 'coat' in order to have a fully formed papillomavirus. The virus-laden cells, by now packed with fully formed new HPV are then shed in the normal process of skin shedding, and are ready to infect the next unsuspecting host.

This mechanism of viral invasion and replication is particularly clever in the way it manages to elude the immune system of the host. The virus infects only the cells of the basal layer, thus evading immunologically competent cells in the upper layers of the skin. Furthermore, viral replication and assembly is only completed in the fully-differentiated cell that is destined to die anyway. For this reason HPV infections generate very poor humoral and cell-mediated immune responses. Infections that are not controlled and persist for a long time may cause severe pathologies and ultimately cancer (Jansen and Shaw 2004).

High and low risk HPV

There are more than 100 types of HPV which infect humans and 35 of these types infect the human genitalia (Kahn and Bernstein 2005). Human papilloma viruses fall into two main categories: cutaneous and mucosotropic. The mucosotropic group is the relevant group for cervical cancer and viruses in this category can be further differentiated into high and low risk.

High risk HPV

HPV strains are named numerically and in the order in which they were discovered. The high risk category includes HPV 16, 18, 31, 33, 35, 39, 45, 51, 52, 56, 58, 59, 68, 73, 82. Cervical cancer can result from infection by any one of these, but types HPV16 and HPV 18 predominate in many western countries, accounting for 50% and 20% of cases of cervical cancer respectively (Munoz et al. 2004). High risk viruses have varying oncogenic potentials, HPV 16 appearing to have one of the highest. After HPV 16 and 18, HPV 45 and 31 are arguably the most common oncogenic subtypes in many developed countries.

HPV prevalence has been found to vary as much as twenty-fold between countries (Clifford et al. 2005). For example, HPV is detected in 2% of Vietnamese women aged 15–69 in Hanoi city (Pham et al. 2003) compared with 90% of women attending an adolescent and STD clinic in Baltimore, MD (Jacobson et al. 2000). Furthermore, different HPV subtypes are found in different proportions according to country (Lowy and Schiller 2006). High risk subtypes account for the following percentages of the total HPV by region:

18% in sub-Saharan Africa
5% in Asia
10% in South America
4% in Europe

The high percentage of high risk virus in Africa and South America explains the increased incidence of cervical cancer within these countries where it is the most common cause of cancer death amongst women (Jacob et al. 2005).

Multitype infections are infections with more than one strain of HPV. These are found in both men and women and tend to be associated with poorer outcomes (Wiley and Masongsong 2006).

Low risk HPV

Low risk HPV strains are not associated with cervical cancer but may still be responsible for considerable physical and psychological morbidity. Low risk strains include HPV 6 and 11 which are responsible for approximately 90% of anogenital warts (Kahn and Bernstein 2005). Genital warts may be found on the vulva, perineum and perianal area, vagina and cervix and also on the penis and scrotum in men (see Chapter 11, Box 11.1).

As well as carrying a physical and psychological cost, HPV infection also has significant economic implications. The overall medical cost of HPV-related conditions in the US population aged 15 to 24 is estimated at $2.9 billion a year plus an additional $108.3 million for medical costs associated with cervical cancer and $123.9 million for treatment of external anogenital warts (Chesson et al. 2004).

Infection with low-risk HPV can also lead to a condition called Recurrent Respiratory Papillomatosis (see Box 1.4). This is a rare but debilitating illness affecting the lungs of children and adults alike and often requires repeated surgical intervention in order to maintain lung patency.

Although principally associated with benign cell proliferation, low risk HPV strains may also act as markers for high risk HPV as the two are often found together in the same lesions.

> **Box 1.4 Recurrent respiratory papillomatosis (RRP)**
>
> Recurrent respiratory papillomatosis is a disease of the respiratory tract caused by HPV. It results in tumour-like lesions which grow on the larynx and in some cases the trachea and lungs. This invariably leads to voice difficulties including hoarseness and vocal fatigue. The lesions can occasionally convert to cancer and if they are left untreated can grow sufficiently to cause suffocation and death.
>
> The incidence of RRP is difficult to determine. One US study estimated it to be 4.3 per 100,000 children and 1.8 per 100,000 adults (Derkay 1995). The precise mode of disease transmission is unclear, although some studies have linked childhood onset RRP to mothers with genital HPV infections (Derkay 2006). Presenting symptoms vary according to the location of the lesion but may be dysphonia, stridor or less commonly cough, recurrent pneumonia, failure to thrive, dyspnoea, dysphagia and rarely acute, life-threatening events. Typically, symptoms may be present for a year until diagnosis is made (Derkay 2006).
>
> The current mainstay of treatment is surgery, involving debridement of the airways to maintain patency. Until recently, laser has been favoured over cold knife techniques, although the use of a microdebrider may supersede this. As many as 20% of patients will require adjuvant therapy with systemic antivirals or interferon (Derkay 2006). It is to be hoped that the newly-developed HPV vaccines such as Gardasil will also have a part to play in the management of RRP.
>
> http://www.rrpwebsite.org/whatis_rrp.shtml (accessed 18/6/07)

HPV infection symptoms

Aside from HPV 6 and 11, which are associated with the development of genital lesions and genital warts, the majority of HPV infections are asymptomatic and not linked with any gynaecologic examination findings apart from perhaps a slightly higher incidence of cervical erythema. An association between detection of HPV DNA and vaginal discharge, itching, burning, or systemic symptoms has not been found (Mao et al. 2003).

Incidence of and risk factors for HPV infection

HPV is transmitted through sexual contact and is thought to infect three quarters of the reproductive-age population (Scheurer et al. 2005). It is the most commonly diagnosed sexually transmitted infection in developed countries, with an estimated 30 million new cases worldwide each year (Scheurer et al. 2005). Between 64% to 82% of sexually active adolescent girls test positive for HPV (Kahn and Bernstein 2005, Wiley and Masongsong 2006) and the estimated lifetime risk of women acquiring one or more genital HPV infections is at least 75% (Scheurer et al. 2005). As well as being the most common sexually transmitted infection among adolescent girls and young women, HPV is also widely prevalent in young men.

A number of risk factors have been linked with HPV infection. Those which have consistently been found to be associated with an increased risk are age and number of current and previous sexual partners (Scheurer et al. 2005). These and some other risk factors are discussed below.

Age

The highest rates of genital HPV infection occur between 15 and 25 years, then decline steadily after the age of 40 (Wiley and Masengong 2006). In some populations, there is an increase in non-oncogenic HPV infections in post-menopausal age groups (Herrero et al. 2000). This is possibly the result of acquired immunity, hormonal factors and a lower number of sexual partners (Scheurer et al. 2005).

Number of sexual partners

Genital HPVs are rarely detected in children and in women who are not sexually active but as soon as sexual activity is initiated, incidence rises sharply. The most significant predictor for acquiring infection appears to be the lifetime number of sexual partners. However, because the infection is so prevalent, even having had only one sexual partner carries some risk for infection. Ley and colleagues found that 21% of young women reporting one penetrative male intercourse partner tested positive for HPV DNA (Ley et al. 1991).

Oral contraceptives

A number of studies have found an association between use of oral contraceptives and HPV infection independent of sexual behaviour and other risk factors. The relationship appears particularly significant amongst adenocarcinomas (Madeleine et al. 2001). The mechanism is not really understood but could be related to hormonal influences.

Immunosuppression

People who are immunosuppressed, such as chemically suppressed transplant recipients or patients infected with HIV have higher rates of HPV infection and HPV-associated disease. Immunogenetic factors may play a role in the ability of the immune response to clear HPV infection.

A number of other factors have been associated with an increased risk of HPV infection in some but not all studies. These include:

- herpes simplex virus and vulvar warts
- a history of anal intercourse
- early age at first intercourse
- black or Hispanic women
- tobacco users

(Dell et al. 2000, Scheurer et al. 2005)

Prevention of HPV transmission

Primary prevention of HPV infection needs to address sexual practices – particularly amongst adolescents – reinforcing the asymptomatic nature of HPV infection, the importance of screening and the high risk associated with certain behaviours (e.g. early sexual debut and having many male sexual partners).

Such education programmes would need to involve both males and females – differences in male sexual behaviour could actually explain the differences in cervical cancer rates globally better than the sexual behaviour of women (Castellsague et al. 2002). Men frequently report having had a greater frequency of lifetime sexual partners, more concurrent partners and more contact with sex workers and prostitutes than women (Scheurer et al. 2005).

HPVs are not independently motile agents and it is unlikely that they will make their way to internal genital sites in the absence of penetrative sexual activities. Nonetheless, even non-penetrative intimate touching carries a risk for infection on external sites. Winer and colleagues reported nearly 10% of initially virginal women who subsequently engaged in any kind of non-penetrative intimate sexual touching of the external genital surfaces tested positive for HPV DNA. In contrast, only approximately 1% (one of 76) of initially virginal women foregoing intimate touching tested similarly positive (Winer et al. 2003).

Evidence about the effectiveness of condoms in preventing HPV infection is inconclusive. Because the virus is often found on areas of the skin not covered by a condom and because condoms may only be applied after some intimate touching has occurred, their efficacy is at best limited. They do, however, clearly protect against pregnancy and other sexually transmitted diseases and thus should still be advocated for these reasons. It has also been suggested that the role of spermicides may be significant in prevention of the spread of the disease (Jacob et al. 2005, Wiley and Masongsong 2006).

Progression of HPV infection and cervical cancer

The natural history of HPV infection is still not well understood. It is a difficult virus to study because infections may have a short duration and are asymptomatic. There is currently no routine screening for HPV and so it is unclear whether detected infections are recently acquired or long term. It is therefore difficult to obtain data about the progression of infection (Scheurer et al. 2005).

It has already been mentioned that in the majority of women HPV infection is mild, transient and resolves spontaneously, causing no or low grade cellular changes – even in the presence of quite high viral loads (Moscicki 1998, Cooper et al. 2003). However, in a proportion of women it will persist and progress. High risk HPV infections that persist for more than three years are unlikely to resolve spontaneously and convey significant risk of development into high grade squamous intraepithelial lesions. It is estimated 15% of LSIL will progress to HSIL (Cooper et al. 2003).

HSIL, in turn, may behave in a number of ways. As with LSIL, some cases of HSIL resolve if left untreated. Modelling data from the UK suggest at least 80% of HSIL will regress without intervention (Raffle et al. 2003). Another study found one third of women with CIN2 and almost 20% with CIN3 had regressed spontaneously within 12 months (Nobbenhuis et al. 2001). Wright et al. (2003) in their review of the published natural history literature found:

- 43% of CIN2 regresses, 35% persists as CIN2 and 22% progresses to CIN3 or invasive cancer (over an undefined time period)
- 32% of CIN3 regresses, 56% persists as CIN3 and 14% progresses from CIN3 to cancer

Progression can take many years, with statistical models estimating the average interval between HSIL and cancer to be 10 to 15 years. This is in keeping with population statistics. HSIL is most commonly diagnosed among women of 25–29 years, whereas cancer peaks two decades later at 44–49 years (Gustafsson et al. 1997).

Carcinoma in situ (CIS) is thought to present another stage in the dysplastic continuum occurring between HSIL and invasive cancer. Like HSIL, the nature of CIS is probably unpredictable, with some lesions inherently more aggressive than others. CIS is generally diagnosed in women who are 10 to 12 years younger than those diagnosed with invasive cancer, although the exact amount of time necessary for progression is difficult to determine and could be anything from 2 to 20 years (Chang 1990). CIS is treated in a similar way to HSIL.

Ascertaining the mechanism of progression of cervical dysplasia is difficult to do ethically, as illustrated by a New Zealand study of CIS involving a cohort of women who were basically left untreated. This much publicised case initiated the cervical screening programme in New Zealand and is discussed in Box 1.5.

On a cellular level it is now widely believed that cervical dysplasia results from HPV DNA integration into the host cervical cells (Cooper et al. 2003). However, the changes from high grade dysplasia to invasive cancer require additional genetic events thought to

---

Box 1.5 The National Women's Hospital Experiment – CIS and invasive cancer

If a physician does not worry too much about the disease then neither will the patient.
(Dr Green, quoted in Coney 1988)

Dr Green, whilst working at the above hospital in New Zealand, developed a belief that CIS did not necessarily progress to invasive cancer. Questioning the value of screening programmes and acting contrary to the consensus of medical opinion, he set out to 'show that the lesion is probably benign in the great majority of cases'.

In 1966, and with the approval of the Hospital Medical Committee, he set up an experiment to withhold conventional treatment for CIS in a cohort of women. For inclusion onto the study patients were to have an area of CIS adequately large to allow repeated biopsies and were to show no clinical signs of cervical cancer.

By 1967, Green and his associates had accumulated 576 cases of CIS; 56% of the women had undergone cone biopsy alone and 4% had only had a punch biopsy. It was claimed that after a follow-up period of 13 to 141 months only one patient had developed invasive carcinoma. The conclusion Green drew from this was that CIS had little potential for invasion.

The outcome of the women participating in Green's study was later analysed in a paper by another physician; 131 women who had continuing abnormal cytology were identified and had received the following treatment:

- 88 cone biopsies
- 33 hysterectomies
- 5 punch biopsies only
- 5 wedge biopsies

The margins were found to be positive in almost three quarters of the cone biopsies and two of the hysterectomy specimens, but despite this no further treatment was given. Subsequently, 22% of the women went on to develop invasive carcinoma and almost 70% had persisting CIS.

Green's research and the management of his patients was exposed in a New Zealand magazine and was subsequently the subject of a judicial inquiry. It transpired that the participants in the study were given little information regarding their disease and did not give proper informed consent.

The result of this – the Cartwright Report – made a number of recommendations which were initially directed towards the National Women's Hospital but have now been adopted nationally in New Zealand. The recommendations included increased emphasis on informed consent, increased patient advocacy on health boards, increased teaching of ethical matters in medical schools and the implementation of a national, population-based cervical screening programme.
(Coney 1988, Chang 1990)

---

be mediated by the HPV proteins E6 and E7. These proteins can inactivate tumour suppressor genes p53 and pRb and also bring about the suppression of apoptosis (Mahdavi and Bradley 2005).

The events described above are illustrated in Figure 1.2.

Risk factors in the persistence and progression of dysplasia

Although our understanding of the cellular changes associated with malignant progression has improved in recent years, the question of why some women with neoplasia develop invasive disease whilst others do not has still not been adequately answered.

A number of studies have addressed this issue and whilst failing to elucidate clear causative factors have suggested apparent co-factors. These epidemiological studies indicate that both environmental and host immunologic factors have a role in disease progression (Scheurer et al. 2005, Soto-Wright et al. 2005, Wiley and Masongsong 2006).

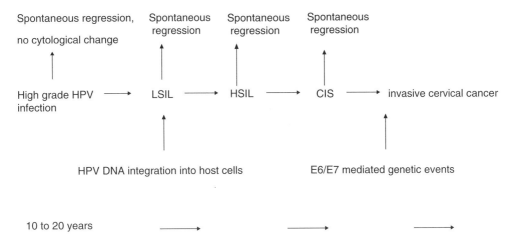

Figure 1.2 The progression to cervical cancer

The single most important factor in the development of cervical cancer appears to be persistent cervical infection with an oncogenic HPV type (especially HPV 16 or 18) (Jacob et al. 2005, Lowy and Schiller 2006). Viral load may also be important – an increased viral load is often associated with more persistent infection. Other postulated risk factors include:

(1) Immune status

Some commentators have suggested that apart from persistent HPV infection, the principal factors which will bring about progression and transformation are related to the hosts' immune status. It is thus a failure in immunosurveillance rather than lifestyle factors which brings about malignant change. Identification of the role of the immune system removes some of the blame from the unfortunate cervical cancer victim who has, for a long time, been stigmatised for having a 'sexually transmitted disease' (Helmerhorst and Meijer 2002).

A number of factors indicate that immune status has a part to play in cervical cancer. Women who are immunosuppressed have two to three times the rate of ASCUS, HPV and CIN compared with women who are not immune compromised (Cox 2005). Organ transplant recipients are at particularly high risk of HPV-related dysplasias and cancer. Although the precise reason for this has not yet been identified, it is generally assumed that the therapeutic immunosuppression to prevent organ rejection increases their vulnerability.

Similarly, a high rate of HPV progression has been observed amongst HIV positive men and women, and is thought to be related to their immunocompromised state (Wiley and Masongsong 2006). This is of particular significance since the introduction of Highly Active Anti-Retroviral Therapy (HAART) which gives HIV/AIDS new status as a chronic disease. The incidence of HPV-related diseases amongst this population has become a significant factor and cervical cancer is now an AIDS defining illness (see Box 1.6).

(2) Smoking

Smoking has the second highest association with the progression of cervical dysplasia after persistent HPV infection (Sellors et al. 2003). The relationship between tobacco, HPV-related dysplasias and cancer has been studied extensively, and although the precise causal carcinogenic mechanism remains unclear, positive associations are consistently reported, to the extent that the United States Surgeon General and International Agency for Research on Cancer have judged that active cigarette smoking is causally associated with cervical cancer (Trimble et al. 2005). There is data to show that women with oncogenic HPV and minimally abnormal cervical smears are up to three times more likely to be diagnosed with greater than CIN3 than non-smokers (McIntyre-Seltman et al. 2005).

Box 1.6 Cervical cancer and HIV/AIDS

HIV positivity renders individuals at a higher risk of HPV infection, cervical intraepithelial neoplasia, progression of neoplasia and cancer. Cervical cancer risk is approximately four-fold higher amongst women with HIV infection and is considered to be an AIDS-defining illness (Ebrahim et al. 2004).

It was anticipated that highly active anti-retroviral therapy (HAART) might have the effect of increasing the incidence of cervical cancer amongst the HIV positive population because more HIV positive people are living for long enough to develop cancers. In fact this has not been the case (Ebrahim et al. 2004). Instead, it would appear possible that HAART has a role in enhancing the regression of CIN in HIV infected women. However, although possibly having a beneficial effect on pre-invasive disease, not all studies have reported a reduction in the incidence of cervical cancer amongst HIV positive women in the HAART era (Ebrahim et al. 2004).

Whilst not at this time classified as an AIDS-defining illness, anal cancer is also found more commonly amongst populations of HIV-positive men who have sex with men (MSM). Anal cancer is also thought to be HPV mediated in a similar way to cervical cancer. In the MSM population it occurs in 35 out of every 100,000 men – a figure comparable with the rate of cervical cancer in women before cervical cancer programmes were instigated (Klenke and Palefsky 2003).

Cigarette smoking is a risk factor for several tumours and is able to induce its carcinogenic effect in sites not directly exposed to cigarette smoke, such as kidney, bladder and cervix. In the uterine cervix it is possible to detect nicotine derivates such as tobacco nitrosamines and it has been hypothesised that smoking is involved in suppression of the local immune response to HPV infection (Matos et al. 2005). Smoking is associated with metaplasia, neoangiogenesis, and proliferation in epithelium as well as overexpression of p53 and markers of cell proliferation (Wiley and Masongsong 2006). A personal history of smoking in addition to second-hand smoke both appear to play a role in the development of cervical cancer precursors (Soto-Wright et al. 2005).

(3) Oral contraceptive use

The duration of oral contraceptive use and risk of cervical cancer have been shown to have a positive correlation in a number of studies (Smith et al 2003, Vessey and Painter 2006). It has been postulated that the addition of progesterone to human papillomavirus-transfected cervical cells, could lead to oncogenic cell transformation (Hellberg and Stendahl 2005).

(4) Parity

High parity and a large number of pregnancies have been correlated with the development of cervical cancer for a long time (Matos et al. 2005). It has been suggested that multiple pregnancies may have a cumulative traumatic or immunosuppressive effect on the cervix, thereby promoting the progression of HPV infection (Matos et al. 2005). Pregnancy could also induce a hormonal effect on the cervix which further increases the risk of oncogenic progression (Matos et al. 2005).

(5) Other factors

Socioeconomic group, genetic factors, HLA type, other sexually transmitted diseases, number of sexual partners, obesity and dietary factors have all been put forward as potential co-factors for the development of high grade dysplasia and cervical cancer, with varying levels of evidence to support them (Carreon et al. 2005, Modesitt et al. 2005, Zelmanowicz et al. 2005).

Cervical cancer

The function of cervical cancer screening programmes is to detect pre-malignant cervical changes before invasive cancer is able to develop. Unfortunately it would seem that most

---

Box 1.7   'He's telling us something.' Women's experiences of cancer disclosure and treatment decision-making in Australia

The psychological impact of a cancer diagnosis can be devastating. Although much of the literature on delivering the diagnosis of cancer implies that the physician imparts this information at a time of absolute certainty about the diagnosis and prognosis, in practice it can be seen that the process is much less straightforward than this. Instead, diagnosis involves the progressive accumulation of information by the treating physician and this in turn involves an ongoing disclosure process rather than simply one consultation.

Markovic et al. (2004) studied the 'cancer disclosure' process, beginning with the patient presenting to their doctor and followed by the ensuing investigative procedures; 27 women with gynaecological cancer were interviewed. The study was conducted in Australia and the sample included Australian-born and immigrant women.

The women had presented with a variety of symptoms, including irregular pre-menopausal or post-menopausal vaginal bleeding, back pain, pain in the abdomen, an enlarged abdomen, a lump or frequency of urination. Typically the woman visited her GP with a specific symptom or mentioned the symptom during a visit for another purpose. This resulted in her being referred for a number of diagnostic procedures, although it did not necessarily mark the commencement of the cancer disclosure process. In Markovic's study, none of the GPs or the specialists conducting the tests raised the possibility of cancer with the women.

This is not to say that the diagnosis was concealed from the women, but rather illustrates that disclosure of a diagnosis of cancer is a multi-layered process. It occurs gradually and involves the participation and interaction of both physician and patient. All the women described their diagnosis being delivered in phases. Initially, physician consultations were characterised by non-disclosure, followed by partial disclosure and finally full disclosure at a time when any ambiguity about what the disease could be had been removed (for example, post-operatively).

---

of the women who develop invasive cancer have 'fallen through the net' with regards to cervical screening. Current estimates suggest that 50% of women diagnosed with cervical cancer have never had a cervical smear and 10% have not had one in the last ten years (Nuovo et al. 2001). Many of these women will have already developed advanced stage disease.

Early stage cervical cancer is generally asymptomatic. It is only as the disease progresses that symptoms occur. Cervical cancer symptoms include post-coital, intermenstrual or post-menopausal bleeding, offensive vaginal discharge, bladder and bowel symptoms. Diagnosis may be complicated in women who cease sexual intercourse in their middle or later life thus 'masking' the symptom of post-coital bleeding. Sometimes the decision to stop intercourse is in fact precipitated by post-coital bleeding. Similarly, other women may cease cervical screening post-menopausally or on ceasing sexual activity, erroneously thinking they are no longer at risk.

Diagnostic and staging investigations

Early stage (asymptomatic) cervical cancer is only likely to be detected through cervical cytology and colposcopy (see Chapter 2). After this a range of investigations will be performed in order to definitively diagnose and stage the disease. These will include many, if not all of those listed below:

- pelvic examination under anaesthetic (EUA)
- sigmoidoscopy
- cystoscopy

- computerised axial tomography scanning (CAT)
- magnetic resonance imaging scanning (MRI)
- intra-venous urogram or pyelogram (IVU or IVP)
- blood tests
- chest X-ray
- PET scanning

There are a number of staging systems for cervical cancer, but the one which is most widely employed was determined by the International Federation of Gynecology and Obstetrics (FIGO) in the late 1950s, and is known as the FIGO system. Basically stage I tumours are confined to the cervix, whereas stage II to IV extend beyond the cervix (See Table 1.4 and Figure 1.3). According to the FIGO report of 2006, globally 42% of cervical cancer cases are diagnosed at stage I, 30% at stage II, 21% at stage III and 6% at stage IV (Quinn et al. 2006).

FIGO staging is clinically based, principally reliant on determinations made by physical examination, EUA, colposcopy, cystoscopy, sigmoidoscopy, IVP and chest X-ray (Moore 2006). Although it is a system which is widely used throughout the world, it is not without its critics. Opponents feel that it is inaccurate and that modern medical imaging methods such as CT, MRI and PET scanning should be employed in addition to the investigations

Table 1.4 FIGO classification system for cervical cancer
http://www.cancerhelp.org.uk/help/default.asp?page=2772#0 (accessed 18/6/07)

Stage 0
This is more commonly referred to as carcinoma in situ. A carcinoma in situ is one that only involves cells in the tissues in which it began but has not spread beyond this. Carcinoma in situ is a phenomenon which has been observed in other cancers for which there are screening programmes such as breast cancer.
CIS is generally treated in the same way as CIN3.

Stage I
Stage 1 describes an invasive cancer which is confined to the cervix. It is divided into stage 1A and stage 1B, each of which is further subdivided into two groups:
Stage IA (microscopic disease)
   (i) IA1: cancer has invaded cervix tissue by less than 3 mm and is less than 7 mm wide (also known as *microinvasive* cervical cancer).
   (ii) IA2: the cancer infiltrates to a depth of 3 to 5 mm but is less than 7 mm wide.
Stage IB (usually macroscopic disease)
   (i) IB1: the cancer is no larger than 4 cm and still localised to the cervix.
   (ii) IB2: the cancer is larger than 4 cm and still localised to the cervix.

Stage II
The cancer has begun to spread beyond the cervix but not to the pelvic sidewall. It may involve the upper part of the vagina but not the lower third.
Stage IIA involves the upper two-thirds of vagina, no parametrial involvement.
Stage IIB obvious parametrial involvement.

Stage III
The cancer has extended though the cervix on to the pelvic wall. On rectal examination there is no cancer-free space between tumour and pelvic sidewall. The tumour involves the lower third of the vagina. All patients with hydronephrosis or a non-functioning kidney are counted as stage III unless known to be the result of other causes.
Stage IIIA: involvement of the lower third of the vagina; no extension to pelvic sidewall.
Stage IIIB: extension to pelvic sidewall and/or hydronephrosis or non-functioning kidney.

Stage IV
The carcinoma extends beyond the true pelvis or clinically involves mucosa of bladder or rectum. Bullous oedema does not allow a case to be designated as stage IV.
Stage IVA: locally invasive.
Stage IVB: spread to distant organs.

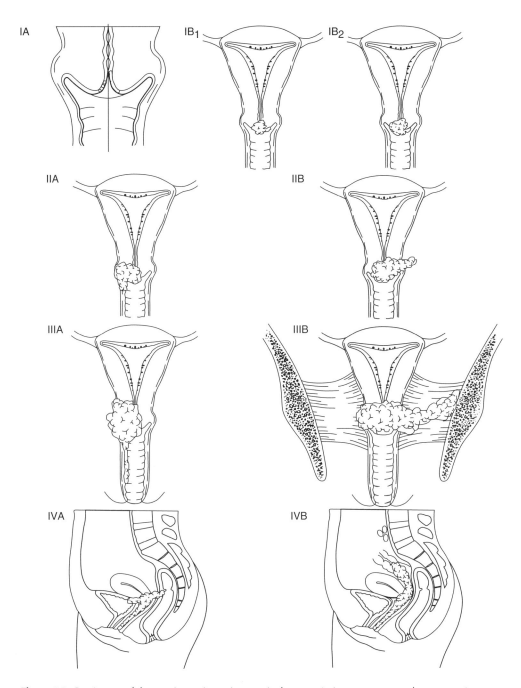

Figure 1.3 Carcinoma of the cervix uteri: staging cervical cancer (primary tumour and metastases)

described above (Choi 2004, Soutter et al. 2004, Rojas-Espaillant and Rose 2005). Whilst these imaging modalities have indeed been shown to have a role in determining disease status in cervical cancer, they also have their limitations. For example, the sensitivity of CT and MRI in identifying nodal disease has been estimated to be as low as 34% (Heller et al. 1990).

However, this is not the main reason for excluding advanced imaging techniques from the FIGO staging system. Instead, these methods are excluded because they are not readily available in many developing nations. Cervical cancer is not simply a disease of industrialised nations – on the contrary, it is much more of a problem in developing countries (see Chapter 9). The principal function of FIGO staging is to facilitate data collection and comparative reporting of results, not to assign treatment (Moore 2006). In order to allow worldwide comparison between cohorts of women with the disease, the tools required for staging must be accessible to less affluent nations.

And so, in summary, whilst the treating doctor is free to perform whatever investigations are deemed necessary to diagnose and treat the cervical cancer, if the FIGO system is used, any additional information afforded by supplementary testing should not be taken into account in determining its stage.

Prognosis

As with most cancers, stage at diagnosis is the most important prognostic factor in cervical cancer (Garg et al. 2006). Women diagnosed with early stage disease (1A to 1B1) have survival rates of 85 to 100% (Waggoner 2003, Rojas-Espaillant and Rose 2005). Stage IIa tumours also have a good prognosis, with a five-year survival of approximately 90% (Hopkins and Morley 1993). However, once the tumour spreads further than this the prognosis is poorer. The estimated five-year disease-free survival rate after therapy for stage IB2 and IIB disease is 50–70%, for stage III disease is 30–60% and for stage IV disease is 5–15% (Waggoner 2003).

Amongst patients with early stage disease who are treated surgically, a number of other factors have been shown to influence the prognosis of patients diagnosed with cervical cancer including:

(1) Regional lymph node involvement
    Inextricably linked with tumour stage, lymph node involvement is the next most important prognostic factor. Indeed, most of the other factors listed below principally impact survival by increasing the incidence of nodal metastasis. Lymph node involvement is associated with a poor prognosis. Patients with negative nodes will have an 85–90% five year survival rate. This figure falls to 20–74% for patients with positive nodes, depending on the number of nodes involved, their location and the size of the metastases (Hatch 1994).
    Lymphatic spread is generally via the parametrial, external iliac, obturator and hypogastric (internal iliac) nodes to the common iliac and eventually paraaortic lymph nodes.

(2) Tumour size
    For some time it has been recognised that a large tumour is associated with a significantly poorer prognosis amongst women with cervical cancer (Soutter et al. 2004). Burghart et al. (1992) illustrated that women with a tumour volume smaller than 2.5 cm^3 had a five-year survival of 91%, while those with larger tumours (10–50 cm^3) had a five-year survival rate of 70%. The extent of nodal metastases appears to be directly proportional to tumour size.

(3) Parametrial invasion
    Deep cervical-stromal invasion, or extension of the cancer to the vaginal or parametrial margins is a poor prognostic sign. The mode of dissemination into the parametrium is not fully understood and could be through metastatic spread rather than simply by local invasion.

(4) Lymph vascular space involvement
  The significance of lymph vascular invasion (LVSI) is controversial, but is thought to signify a high possibility of node positivity and is therefore often used as an indication for lymph node dissection. LVSI is considered to be a poor prognostic factor (Morice et al.).

Conclusion

Cervical cancer is a significant public health issue, particularly in the developing world. It is triggered by HPV infection, which results in various stages of pre-cancerous neoplasia before progressing to invasive cancer. Early detection and treatment of such abnormalities can prevent the development of cancer and is the principle behind cervical screening. Unfortunately, a proportion of women do not participate in such programmes either through choice or lack of availability. Such women are at increased risk of developing advanced cervical cancer. The management of invasive disease is discussed in chapter 2 and in the following 3 chapters.

Frequently asked questions

(1) If I have sex, could I be re-infected with HPV and would that make my cancer recur?
  You cannot develop a second primary cervical cancer if your cervix has been removed in your treatment. Furthermore, you may have acquired some immunity to the HPV strain that originally infected you. However, if your cervix remains in situ there could be a theoretical possibility of developing a second primary cervical cancer from another HPV type. Remember, the disease will generally evolve over many years and should therefore be detected through regular cervical screening. There is also a low but increased risk of acquiring other HPV related cancers such as vulval or anal cancer (Edgren 2007). You may wish to discuss this risk with your doctor when you attend for follow-up visits.
(2) My mother died of cervical cancer. Does that increase my risk? Or the risk of my children?
  No, there is not considered to be a familial link for squamous cell carcinoma although associations have been drawn between cervical adenocarcinoma and hereditary non-polyposis colon cancer.
(3) Is cervical cancer associated with being overweight?
  No, there is no link between cervical cancer and obesity.
(4) Is cervical cancer less common amongst women whose partners are circumcised?
  There does now appear to be data to suggest that male circumcision reduces the likelihood of males carrying HPV and affords some protection for their partners against cervical cancer (Castellsague et al. 2002)
(5) Are condoms effective in reducing the incidence of cervical cancer?
  Whether condoms protect the cervix remains controversial, and many individuals who claim to use condoms use them inconsistently and often not during foreplay. It is unlikely that use of a condom will prevent HPV infection altogether (Frazer et al. 2006).
(6) I have been diagnosed with an HPV infection. Does this mean that my partner has been unfaithful?
  HPV can remain latent for months or years and so infection does not indicate infidelity has occurred.
(7) How many women with high risk HPV will develop persistent lesions?
  Between 5–10% of women with high risk HPV will develop persistent lesions (Walboomers et al. 1999).

(8) I have tested positive for the HPV virus. Is there any treatment?
No, there is not any treatment because the virus resolves spontaneously over time with most women. Ongoing monitoring is considered sufficient action in the case of HPV positivity to ensure that any cytological changes to the cervix are detected early (NHSCSP 2004).
(9) Should my husband be tested for the virus?
Currently there is no HPV testing for males. Many normal, healthy males will be positive for the virus and the benefits of testing most heterosexual men are unclear (NHSCSP 2004).

Resources

National Health Service (NHS) Cancer Screening Programme: http://cancerscreening.org. uk/index.html
British Society for Clinical Cytology: http://www.clinicalcytology.co.uk/index.asp
National Association of Cytologists: http://www.nac.org.uk/index.php
British Society for Colposcopy and Cervical Pathology: http://www.bsccp.org.uk/
National Health Service Cervical Screening Programme (NHSCSP): http://www.cancer-screening.nhs.uk/
National Institute for Health and Clinical Excellence (NICE): http://www.nice.org.uk/
National Cervical Screening Program, Australia: http://www.breastscreen.info.au/internet/screening/publishing.nsf/Content/home
Imperial Cancer Research Fund: http://www.cancerhelp.org.uk/help/default.asp?page=2739
National Cancer Institute: http://www.cancer.gov/
European Cervical Cancer Association: http://www.ecca.info/webECCA/en/

References

Anderson CE, Lee AJ, McLaren KM, et al. (2004) Level of agreement and biopsy correlation using two- and three-tier systems to grade cervical dyskaryosis. *Cytopathology*, volume 15 (5), p. 256–262
ASCUS-LSIL Triage Study (ALTS) Group (2003) Results of a randomized trial on the management of cytology interpretations of atypical squamous cells of undetermined significance. *Am J Obstet Gynecol*, 188, 1383–1392
Burghardt E, Baltzer J, Tulusan AH and Haas J (1992) Results of surgical treatment of 1028 cervical cancers studied with volumetry. *Cancer*, 70, 648–655
Cancer Council (2006) Fact sheet: Cervical cancer: http://www.cancercouncil.com.au/editorial. asp?pageid=54&fromsearch=yes (accessed 17/6/07)
Cancer Research UK (2006) Cervical cancer statistics: http://info.cancerresearchuk.org/cancerstats/ types/cervix/ (accessed 17/6/07)
Carreon JD, Martin MP, Hildesheim A, et al. (2005) Human leukocyte antigen class I and II haplo-types and risk of cervical cancer. *Tissue Antigens*, volume 66 (4), p. 321–324
Castellsague X, Bosch FX, Munoz N, et al. (2002) Male circumcision, penile human papillomavirus infection, and cervical cancer in female patients. *New England Journal of Medicine*, 346, 1105–1112
Chang AR (1990) Carcinoma in situ of the cervix and its malignant potential. A lesson from New Zealand. *Cytopathology*, 1, 321–328
Chesson HW, Blandford JM, Gift TL, Tao G and Irwin KL (2004) The estimated direct medical cost of sexually transmitted diseases among American youth 2000. *Perspect Sex Reprod Health*, 36, 11–19
Choi SH, Kim SH, Choi HJ, Park BK and Lee HJ (2004) Preoperative magnetic resonance imaging staging of uterine cervical carcinoma; results of prospective study. *J Comput Assist Tomogr*, 28 (5), Sept/Oct, 620–627

Clifford GM, Gallus S, Herrero R, et al. (2005) Worldwide distribution of human papillomavirus type in cytologically normal women in the International Agency for Research on Cancer HPV prevalence surveys: a pooled analysis. *Lancet*, 366, 991–998

Coney S (1988) *The Unfortunate Experiment; the Full Story behind the Inquiry into Cervical Cancer Treatment*. Penguin, Auckland, NZ: http://www.womens-health.org.nz/cartwright/unfortunate (accessed 7/7/08)

Cooper K, Evans M and Mount S (2003) Biology and evolution of cervical squamous intraepithelial lesions: a hypothesis with diagnostic prognostic implications. *Advances in Anatomical Pathology*, 10 (4), 200–203

Cox JT (2005) Management of women with cervical cytology interpreted as ASC-US or as ASC-H. *Clinical Obstetrics and Gynaecology*, 48 (1), 160–177

Dell DL, Chen H, Ahmad F and Stewart DE (2000) Knowledge about human papillomavirus among adolescents. *Obstet Gynecol*, 96, 653–656

Derkay CS (1995) Task force on recurrent respiratory papillomas. A preliminary report. *Arch Otolaryngol Head Neck Surg*, 121, 1386–1391

Derkay CS and Darrow DH (2006) Recurrent respiratory papillomatosis. *Annals of Otology, Rhinology & Laryngology*, 115 (1), Jan, 1–11

Ebrahim SH, Abdullah AS, McKenna M and Hamers FF (2004) AIDS-defining cancers in Western Europe, 1994–2001. AIDS *Patient Care & Stds*, 18 (9), 501–508

Ferlay J, Bray F, Pisani P and Parkin DM (2004) *GLOBOCAN 2002: Cancer Incidence, Mortality and Prevalence Worldwide, IARC CancerBase*, no 5, version 2.0. IARC Press, Lyon

Frazer IH, Cox JT, Mayeaux EJ, et al. (2006) Advances in prevention of cervical cancer and other human papillomavirus-related diseases. *Paediatric Infectious Disease Journal*, 25 (2) Supplement, February, S65–S81

Garg K, Rabban J, Chen L and Zaloudek C (2006) Microinvasive carcinoma of the cervix. *Pathol Case Review*, 11 (3), May/June, 121–129

Grimes DA (1999) Role of the cervix in sexual response: evidence for and against. *Clinical Obstetrics & Gynecology*, 42 (4), 972–978

Gustafsson L, Ponten J, Bergstrom R and Adami HO (1997) International incidence rates of invasive cervical cancer before cytological screening. *International Journal of Cancer*, 71, 159–165

Hatch KD (1994) Cervical cancer, in Berek JS and Hacker NF (eds) *Practical Gynaecologic Oncology*, 2nd edn. Williams and Wilkins, Baltimore. pp. 243–283

Health and Social Care Information Centre Statistics (2005) *Cervical Screening Programme, England 2004–2005*. Health and Social Care Information Centre Bulletin 2005/09/HSCIC: http://www.ic.nhs.uk/pubs/cervicscrneng2005/sb0509.pdf/file (accessed 17/6/07)

Hellberg D and Stendahl U (2005) The biological role of smoking, oral contraceptive use and endogenous sexual steroid hormones in invasive squamous epithelial cervical cancer. *Anticancer Research*, 25 (4), 3041–3046

Heller PB, Malfetano JH, Bundy BN, et al. (1990) Clinical-pathologic study of stage IIB, III, and IVA carcinoma of the cervix: extended diagnostic evaluation for paraaortic node metastasis. A Gynecologic Oncology Group study. *Gynecol Oncol*, 38, 425–430

Helmerhorst TJM and Meijer JLM (2002) Cervical cancer should be considered as a rare complication of oncogenic HPV infection rather than an STD. *Int J Gynaecol Cancer*, 12, 235–236

Herrero R, Hildesheim A, Bratti C, et al. (2000) Population-based study of human papillomavirus infection and cervical neoplasia in rural Costa Rica. *J Natl Cancer Inst*, 92, 464–474

Herrington CJ (1999) Do HPV-negative cervical carcinomas exist? revisited (ed.). *Journal of Pathology*, 189 (1), 1–3

Hopkins MP and Morley GW (1993) Prognostic factors in advanced stage squamous cell cancer of the cervix. *Cancer*, 72, 2389–2393

IARC Working Group (1995) IARC monographs on the evaluation of carcinogenic risks to humans: human papillomaviruses. International Agency for Research on Cancer, Lyon, France. 64

Jacob M, Bradley J and Barone M (2005) Human papillomavirus vaccines: what does the future hold for preventing cervical cancer in resource-poor settings through immunization programs? *Sexually Transmitted Diseases*, 32 (10), Oct, 635–640

Jacobson DL, Womack SD, Peralta L, et al. (2000) Concordance of human papillomavirus in the cervix and urine among inner city adolescents. *Pediatr Infect Dis J*, 19, 722–728

Jansen KU and Shaw AR (2004) Human papillomavirus vaccines and prevention of cervical cancer. *Annual Review of Medicine*, 55, 319–331

Johnson J and Patnick J (2000) Achievable standards, benchmarks for reporting, and criteria for evaluating cervical cytopathology. NHSCP Publication number 1, May

Kahn JA and Bernstein DI (2005) Human papillomavirus vaccines and adolescents. *Current Opinion on Obstetrics and Gynaecology*, 17, 476–482

Klenke BJ and Palefsky JM (2003) Anal cancer: an HIV-associated cancer. *Hematology/Oncology Clinics of North America*, 17, 859–872

Ley C, Bauer HM, Reingold A, et al. (1991) Determinants of genital human papillomavirus infection in young women. *J Natl Cancer Inst*, 83, 997–1003

Lowy DR and Schiller JT (2006) Prophylactic human papillomavirus vaccines. *Journal of Clinical Investigation*: http://www.jci.org, 116 (5), May, 1167–1173

McIntyre-Seltman K, Castle PE, Gido R, Schiffman M and Wheeler CM (2005) Smoking is a risk factor for cervical intraepithelial neoplasia grade 3 among oncogenic human papillomavirus DNA-positive women with equivocal or mildly abnormal cytology. *Cancer Epidemiology, Biomarkers and Prevention*, 14 (5), May, 1165–1169

Madeleine MM, Daling JR, Schwartz SM, et al. (2001) Human papillomavirus and long-term oral contraceptive use increase the risk of adenocarcinoma in situ of the cervix. *Cancer Epidemiology, Biomarkers & Prevention*, 10 (3), 171–177

Mahdavi A and Bradley JM (2005) Vaccines against human papillomavirus and cervical cancer; promises and challenges. *Oncologist*, 10, 528–538

Mao C, Hughes JP, Kiviat N, et al. (2003) Clinical findings among young women with genital human papillomavirus infection. *American Journal of Obstetrics & Gynecology*, 188 (3), 677–684

Markovic M, Manderson L, Wray N and Quinn M (2004) 'He's telling us something.' Women's experiences of cancer disclosure and treatment-making in Australia. *Anthropology and Medicine*, 11 (3), Dec, 327–341

Matos A, Moutinho J, Pinto D and Medeiros R (2005) The influence of smoking and other co-factors on the time to onset to cervical cancer in a southern European population. *European Journal of Cancer Prevention*, 14 (5), Oct, 485–491

Miller AB (1992) *Cervical Cancer Screening Programmes: Managerial Guidelines*. WHO, Geneva

Modesitt SC and van Nagell JR (2005) The impact of obesity on the incidence and treatment of gynecologic cancers: a review. *Obstet Gynaecol Surv*, 60 (10), Oct, 683–692

Moghissi KS (1972) The function of the cervix in fertility. *Fertil Steril*, 23 (4), April, 295–306

Moore DH (2006) Cervical cancer. *Obstet Gynaecol*, 107 (5), 1152–1161

Morice P and Castaigne D (2005) Advances in the surgical management of invasive cervical cancer. *Current Opinion in Obstetrics and Gynaecology*, 17 (1), 5–12

Moscicki AB (1998) Genital infections with human papillomavirus (HPV). *Pediatric Infectious Disease Journal*, 17 (7), July, 651–652

Munoz N, Bosch FX, Castellsague X, et al. (2004) Against which human papillomavirus types shall we vaccinate and screen? The international perspective. *International Journal of Cancer*, 111, 278–285

National Health and Medical Research Council (NHMRC) (1994) *Guidelines for the Management of Women with Screen Detected Abnormalities*. Australian Government Publishing Service, Canberra, p. 20

National Health and Medical Research Council (NHMRC) (2005) Screening to prevent cervical cancer: guidelines for the management of asymptomatic women with screen detected abnormalities: http://www.nhmrc.gov.au/publications/synopses/wh39syn.htm (accessed 18/6/07)

NHS Cancer Screening Programmes (NHSCSP) (2004) *Cervical Cancer: a Pocket Guide*. DOH Publications, London

Nobbenhuis MAE, Helmerhorst TJM, van den Brule AJC, et al. (2001) Cytological regression and clearance of high risk human papillomavirus in women with abnormal cervical smear. *Lancet*, 358, 1782–1783

Nuovo J, Melnikow J and Howell LP (2001) New tests for cervical cancer screening. *American Family Physician*, 64, 780–786

Office for National Statistics (1999) *Cancer 1971–1997*. Office for National Statistics, London

Parkin DM (1997) The epidemiological basis for evaluating screening policies, in Franco E and Monsonego J (eds) *New Developments in Cervical Cancer Screening and Prevention*. Blackwell Science, Oxford

Pham TH, Nguyen TH, Herrero R, et al. (2003) Human papillomavirus infection among women in South and North Vietnam. *Int J Cancer*, 104, 213–220

Pisani P, Parkin DM, Munoz N and Ferlay J (1997) Cancer and infection: estimates of the attributable fraction in 1990. *Cancer Epidemiology Biomarkers and Prevention*, 6 (6), 387–400

Quinn M, Babb P, Brock A, et al. (2001) *Cancer Trends in England & Wales 1950–1999*. Vol. SMPS no. 66. TSO, London

Quinn MA, Benedet JL, Odicino F, et al. (2006) Carcinoma of the cervix uteri. FIGO annual report. *International Journal of Gynaecology and Obstetrics 95*, 26, Supplement 1, S43–S101

Rana DN, Marchall J, Desai M, et al. (2004) Five year follow-up of women with borderline and mildly dyskaryotic cervical smears. *Cytopathology*, 15, 263–270

Raffle AE, Alden B, Quinn M, Babb PJ and Brett MF (2003) Outcomes of screening to prevent cancer: analysis of cumulative incidence of cervical abnormality and modelling cases and deaths prevented. *British Medical Journal*, 326 (7395), 901

Richart RM (1973) Cervical intraepithelial neoplasia. *Pathol Annu*, 8, 301–328

Rojas-Espaillant LA and Rose PG (2005) Management of locally advanced cervical cancer. *Curr Opin Oncol*, 17 (5), Sep, 485–492

Sankaranarayanan R and Ferlay J (2006) Worldwide problem of gynaecological cancer: the size of the problem. *Best Practice and Research Clinical Obstetrics and Gynaecology*, 20 (2), 207–225.

Scheurer ME, Tortolero-Luna G and Adler-Storthz K (2005) Human papillomavirus infection; biology, epidemiology and prevention. *International Journal of Gynaecological Cancer*, 15, 727–746

Schiffman M and Castle PE (2003) Human papilloma virus epidemiology and public health. *Arch Pathol Lab Med*, 127, 930–934

Schneider, V (2003) Symposium part 2: should the Bethesda System Terminology be used in diagnostic surgical pathology? Counterpoint. *International Society of Gynecological Pathologists*, 22 (1), Jan, pp. 13–17

Schorge JO, Knowles LM and Lea JS (2004) Adenoma of the cervix. *Current Treatment Options in Oncology*, 5, 119–127

Sellors JW and Sankaranarayanan R (2003) *Colposcopy and Treatment of Cervical Intraepithelial Neoplasia. A Beginner's Manual*. International Agency for Research on Cancer (IARC), Lyon

Smith HO, Tiffany MF, Qualls CR and Key CR (2000) The rising incidence of adenocarcinoma relative to squamous cell carcinoma of the uterine cervix in the United States: a 24-year population-based study. *Gynaecol Oncol*, 78, 97–105

Smith JHF (2002) Bethesda 2001. *Cytopathology*, 13 (1), Feb, 4–10

Smith JS, Green J, Berrington De Gonzalez A, et al. (2003) Cervical cancer and use of hormonal contraceptives: a systematic review. *Lancet*, 361 (9364), 1159–1167

Soto-Wright V, Samuelson R and McLellan R (2005) Current management of low-grade squamous intraepithelial lesion, high grade squamous intraepithelial lesion and atypical glandular cells. *Clin Obstet Gynaecol*, 48 (1), March, 147–159

Soutter WP, Hanoch J, D'Arcy T, Dina R, McIndoe GA and DeSouza NM (2004) Pretreatment tumour volume measurement on high-resolution magnetic resonance imaging as a predictor of survival in cervical cancer. *BJOG*, 111 (7), July, 741–747

Stoler MH and Schiffman M (2001) Interobserver reproducibility of cervical cytology and histologic interpretations. Realistic estimates from the ASCUS-LSIL Triage Study. *JAMA*, 285, 1500–1505

Trimble CL, Genkinger JM, Burke AE, et al. (2005) Active and passive cigarette smoking and the risk of cervical neoplasia. *Obstetrics & Gynecology*, 105 (1), 174–181

US Department of Health and Human Services, Public Health Services, National Toxicology Program (2004) *Report on Carcinogens*, 11th edn, US Department of Health and Human Services, Washington, DC

Vessey M and Painter R (2006) Oral contraceptive use and cancer. Findings in a large cohort study, 1968–2004. *British Journal of Cancer*, 95 (3), 385–389

Walboomers JM, Jacobs MV, Manos MM, et al. (1999) Human papillomavirus is a necessary cause of invasive cervical cancer worldwide. *J Pathol*, 189, 12–19

Wiley D and Masongsong E (2006) Human papillomavirus: the burden of infection. *Obstetrical and Gynaecological Survey*, 61 (6), supplement 1, S3–S14

Winer RL, Lee SK, Hughes JP, et al. (2003) Genital human papillomavirus infection: incidence and risk factors in a cohort of female university students. *Am J Epidemiol*, 157, 218–226

Wright TC, Cox JT, Massad LS, Carlson J, Twiggs LB, Wilkinson EJ for the 2001 ASCCP-sponsored Consensus Workshop (2003) 2001 Consensus guidelines for the management of women with cervical intraepithelial neoplasia. *Am J Obstet Gynaecol*, 189 (1), 295–304

Yang BH, Bray FI, Parkin DM, et al. (2004) Cervical cancer as a priority for prevention in different world regions: an evaluation using years of life lost. *Int J Cancer*, 109 (3), 418–424

Zelmanowicz AM, Schiffman M, Herrero R, et al. (2005) Family history as a co-factor for adenocarcinoma and squamous cell carcinoma of the uterine cervix: results from two studies conducted in Costa Rica and the United States. *International Journal of Cancer*, 116 (4), 599–605

Chapter 2

Pre-invasive disease, colposcopy and adenocarcinoma

'My GP said "it might be cancer in ten years time but then again it might not". But you remember her saying "in ten years time" whereas you don't remember "it might not."'

(Patient quote from Lagro-Jansen and Schijf 2005)

Introduction

The first part of this chapter will look more closely at the practical aspects of abnormal cervical cytology management, beginning with a discussion of the cervical smear-taking procedure and the development of liquid based cytology. The next step in the assessment of many cervical abnormalities is colposcopy. The role of colposcopy in cervical screening programmes is described and the evolution of the nurse colposcopist explored.

Chapter 1 focused exclusively on squamous cell carcinoma, which is by far the most common type of cervical cancer, occurring in 80% of cases. The next most common form of cervical malignancy is adenocarcinoma. Whereas the cervical smear test has been found to be invaluable in the detection of pre-cancerous squamous cell lesions, its role in the detection of the less common glandular lesions associated with adenocarcinoma is not as helpful. The final part of the chapter looks at atypical glandular cells and the diagnosis and management of adenocarcinoma.

Cervical cytology testing

As discussed in Chapter 1, the key to early detection of cervical abnormalities lies with being able to monitor and evaluate changes in the cervical epithelium – usually by obtaining samples of epithelial cells and looking at them under a microscope (cervical cytology). A number of different strategies have been developed in order to collect cervical cells but by far the most prevalent and established in the western world is the cervical smear test. The cervical smear is also referred to as the Pap smear because it was developed in the 1940s by Papanicolaou. The procedure for performing a cervical smear is described in Box 2.1.

Box 2.1 The cervical smear – obtaining an optimal sample

There are two important components in ensuring accurate Pap smear reports – rigorous cytological examination and a good smear taking technique (National Health and Medical Research Council, Australia (NHMRC) 2005).

A good smear sample needs to contain sufficient metaplastic squamous cells from the transformation zone and also some endocervical cells to ensure that the upper reaches of the transformation zone have been reached. To help ensure that an adequate specimen is obtained, it is preferable to avoid smear-taking at certain times, specifically:

- during menstruation
- if obvious vaginal infection is present
- within 24 hours of use of vaginal creams or pessaries

(NHMRC 2005)

Table 2.1 summarises the procedure for taking a cervical smear (NHSCSP 2006a). It compares the procedures for conventional cytology with liquid based cytology, although in practice for the patient both will feel very similar.

Cervical cytology: conventional smear versus liquid based cytology (LBC)

Although the cervical smear test has been used for many years, it is not failsafe. One of the main criticisms against it is that it lacks sensitivity. Test sensitivity and specificity are further discussed in Chapter 8, but basically the term sensitivity refers to the proportion of truly diseased persons in the screened population who are identified by the test. In other words it is the propensity of the test to avoid false negatives (Karnon et al. 2004). False negative rates for cervical smear tests vary from 10% to 80%.

Within many screening programmes there have been 'scares' related to poor sensitivity. For example, in the UK National Health Service Cervical Screening Programme (NHSCSP) 8000 cervical smears taken at James Paget Hospital in Norfolk had to be re-checked in the late 1990s. In 1998, a further 1000 women were recalled to St Georges Hospital in South London because of concerns about the accuracy of their cervical screening (Jolley 2004).

False negatives can arise from a number of sources:

(1) Laboratory factors: abnormal cells are present in the specimen but these have not been detected or interpreted correctly by the laboratory. It has been estimated that anything from 5% to 50% of cervical slides are falsely reported as negative or are under-reported (Baker et al. 1999).

(2) Biological factors: rapid progression of the disease such that the lesion itself was not present at the time of sampling – this is thought to be uncommon (Karnon 2004).

(3) Collector factors: most of the false negatives are secondary to clinical sampling (usually failure to obtain adequate material from the diseased area) (Raab 2006). Additionally, a proportion of cervical smears will be unevaluable. Within the UK, approximately 9% of cervical smears are classified as 'inadequate' (Health and Social Care Information Centre Statistics 2006). A number of factors may make a smear test inadequate. These include:

(a) insufficient or unsuitable material
(b) inadequate fixation of smear
(c) poor spreading of smear
(d) smear consisting mainly of blood and pus or inflammatory exudates

(Bankhead et al. 2003)

In the late 1990s it was decided by the NHSCSP that the cervical cytology shortcomings (particularly the high incidence of unevaluable smears) needed to be addressed. An investigation into alternative technologies was instigated and a number of studies were set up to evaluate the comparative effectiveness of liquid based cytology (LBC). In 2003 the National Institute of Clinical Excellence (NICE) stated that national implementation of LBC would significantly reduce the number of unevaluable smears. LBC was thought to be up to 12% more sensitive than conventional cervical smears, with the potential to decrease the number of inadequate samples from 9.1% to 1.6% with LBC (NICE 2003, Karnon 2004). Thus, the decision was made to replace the Pap smear with LBC testing over the forthcoming years (Karnon 2004).

Liquid based cytology is simply a new way of processing the cervical sample. The cells are collected as before but rather than 'smearing' them straight on to a slide, the head of the collecting brush is broken off into a preservative fluid (see Table 2.1). The result is a suspension of cells which is then centrifuged to remove contaminants before the slide is prepared. Cytoscreen, Surepath, Labonard Easy Prep and Thin Prep are all different LBC techniques.

Other advantages of LBC samples over conventional cytology are that:

- cellular preservation is improved
- the samples stain better
- samples can be preserved for future Human Papilloma Virus (HPV) testing

Table 2.1 Procedure for taking a cervical smear

Conventional cytology	Liquid based cytology (LBC)
Assess patient and provide appropriate interventions regarding: • educational needs (is it first smear?) • cultural requirements (e.g. need for a chaperone?)	As with conventional cytology.
Consent – written consent not necessarily required but a minimum of oral consent. Non-compliance with procedure indicates a withdrawal of consent.	As with conventional cytology.
Warm speculum and insert into vagina with appropriate lubrication.	As with conventional cytology.
A Cervex-Brush®, plastic or wooden spatula may be used depending on: the state of the os, the shape and contours of the cervix, the need to sample the whole transformation zone, any unusual features.	Insert central bristles of Cervex-Brush® into endocervical canal so outer bristles are in full contact with ectocervix.
For use of a Cervex-Brush® refer to LBC. If spatula is used introduce into the cervix and rotate more than one complete turn to ensure sampling of the whole of the cervix. Cervical mucus can reduce the quality of the smear and should be removed where possible.	Rotate brush five times clockwise, (bristles are designed for clockwise rotation only).
Cells should be transferred onto a glass slide immediately: • for an extended tip spatula transfer from both sides of the sampler using straight sweeps • for a Cervex-Brush® use a 'paint brush' action, sweeping both sides of the brush along the slide	
Immediately fix the sample by immersing in alcohol or applying the fixative from a dropper or spray. Leave slide in a horizontal position to dry for about 15 minutes. Do not place in refrigerator.	Fix sample immediately as per fixative instructions.
Remove speculum and complete consultation.	Remove speculum and complete consultation.

Not all countries have opted to completely switch to LBC, but in many it may be offered as an alternative to the traditional cervical smear. Indeed, some argue that there is inadequate evidence to support its superiority to conventional cytology and that further research is required (Arbyn et al. 2008).

An abnormal smear – what next?

As discussed in Chapter 1, there are many grades of cervical abnormality, each one calling for a different clinical response. Box 2.2 lists the range of abnormal cytology results which may be diagnosed on a cervical smear report and the subsequent action required. It will be seen that follow-up practices vary between different countries and different screening programmes.

Where closer examination of the cervix is required, the next step is to perform a colposcopy. The following section explains the term colposcopy and discusses the situations in which it is indicated. The informational needs of a patient undergoing colposcopy and the role of the nurse in this field are also discussed.

Colposcopy

Colposcopy is examination of the cervix using a scope which allows visualisation and magnification of the cervix and the collection of biopsies. The aim of colposcopy is to assess the nature, severity and extent of any abnormality detected in the cervical smear, and where appropriate to take specimens for cervical histology.

The first colposcopy was performed in 1925 by Hinselmann. He observed that cervical cancer started as minute ulcers which could be recognised by means of suitable illumination and magnification. He developed the colposcope which provides three-dimensional images which can be magnified from 4 to 40 times (Farley 2005).

Colposcopy gained momentum globally in the 1970s, with one of its main objectives being the prevention of unnecessary cone biopsies. Cone biopsies are discussed in greater detail below but involve removal of a relatively large quantity of cervical tissue and may be associated with significant side effects. Cone biopsies in the 1970s were often found on laboratory analysis to contain little or no abnormal pathology. There was concern that these invasive procedures were being unnecessarily performed on young, reproductive-aged women to the possible detriment of their childbearing ability (Benedet et al. 2004).

The colposcope is both a diagnostic and therapeutic tool. As well as allowing the cervix to be examined and biopsied, it also allows visualisation of the cervix to facilitate treatment. Sometimes the two procedures will be combined in one visit (see 'See and Treat' colposcopy). However, for the most part an initial colposcopy will be performed to assess the extent of any cervical abnormality, and treatment will be carried out at a subsequent appointment. Therapeutic and diagnostic colposcopies are principally carried out in gynaecological clinics and primary care facilities.

When is a colposcopy performed?

Despite the fact that cervical screening programmes are now relatively mature and would appear to provide a perfect forum for randomised, controlled trials, there are still many screening issues which remain the subject of debate. The exact indication for performing a colposcopy is one such issue. Although clearly warranted in some situations, there are others in which its advantage over conventional cytology testing is yet to be confirmed.

Within the UK, over 129,000 referrals for colposcopy were reported between 2005–2006, 80% of which were triggered by a screening test and 17% were clinically indicated. Of women referred for a colposcopy after a screening test over a third followed findings

Box 2.2 Possible cervical smear test results and action to be taken

Smear result	Action – Australia (NHMRC 1994)	Action – UK NHSCSP
Negative	Return to recall.	Return to recall.
Negative but with incidental observations		Return to recall and treat any infections as appropriate.
Inadequate results/sample/Unsatisfactory result	Repeat smear within six months (ideally 6–12 weeks later).	Repeat smear.
Borderline nuclear changes/ ACS-US/ASC-H	Repeat smear in 1 year.	Repeat test in six months. After three consecutive negative tests woman can return to normal recall. If three borderline tests proceed to colposcopy.
Mild dyskaryosis/LSIL	Repeat smear in 12 months – if still LSIL then proceed to colposcopy. If repeat smear normal – another smear in 12 months. After two further negative smears proceed to normal screening intervals.	Colposcopy or repeat smear in six months.
LSIL + age > 30 and no negative history of normal smears in last three years (Australia)	Immediate colposcopy or repeat smear in six months.	
Moderate dyskaryosis/ HSIL	Colposcopy. Histological confirmation of a high grade lesion is recommended before treatment.	Colposcopy
Severe dyskaryosis/ HSIL	Colposcopy. Histological confirmation of a high grade lesion is recommended before treatment.	Colposcopy
Severe dyskaryosis/? Invasive carcinoma HSIL +? invasive component	Colposcopy within two weeks.	Urgent colposcopy.
Squamous cell carcinoma	Colposcopy within two weeks.	Urgent colposcopy.

of moderate dyskaryosis (HSIL) and a slightly smaller proportion followed findings of severe dyskaryosis (HSIL) or worse (Health and Social Care Information Centre Statistics 2006). It is generally accepted that cytology indicating HSIL suggests the need for immediate colposcopy. Women with HSIL have a 62–89% chance of having high grade CIN and a 0–3% chance of invasive cancer, depending on the severity of the cytology (Victorian Cervical Cytology Registry 2002).

However, whether or not colposcopy is necessary for low grade or borderline lesions is less clear. In most cases LSIL do not require any intervention. According to one meta-analysis more than two thirds of ASCUS/ borderline changes and almost half of LSIL/mild dyskaryosis regress spontaneously over a period of up to 24 months (Melnikow et al. 1998).

However, a minority of low grade lesions are known to harbour high grade CIN or even invasive cancer which is not detected by cervical cytology testing alone. Between 5% and 17% of women with ASC-US and 15–30% of women with LSIL are expected to have CIN 2 or 3 on biopsy (Lindique 2005). The sheer number of low grade lesions diagnosed each year (more than a quarter of a million in the UK (Bentley 2006)), means that there are relatively large numbers of high risk women 'hidden' amongst the low grade dysplasia population. The question is whether or not to further investigate all low grade lesions with colposcopy, recognising the fact that in the majority of cases the procedure would be unnecessary.

Different countries have tackled this issue in different ways. Scheungraber et al. (2004) requested national guidelines from 38 cervical pathology/colposcopy specialists in different countries in order to compare when colposcopy was performed. Of the 23 that responded it was found that practices varied significantly. For example, in Australia it is considered that ASC-US and LSIL can be safely managed by repeat cytology at 12 and 24 months (National Health and Medical Research Council (NHMRC) 2005). Conversely, the NHSCSP suggests that ideally women with mild dyskaryosis require a colposcopy, although they qualify this statement by saying that repeat cytology testing is also adequate (NHSCSP 2004).

In the USA, a 30 million dollar study was set up by the National Cancer Institute (NCI) in order to investigate this and other factors in the management of women with equivocal and low grade cervical smear abnormalities. The Atypical Squamous Cells of Undetermined Significance/Low Grade Squamous Intraepithelial Lesion (ASCUS/LSIL) Triage Study (ALTS) looked at the role of HPV testing in the follow-up of women with cervical neoplasia (Solomon et al. 2001). It determined that in the presence of high risk HPV subtypes, colposcopy should be performed for LSIL but in the absence of high risk HPV repeat cytology alone was probably adequate.

It is interesting to note that despite this recommendation, a random sample of American College of Obstetrician and Gynecologist (ACOG) fellows indicated that most of the survey participants continued to perform colposcopy for any ASC-US result, regardless of HPV status (Noller 2003, Cox 2005). This is probably a reflection of the litigious climate in the USA which is also a growing concern in many other western countries.

Within the UK, the evidence to support HPV testing for low grade abnormalities was considered to be insufficient to incorporate it into the NHSCSP. The Medical Research Council is currently conducting a trial into HPV testing called the Trial of Management of Borderline and Other Low Grade Abnormal smears (TOMBOLA: see www.tombola.ac.uk).

Within cervical screening programmes there are a few situations in which colposcopy is generally accepted to be better than an ordinary cervical smear and has replaced it. These include the screening of:

(1) high risk groups of women (e.g. the immunosuppressed such as women post-organ transplant or with HIV)
(2) women whose cervical smear samples are repeatedly reported as inadequate
(3) a persistent unsatisfactory smear
(4) atypical glandular cytology (AGC)

Box 2.3 shows some other indications for colposcopy as outlined by the National Health Service Cervical Screening Programme (2004).

Box 2.3 Screening indications for colposcopy (National Health Service Cervical Screening Programme 2004)

Under normal circumstances women should be referred for colposcopy if they have:

(1) Three consecutive inadequate samples.
(2) Three cervical smears showing borderline nuclear changes.
(3) Endocervical cell changes.
(4) Three abnormal smears of any grade in a period of ten years, even if returned to recall on one or more occasions in that period.
(5) Mild dyskaryosis on a cervical smear; it is also considered acceptable to have a repeat cervical smear.
(6) All women with moderate dyskaryosis should proceed to colposcopy within four weeks of referral.
(7) All women with severe dyskaryosis should proceed to colposcopy within four weeks of referral.
(8) Women with possible invasive disease should be seen urgently – preferably within two weeks of referral – for colposcopy.
(9) Women with a cervical smear showing glandular neoplasia – preferably within two weeks of referral.
(10) All women with an abnormal cervix.
(11) All women with symptoms of cervical cancer (e.g. postcoital bleeding in women over 40 years, intermenstrual bleeding, persistent vaginal discharge.
(12) Previous treatment for CIN if they have a cytology report of mild dyskaryosis or worse.

How is a colposcopy performed?

The woman is placed into the lithotomy position and a speculum is inserted into her vagina. Before any cervical examination is commenced, the external genitalia and vaginal walls should be examined for signs of warty pre-malignant disease (Lindique 2005). Sometimes a cervical smear will be taken before the colposcopy although the usefulness of this practice has been questioned (Rieck et al. 2006).

A comprehensive colposcopic examination involves four steps (Farley 2005):

(1) Inspection of the unprepared cervix with the naked eye.
(2) Inspection of the cervix with the colposcope, usually after the application of dilute acetic acid. The dilute acetic acid removes mucous, dehydrates and desiccates cells and highlights abnormal epithelium by making it appear white, a process known as aceto-whitening (Smith 2000).
(3) Inspection of the cervix with colposcope after application of Lugol's iodine. This stage is not always necessary and its added benefit has been questioned by some (Bosze 2006).
(4) Biopsy. After adequate assessment has been made of the cervix visually, punch biopsies may be performed, although sometimes they are omitted when high grade dysplasia is suspected. This is because it is possible to miss the area of highest grade abnormality.

While it may be reassuring to have confirmation of the presence of cervical disease prior to treatment, some consider punch biopsy to be a potentially misleading investigation. It is thus argued by some that if excisional treatment is planned, the decision of whether or not to proceed should be based on cytologic and colposcopic findings alone (Byrom et al. 2006).

Limitations of colposcopy

The sensitivity of colposcopy is variable and contingent on the practitioner (Ferris et al. 2005). Its accuracy can be measured by comparing colposcopy findings with the eventual

---

> **Box 2.4 Endocervical curettage (ECC)**
>
> One of the reasons that colposcopy can fail to identify invasive cancer is that the endocervical canal is not visualised during the procedure. In order to overcome this difficulty the procedure of endocervical curettage was introduced to be performed at the same time as the colposcopy. The entire length of the cervical canal was curetted (i.e. the mucous membrane was scraped) using either a curette or more recently an endocervical cytobrush.
>
> ECC was used for many years in the absence of large, randomised controlled trials to determine its efficacy. The data which does exist to support the practice is limited, particularly for use in women under the age of 40 (Solomon et al. 2007). Today in many centres it has therefore been abandoned. Most colposcopists instead use an endocervical speculum which allows examination of the lower endocervical canal, reducing the necessity for ECC. Most patients with suspected glandular abnormalities are treated with excisional techniques, also rendering ECC unnecessary.
>
> (Abu and Davies 2005)

---

histology findings. A meta-analysis in 2002 found that colposcopy was accurate in 89% of cases (Olaniyan 2002). It was considered to be more accurate in detecting high grade disease (although the ALTS study failed to corroborate this). In the ALTS study, only 53.6% of the CIN3 cases identified during follow-up had been detected at the 'immediate' colposcopy (ALTS Group 2003). The accuracy of colposcopy in detecting micro-invasive and invasive cancer has also been shown to be low on some occasions. (Farley 2005).

In order to improve the accuracy of colposcopy some centres in the past performed an additional procedure known as endocervical curettage (see Box 2.4).

Most countries now have stringent training courses for colposcopists. Training and maintaining skills requires a high volume of patients and good interactive correlation with cytologists and histopathologists. Ongoing multidisciplinary communication facilitates confirmation that what is seen colposcopically correlates with the final cytologic and histopathologic diagnosis (Mitchell 1993).

Nursing care of a patient undergoing a diagnostic colposcopy

Colposcopy is a distressing procedure for most women (Rostad 2002). There are two reasons for this. First, it indicates that a cervical abnormality is present with its inevitable associations with cancer. Second, it is invasive and discomforting. There is some data to suggest that anxiety is associated more with fear of the procedure than the actual results (Marteau et al. 1990).

Many women lack understanding of what happens during colposcopy – a factor which exacerbates anxiety levels (Marteau et al.1990). This being the case, the principal strategy available to nurses has traditionally been to help alleviate anxiety by the provision of information (Howells et al. 1999, Freeman-Wang et al. 2001).

The question is what kind of information do women seek? A study by Byrom et al. (2003) indicated that much of the printed information women were being given was inadequate. A qualitative study by Neale et al (2003) identified a number of areas in which women requested the need for further information. Common questions which arose included:

(1) What will happen during the colposcopy?
(2) What will be found?
(3) How will I feel afterwards?
(4) What am I allowed to do?

Many women expressed concerns about the waiting times involved between receiving their abnormal cytology report and undergoing a colposcopy. This is a theme which has been consistently raised as a source of anxiety and possibly reflects more weighty fears about the biopsy results and cancer (Posner and Vessy 1988). Within the UK between 2005 and 2006, of the women requiring colposcopy only 15% were offered an appointment within two weeks, 43% within four weeks and 83% by eight weeks from referral (NSHSC 2006). These waiting times indicate a failure to achieve National Health Service Cervical Screening Programme goals and reflect the high demand on colposcopy services within the UK (NHSCSP 2004, Bentley et al. 2006).

Who carries out colposcopies?

Initially, this was considered the role of the doctor, but increasingly it is being delegated to specially trained colposcopists, many of whom are nurses. In part this is a pragmatic decision, arising out of a need to reduce doctors' hours. It has received a mixed response from the nursing fraternity, some of whom feel that the nurse's role is becoming over medicalised (Jolley and Wright 2006).

Colposcopy nurses have been practising for many years, assisting with the colposcopy procedure and in the care of the patients undergoing colposcopy. The nurse colposcopist, however, is a much more recent development. In the UK, the first was accredited by the British Society for Colposcopy and Cervical Pathology (BSCC) in 1996. There are now over 120 nurse colposcopists in the UK with a further 90 in training (Jolley and Wright 2006). The training nurses receive is the same as the doctors' with an additional input in cytology and histopathology. Nurses participate in every stage of colposcopy – both diagnostic and therapeutic (Huff 2005).

The principles behind the extended role of the nurse are examined in Box 2.5. There are now a number of studies evaluating the impact of nurses taking on roles that were previously held by other health professionals – principally doctors. These have consistently shown the potential for specialist nurses to provide a service which is at least of equivalent quality to that of their predecessors (Hill et al. 1994, Sharples et al. 2002). For example, Aubrey and Yoxall (2001) examined the skills of the advanced neonatal nurse practitioner in their unit and found that they were comparable with the specialist registrar. In addition, they had faster intubation times and babies were found to receive surfactant more quickly and were found to be warmer when treated by the specialist nurse.

There is only a small literature concerning the efficacy of nurse colposcopists. Smith (2000) cites a number of advantages of having nurses perform colposcopy including:

- greater continuity of care
- improved patient contact
- greater choice for patients
- improved flexibility of clinic times
- greater involvement and job satisfaction for nurses

Morris et al. (1998) compared cervical dysplasia evaluation and treatment techniques of eleven gynecologists and six nurse practitioners and found nurse practitioners to be viable alternative providers to doctors in the evaluation and treatment of cervical dysplasia. McPherson audited their nurse colposcopist in New Zealand and found an 82% histology: cytology: colposcopy correlation was achieved by the nurse in the third phase of his/her training programme. These results are comparable with other reported studies involving medical and nurse colposcopists. Todd et al. (2002) also examined the role of nurse colposcopist in a London hospital and found the service to be equivalent to medical practitioners.

Box 2.5 The extended role of the nurse

Nurses have adopted extended roles in something of an ad hoc way throughout the world, in general to meet local service requirements. Thus, the advanced nurse practitioner has in many cases been a reactive not a proactive position role. Castledine (2003) outlines criteria for advanced nursing practitioner:

(1) autonomous practitioner
(2) experienced and knowledgeable
(3) researcher and evaluator of care
(4) expert in health and nursing assessment
(5) expert in case management
(6) consultant, educator and leader
(7) respected and recognised by others in the profession

The extended role of the nurse has been embraced in both the UK and Australia. The nurse practitioner is defined by the ANMC (Australian Nursing and Midwifery Council):

> A nurse practitioner is a registered nurse educated to function autonomously and collaboratively in an advanced and extended clinical role. The nurse practitioner role includes assessment and management of clients using nursing knowledge and skills and may include but is not limited to the direct referral of patients to other healthcare professionals, prescribing medications, ordering diagnostic interventions.
>
> The nurse practitioner's role is grounded in the nursing profession's values, knowledge, theories and practice and provides innovative and flexible healthcare delivery that complements other healthcare providers. The scope of practice of the nurse practitioner is determined by the context in which the nurse practitioner is authorized to practice.
>
> (ANMC 2004).

Within the UK, the Nursing and Midwifery Council defines an advanced practitioner as:

> A registered nurse who has command of an expert knowledge and clinical competence, is able to make complex clinical decisions using expert clinical judgement, is an essential member of an interdependent healthcare team whose role is determined by the context in which he/she practises.
>
> (NMC 2004)

Whatever the semantics within different countries, advanced nursing practice worldwide shares certain characteristics which are central to the concept of the extended role of the nurse. These include post-graduate education and preparation, possession of expert clinical skills, independence and autonomy in the organisation of clinical practice, role eclecticism, ability to function in collegiate relationships with other healthcare providers and a world view of advanced practice which guides thinking. (NCPDNM 2005).

Management of high grade CIN

The type of treatment required for cervical abnormalities is determined by evaluation of the cytology report, colposcopic assessment and assessment of any histology specimens which may have been obtained during the colposcopy procedure. A number of other patient factors will also be taken into account, including:

- age
- parity
- desire for further children
- menstrual status
- general health
- immune status
- availability for follow-up and return visits

(Lindique 2005)

Two categories of therapy are available: ablative and excisional.

Ablative techniques

Ablative therapies have been widely used in the past because they cause comparatively few side effects. As their name suggests, they are basically methods of destroying the abnormal tissue at the transformation zone. There are a number of different types of ablative techniques. The most common techniques are laser ablation, which uses a laser, and cryotherapy which uses refrigerated gas. Cold coagulation, rather misleadingly, removes cells by heat (not cold) and is a third commonly-used ablative strategy.

Laser ablation is reported as having a success rate of approximately 95% and cryotherapy between 77% and 93%, although cryotherapy appears to be less effective treating high stage disease (Martin-Hirsh et al. 1999). Cryotherapy is the least costly option and is therefore more prevalent in low-resource settings (Kleinberg et al. 2003).

The major disadvantage shared by all the ablative strategies is that they leave no tissue specimen for histology. For this reason their use is restricted to situations in which:

(1) The cervix has been assessed by an experienced colposcopist and the entire transformation zone visualised.
(2) A targeted biopsy has confirmed the lesion.
(3) There is no evidence of an invasive cancer on cytology, colposcopic assessment or biopsy.
(4) There is no evidence of a glandular lesion on cytology or biopsy.

In recent years improvements to non-ablative methods have led to a marked reduction in the use of destructive strategies, specifically with the development of the Large Loop Excision of the Transformation Zone (LLETZ) procedure. This is described more fully below.

Excisional techniques – cervical conisation

This refers to cervical procedures in which a 'cone' of the cervix is removed. There are basically three methods:

• laser
• Large Loop Excision of the Transformation Zone (LLETZ) procedure, (also known – mainly in the USA – as Loop Electrosurgical Excisional Procedure)
• cold knife cone biopsy (this is described more fully in 'surgical techniques' on page 38)

These strategies can be diagnostic and/or therapeutic because they remove a piece of tissue which is evaluable by the histopathologists (Dresang 2005)

Laser conisation

A highly focused laser spot is used to take the cone biopsy. Haemostasis is achieved using the laser but a disadvantage of this technique is that the biopsy specimen can become damaged from the heat of the laser making it unreadable histopathologically. Treatment success rate is reported as 93–96%, and it is considered a less-traumatic alternative to a cold knife approach (Martin-Hirsch et al. 1999).

Large Loop Excision of the Transformation Zone (LLETZ)

The LLETZ procedure has largely replaced cold knife cone biopsy. It uses a wire loop electrode on the end of an insulating handle powered by electricity. The current is designed to cut and achieve coagulation simultaneously without causing heat damage to the tissue which is excised. It is generally performed under local anaesthetic and is cited as having a success rate of over 95% in a number of studies (Martin-Hirsch et al. 2004).

The low level of complications associated with the LLETZ procedure, coupled with general concerns about the accuracy of punch biopsies for cervical abnormalities (punch biopsies may miss the affected area) means that LLETZ is sometimes performed in the absence of punch biopsy. This is particularly common where there is clinical suspicion of high grade disease. Indeed, in recent years there has been concern about the proportion of LLETZ biopsies that contain no CIN, with reports of negative biopsy rates of between 4.7% and 41% (Mossa et al. 2005).

Side effects of treatment

Excisional treatments carry more toxicity than ablative ones and cold knife biopsy is associated with the most side effects of all and is examined more fully in the following section. Although LLETZ procedures are described as having low morbidity rates, they are not without toxicity altogether. Dunn et al. (2004) looked at morbidity after LLETZ in 557 patients and found an overall complication rate of 9.7% – of which 0.6% were major complications and 9.1% minor.

Minor complications included abdominal pain, vaginal bleeding, vaginal discharge and bladder spasm. The major complications included one patient who suffered a bowel injury, one who had transient chest pain and one with vaginal bleeding requiring surgical ligation.

Potential side effects from excisional and ablative treatments are discussed below and some of the information which may be helpful when caring for a woman who is about to undergo treatment for CIN is given in Box 2.6.

Box 2.6 Out-patient care of a patient receiving treatment for high grade CIN

With the exception of a hysterectomy and possibly a cone biopsy, generally patients will receive high grade CIN therapy as day cases. Most women will be discharged home feeling well, although it is generally recommended to:

- take the day off work
- arrange for a friend to collect you from the hospital

Expected side effects:

- period-type pain for the rest of the day, possibly feeling a little worse as the anaesthetic wears off
- light bleeding or discharge for a few days, no heavier than a light period. Should settle in two weeks but may persist for 4–6 weeks

Unexpected side effects (contact GP or gynaecologist):

- heavier bleeding
- offensive-smelling discharge

Discharge advice:

- avoid sexual intercourse for 3–4 weeks until the cervix has healed
- avoid use of tampons for a similar duration
- follow-up advice will necessitate repeat cervical cytology the frequency of which is dependent on the CIN stage – discuss with your gynaecologist

http://www.cancerbackup.org.uk/Aboutcancer/Screening/Cervicalscreening/TreatingCIN

Potential side effects from excisional and ablative treatments for CIN include:

(1) Pain

Pain may occur during or post-procedure. Usually the procedure is tolerated with minimal anaesthetic. Some studies have examined the role of topical and inhalational analgesia during LLETZ with possible benefit (Cruickshank et al. 2005, Farley et al. 2005). Pain post-procedure is generally mild 'period-like', and does not persist for long. Patients should be advised to seek medical help if they experience pain any more severe than this.

(2) Haemorrhage

Light, bloodstained discharge for a few weeks post-procedure is normal. Heavier bleeding is less usual but generally improves with rest. Sometimes the usual menstrual pattern is disturbed. The risk of haemorrhage can be minimised by avoiding coitus for three weeks post-procedure and also avoiding the insertion of tampons, etc. In the rare case of severe bleeding, occasionally hospital admission is necessary for observation, bed rest, packing or suturing under anaesthesia.

(3) Infection

Sometimes secondary bleeding commencing a couple of weeks after the procedure is related to infection, in which case treatment with antibiotics might be helpful (Jolley and Wright 2006).

(4) Cervical stenosis

This is a rare side effect and is a greater risk in women older than 40 years (Houlard et al. 2002). The risk may be reduced by using vaginal oestrogen cream post-operatively. Management depends on the menopausal status of the patient, desire for preservation of fertility, histopathology and presence or absence of symptoms. Potential options include observation with or without ultrasound, cervical dilatation or hysterectomy.

(5) Complications with pregnancy

There is data to suggest that a LLETZ procedure can result in pregnancy-related complications. Kyrgiou at al. (2006) in a systematic review of the literature found it to be significantly associated with preterm delivery, low birthweight and premature rupture of the membranes.

Surgical techniques: cold knife cone biopsy and hysterectomy

Initially, cold knife cone biopsy was the main cervical conisation option before colposcopy and LLETZ. It is an excisional technique which removes a significant length of tissue along the cervical canal (from 1.5 to 3 cm). It uses a traditional surgical approach, cutting the tissue with a knife, and is usually performed under general anaesthetic.

Specific indications for cold knife cone biopsy today are:

(1) failure to visualise the upper limit of the cervical transformation zone in a woman with a high grade squamous abnormality on her referral smear
(2) suspicion of an early invasive cancer on cytology, biopsy or colposcopic assessment
(3) suspected presence of an additional glandular abnormality (e.g. adenocarcinoma in situ) on cytology or biopsy (i.e. a mixed lesion)

Its success is cited to be 90–94% in non-randomised studies (Martin-Hirsch et al. 1999). Women over 50 with a high grade squamous abnormality more frequently require cold knife cone biopsy. Potential post-procedural problems are similar to those described for the other conisation strategies described above except that there is a greater risk of bleeding and of fertility issues.

Bleeding is a particular problem after a large resection. One study indicated bleeding occurred in 10–15% cases of cold knife conisation as opposed to 2% of cases after LEEP (Montz 2000). Because of this risk of haemorrhage, the cervix may be packed with gauze post-procedure and occasionally pharmacological measures will be needed to arrest the bleeding such as tranexamic acid or vasopressin (Martin-Hirsch and Kitchener 1999). Cold knife conisation has also been found to be associated with a significantly higher rate of preterm delivery, low birthweight and caesarean section (Kyrgiou at al. 2006).

Situations in which cold knife cone biopsy might be indicated are if adequate resection margins are required which may not be attainable with loop excision techniques, for example if:

- the squamo-columnar junction is not visible
- there is suspicion of invasive disease
- there is suspicion of glandular intra-epithelial neoplasia

(Martin-Hirsch and Kitchener 1999)

Hysterectomy is widely used in the management of invasive cancer and is discussed more fully in Chapter 3. It is not often used for the treatment of CIN, but may be advised in certain situations, particularly amongst older women who have completed their family. A hysterectomy might be indicated:

- in the presence of co-existent benign disease (fibroids, prolapse, endometriosis)
- following previous treatment (e.g. cone biopsy) where positive margins are still suspected

Which CIN treatment is the best?

In a meta-analysis by Martin-Hirsch et al. (1999) there was deemed to be inadequate data to definitively nominate one technique against another. The toxicity profiles were, however, considered to be significant in choosing a therapy. The review indicated that laser ablation caused more peri-operative severe pain, and possibly more haemorrhage compared with loop excision. Laser conisation takes longer to perform, requires greater operative training and investment in expensive equipment, produces more peri-operative pain, and more severe thermal artefact than loop excision. LLETZ is associated with decreased blood loss, reduced operative time and is tissue sparing when compared with cold knife cone biopsy or CO_2 laser (Lewis and Lashgari 1994). It was thus concluded that LLETZ might be a preferred choice for many indications.

'See and treat' colposcopy

Following a diagnosis of abnormal cervical cytology, multiple clinic visits may be required, sometimes over a period of months (Dainty et al. 2005). Separate appointments may be made for colposcopic assessment, then treatment, then follow-up. Sometimes there are also supplementary visits to obtain histology results. Each of these consultations can be anxiety-provoking and time-consuming. They also have the potential to 'lose' patients who drop out of treatment or follow-up. It is estimated that between biopsy and returning for treatment 25–70% of patients may be lost to the system (Dainty et al. 2005, Lindique 2005). According to Health and Social Care Information Centre Statistics (2006) out of every ten 'new' and 'return for treatment' appointments, eight were attended, one was cancelled by the patient and in one the patient failed to turn up without reason. Only 67% of follow-up appointments were attended.

Because of this, some centres have developed 'see and treat' clinics. In these clinics, instead of having first a diagnostic colposcopy and then a therapeutic intervention, women are seen and treated immediately if intervention is deemed necessary. This strategy is particularly useful in cases when non-attendance for future follow-up is predicted to be a problem (for example, in developing countries). However, there are also some problems with the 'see and treat' model. The most common criticism is that there is a potential for over-treatment. To quote from Benedet et al. (2004):

> This form of 'see-and-treat' colposcopy, in which an abnormal Pap test is followed by colposcopy and immediate excision, potentially brings the clinician back full circle, negating the need for colposcopic proficiency, and results in a high rate of surgical procedures, often with minimal or no pathology.

The psychological effects of 'see and treat' colposcopy are unclear, with the research in this area conflicting. Some studies associate it with higher and others with lower levels of anxiety (Freeman-Wang et al. 2001, Orbell et al. 2004).

For this reason, some organisations, such as the Royal Australian and New Zealand College of Obstetricians and Gynaecologists (RANZCOG) caution against the 'see and treat' system, suggesting it is reserved for specific situations such as:

- colposcopic indication of significant high grade lesion
- major concern about patient compliance
- logistical problems – for example the patient lives a long way from treatment centre

Another possible solution is a 'one stop' colposcopy clinic. Here, colposcopy biopsy results are made available in two hours and the woman has the option of immediate treatment if necessary. However, such a clinic requires a high investment in technology and is therefore costly to set up (Jolley and Wright 2006).

Adenocarcinoma of the cervix

Chapter 1 discussed the most common form of cervical carcinoma, which is squamous cell carcinoma and accounts for the majority of cervical cancer cases. The following section will review the diagnosis and management of adenocarcinoma, which although only accounting for the minority of cervix cancer cases is becoming an increasingly important topic within gynaecological oncology.

Diagnosis

As opposed to squamous cell carcinoma of the cervix, which has been declining in recent decades, the incidence of adenocarcinoma of the cervix has increased. Cervical adenocarcinoma accounts for almost a quarter of all cervical cancers diagnosed in the USA and has increased by 107% relative to all cervical cancers and 95% relative to squamous cell carcinoma (Schorge et al. 2004).

In part, this could be explained by difficulties in diagnosing adenocarcinoma. Cervical screening would appear to be less effective at detecting glandular lesions, probably because of a combination of cytology sampling difficulties and problems with cytological interpretation. The role of liquid based cytology in the diagnosis of adenocarcinoma is not clear, but is hoped to improve detection.

Box 2.7 Beyond colposcopy

A number of different technologies have been developed which may impact on the use of colposcopy and replace it in some settings – particularly in remote and rural or in poorly resourced areas which are not frequently accessed by experienced colposcopists. These techniques include: cervicography, telecolposcopy, digital image colposcopy, direct visual inspection, and fluorescence spectroscopy.

Cervicography uses a cervicograph apparatus, which consists of a camera and strobe light. It is a technique which allows non-medical staff to collect an image which is essentially a 'snap shot' of the colposcopic appearance. This image can be later analysed by trained personnel (Farley et al. 2005).

Telecolposcopy allows for the transportation and interpretation of the colposcopic image over short or long distances using telemedicine (Farley et al. 2005).

Direct visual inspection (DVI) is a method of visualising the cervix, which has been proposed in areas with limited health care. It may be performed with either dilute acetic acid or with Lugol's solution applied to the cervix, as in colposcopy. The cervix is then visualised with the naked eye alone. This technique may have a role in mass screening campaigns in developing countries which have limited resources (Farley et al. 2005). It is discussed more fully in Chapter 9.

Laser-induced fluorescence spectroscopy is a non-invasive real-time technique for evaluating neoplasia by measuring the autofluorescence of tissue based on the amounts of naturally occurring fluorophores present (Farley et al. 2005). Spectroscopy requires only that a probe be placed on the cervix and so any practitioner able to perform cervical smear screening could one day use fluorescence spectroscopy. The ease of use of fluorescence spectroscopy would permit a large number of trained personnel to use the device and means that results are immediately available (Mitchell et al. 1999).

Furthermore, colposcopy, which has been found to be a helpful diagnostic tool with squamous cell carcinoma, is not thought to be very accurate in the case of glandular lesions. Nevertheless, it is usually performed in the assessment of adenocarcinoma, with the rationale that it can at least exclude a clinically overt carcinoma.

Cold knife cone biopsy is considered the best biopsy strategy for women with suspected glandular abnormality because it allows deeper excision and preservation of the tissue sample for histology.

Natural history

The natural history of adenocarcinoma is less well understood than squamous cell carcinoma. However, just as pre-cancerous cellular abnormalities precede the development of SCC of the cervix, so they are thought to precede adenocarcinoma of the cervix. The grading of glandular lesions is illustrated in Table 2.2 and can be seen to be complicated by more than one classification system.

Risk factors

The risk factors associated with cervical adenocarcinoma are not well understood, but those which are significant for SCC, such as cigarette smoking, seem not to play a major role (Berrington de Gonzalez et al. 2004; Lindstrom et al. 2004). Furthermore, the frequency of HPV reported in glandular dysplasia is highly variable, with positivity for HPV 16 or 18 ranging from 6% to 95% (Zaino 2002). Diabetes mellitus, hypertension, obesity and nulliparity have all been suggested as co-factors (Chargui et al. 2006).

Table 2.2 Classification of glandular lesions

USA (Bethesda System)	UK	Australia (Modified Bethesda system)	World Health Organization (WHO)
atypical glandular cells (AGC) not otherwise specified		atypical endocervical or glandular cells of undetermined significance	glandular atypia
favour neoplasia	low grade cervical glandular intraepithelial neoplasia (CGIN)	possible high grade cervical lesion	endocervical glandular dysplasia
endocervical AIS	high grade CGIN	endocervical adenocarcinoma in situ	adenocarcinoma in situ
adenocarcinoma	adenocarcinoma	adenocarcinoma	adenocarcinoma

Treatment

The diagnostic difficulties detecting adenocarcinoma, coupled with its relative rarity, makes randomised, controlled trials difficult to perform. Much of the data about management is based on retrospective analyses and must therefore be interpreted with caution.

Cervical adenocarcinoma is known for its unfavourable outcome, and it remains controversial whether this is due to a late detection by the cervical smear test or poorer response to therapy (Chargui et al. 2006). At diagnosis, adenocarcinomas tend to be larger and tumour size is a prognostic indicator, with tumours that are larger than 4 cm being associated with the worst outcome (Chargui et al. 2006). This, coupled with a propensity for early lymphatic and haematogenous metastasis, probably contributes to the poorer prognosis.

Once the diagnosis is confirmed management strategies differ according to the degree of invasion and are comparable with therapies for squamous cell disease. Choice of treatment is significantly influenced by the fact that the median age of women with adenocarcinoma of the cervix is mid-thirties. At this age many women will wish to preserve their fertility and so a balance must be struck between eradication of the disease and fertility preservation. (NHSCSP 1999, McCluggage 2003).

Stages of adenocarcinoma

Adenocarcinoma in situ (AIS)

Adenocarcinoma has an in situ phase just as squamous cell carcinoma does. Although the relationship between low grade adenocarcinoma in situ (AIS) and cancer has also not been clearly established, it is now widely accepted that high grade AIS can progress to invasive disease.

Treatment for AIS remains controversial, ranging from large loop excision of the transformation zone to simple or even radical hysterectomy (Krivak et al. 2001, Shipman and Bristow 2001). Although more conservative measures have been adopted in recent years, these must be applied cautiously and in the context of assiduous follow-up. Rates of residual adenocarcinoma in situ after cone biopsy vary from 0% to 40% despite negative margins (Krivak et al. 2001, Shipman and Bristow 2001).

Microinvasive adenocarcinoma

Within the spectrum of glandular cervical neoplasia, early invasive (or microinvasive) adenocarcinoma has been difficult to define histologically. Definitions of the level of invasion have varied from 1 to 5 mm, depending on the study. Once again, simple hysterectomy is generally the therapy of choice, although more conservative therapies are being evaluated. A retrospective review by Ostor (2000) indicated that seven women with microinvasive adenocarcinoma who were treated with conisation alone had not developed recurrent disease after four years' follow-up. Although clearly only a small sample, these results are encouraging for those who wish to adopt fertility sparing strategies.

Nevertheless, some physicians are reluctant to recommend conservative treatment for a number of reasons. These include the risk of non-compliant patient follow-up, concerns about multifocal disease and general discomfort in following patients with this diagnosis (Krivak et al. 2001).

Invasive adenocarcinoma

A diagnosis of invasive carcinoma requires hysterectomy at a minimum and stages IA2 or higher will probably benefit from the addition of adjuvant chemoradiotherapy (Schorge et al. 2004). Cervical adenocarcinomas tend to metastasise to the lymph nodes and have been described as being less sensitive to radiation therapy and to chemotherapy than squamous carcinomas. Some recent reports suggest there is a role for combination chemotherapy in cases of advanced disease (Saito et al. 2004).

Adenosquamous carcinoma

Often adenocarcinoma cells may be found within squamous lesions (Zaino 2002). Adenosquamous tumours contain both malignant squamous and glandular cells and appear to be relatively more frequent in younger women. There is considerable argument about their relative prognosis and further work is required to define true outcome in relation to other tumours.

Diethylstilbestrol (DES) exposure and adenocarcinoma

Diethylstilbestrol is a synthetic oestrogen that was used from the late 1930s to the 1970s in order to prevent miscarriage and other complications of pregnancy. In 1971 the FDA issued a warning about its use after a high incidence of cervical and vaginal adenocarcinoma was observed in young women whose mothers had taken DES during pregnancy. It is thought that 15,000 Australian, 4 million American and 300,000 British women have taken the drug (Fickling 2004).

DES has not been given to pregnant women since this time but still has its legacy. Women who took it have a slightly higher risk of breast cancer than average and are encouraged to have regular mammograms (Palmer et al. 2006). Women exposed to the drug in utero may have structural abnormalities in their reproductive tract, a decreased fertility rate and poor pregnancy outcomes, (although many of them have also had successful pregnancies). They are recommended to have regular gynaecological examinations – either digital or colposcopic – plus annual cytological evaluation. These women have a higher risk of ectopic pregnancy and pre-term delivery and are therefore recommended to have an obstetric consultation if trying to conceive. Male offspring of mothers who took DES also have an increased risk of genital abnormalities and possibly increased risk of prostate and testicular cancer.

Many females who may have been exposed to DES in utero are now of childbearing age. Current researchers continue to look at the effects of DES and at the potential for health problems in a third generation: the grandchildren of women who took DES during pregnancy.

The NHMRC cervical screening guidelines in Australia specifically address the issue of DES exposure and suggest that these women:

(1) Should be offered annual cytological screening and colposcopic examination of both the cervix and vagina.
(2) Should begin screening at any time they request and continue indefinitely.
(3) Should be managed in a specialist centre by an experienced colposcopist, if DES-exposed.

Conclusion

This chapter has reviewed the procedure for taking a cervical smear and for performing a colposcopy. It has looked at the management of high grade neoplasia and discussed some

---

Box 2.8 Cervical neoplasia in pregnancy

Although cervical cancer is cited as being the most common reproductive tract malignancy associated with pregnancy, it is still a rare occurrence (Brown et al. 2005). In spite of this there is a large quantity of literature on the subject, and clearly it is a difficult clinical problem. Effective treatment has to be provided without compromising the pregnancy, especially when it is possible that patients will be deprived of their fertility after the treatment (Germann et al. 2005).

The exact incidence of cervical cancer amongst pregnant women is difficult to establish. One Swedish study found 1.1 cases per 100,000 deliveries (Norstrom et al. 1997). Other estimates are much higher – as high as 1 per 1000 to 2500 live births, with carcinoma-in-situ (CIS) estimated to affect a further 1 in 750 pregnancies (Brown et al. 2005). The number of obstetric deliveries associated with cervical cancer between 1991 and 1999 in California was 434 (Dalrymple et al. 2005). Most of these were not diagnosed until after the delivery.

Management of cervical cancer in pregnancy raises two important questions. First, is the prognosis of cervical cancer different during pregnancy? Second, under which conditions can treatment be delayed in order to give the foetus time to mature (Germann et al. 2005)?

The former of these two questions relates to a common misconception that the immunosuppression that accompanies pregnancy may lead to faster progression of the disease (Muller and Smith 2005). In fact the consensus appears to be that the prognosis of cervical cancer during pregnancy is not any worse than in non-pregnant women (Germann et al. 2005). Whether or not delivery can be delayed is more problematic. This decision is dependent on two factors: the gestational age and the stage of disease.

Pre-invasive cervical abnormalities can be satisfactorily managed with observation using colposcopy and biopsy – the risk of progression into an invasive lesion during that time period is low (Muller and Smith 2005). Even high grade lesions can be followed in this way until the pregnancy is completed unless there is a suggestion of invasive disease. Colposcopy has been described as safe in pregnancy (Brown et al. 2005) and although biopsy may induce bleeding, it has not been cited as resulting in pregnancy losses (Massad et al. 2005). The risk of bleeding increases incrementally each trimester (Muller and Smith 2005).

For micro-invasive disease, cone biopsy has been cited as adequate therapy although it must be accompanied by rigorous follow-up. Cervical conisation in pregnancy has been associated with a number of problems. First of all it may result in significant blood loss – up to half a litre in approximately 10% of patients. It has also been associated with infection, pre-term labour and spontaneous abortion occurring in as many as 18% of women in the first trimester. Because of these toxicities the procedure may be modified to obtain a shallower specimen, obviously increasing the risk of residual disease (Brown et al. 2005). Others recommend delaying excisional strategies until after the pregnancy. Muller and Smith (2005) suggest that if absolutely indicated cone biopsy should be performed between 14 and 20 weeks and may necessitate cervical cerclage (surgically stitching the cervix closed). Conisation should not be performed within four weeks of anticipated delivery because of inadequate healing and the risk of haemorrhage during labour.

Fortunately, most women diagnosed with invasive disease during pregnancy are found to be in the early stages (Muller and Smith 2005). Following a diagnosis of invasive cancer in a pregnancy of less than 20 weeks, some advocate that therapy should be implemented immediately (Brown et al. 2005). If the therapy is surgery or radiotherapy this will unfortunately mean loss of the baby. Radiotherapy will induce abortion at doses of 35 to 40 Gy and at a median of 20 to 24 days or longer if started in the second trimester (Muller and Smith 2005). For some women this is an unacceptable option. In strongly desired pregnancies, the use of neoadjuvant chemotherapy in order to obtain fetal maturity can be considered and there is some, but limited evidence supporting the short-term safety of in-utero exposure of cytotoxic drugs (Sadler and Sykes 2005).

Where the gestation period is greater than 24 weeks, it is generally considered reasonable to delay treatment until after the birth of the child. For patients in this category, a caesarean section is recommended when the foetus is viable. If surgical management of the disease is chosen, radical hysterectomy and pelvic lymphadenectomy can be performed concurrently with the caesarean section (Germann et al. 2005).

In rare cases of advanced cancer in pregnancy the safety of delayed therapy is less clear and management decisions are thus more difficult. Because there is no cure for stage IVb disease then foetal issues will take precedence in this situation.

of the nursing issues associated with this. In the second part of the chapter adenocarcinoma of the cervix has been reviewed, along with the pre-cancerous cervical abnormalities which may precede this. Adenocarcinoma of the cervix appears to be increasing in incidence and is likely to be of growing significance in the future.

Frequently asked questions (see also Chapter 8, Cervical screening)

(1) Can I have a smear during my period?
   The best time is half way between menstrual periods because the cervix can be better viewed. Cervical smears taken during a period may result in an 'unsatisfactory' sample (Sherman et al. 2006).
(2) Can I have sex the night before my smear?
   Spermicides, barrier methods of contraception and lubricant jellies may interfere with the smear results, so avoid sex for 24 hours before smear if one of these is to be used NHSCSP (2006b)
(3) What will happen when I go for a colposcopy?
   A colposcopy is an out-patient procedure. You will be asked to lie on your back and a speculum will be inserted into your vagina. The colposcopist will then look at your cervix and may also apply some agents to help visualise it better. The colposcope doesn't go into your vagina. The procedure may be a little uncomfortable but should not be painful and there shouldn't be any significant after-effects. It may be necessary for biopsies to be taken. Once the results are available (which may take a week or two) you will be contacted regarding whether further treatment is necessary.

Resources

British Society for Clinical Cytology: http://www.clinicalcytology.co.uk/index.asp
National Association of Cytologists: http://www.nac.org.uk/index.php
British Society for Colposcopy and Cervical Pathology: http://www.bsccp.org.uk/
Royal Australian and New Zealand College of Gynaecologists and Obstetricians: http://www.ranzcog.edu.au/
National Health Service Cervical Screening Programme (NHSCSP): http://www.cancer-screening.nhs.uk/
National Institute for Health and Clinical Excellence (NICE): http://www.nice.org.uk/
Australian Society for Colposcopy and Cervical Pathology: http://www.asccp.com.au/
National Cervical Screening Program, Australia: http://www.breastscreen.info.au/internet/screening/publishing.nsf/Content/home
Cancer Research Council: http://www.cancerhelp.org.uk/help/default.asp?page=2739
DES Action UK: http://www.des-action.org.uk/

References

Abu J and Davies Q (2005) Endocervical curettage at the time of colposcopic assessment of the uterine cervix. *Obstetrical & Gynecological Survey*, 60 (5), 315–320

Arbyn M, Bergeron C, Klinkhamer P, et al. (2008) Liquid compared with conventional cervical cytology. A systematic review and meta-analysis. *Obstetrics and Gynaecology*, 111 (1), 167–177.

ASCUS-LSIL Triage Study (ALTS) Group (2003) Results of a randomized trial on the management of cytology interpretations of atypical squamous cells of undetermined significance. *Am J Obstet Gynecol*, 188, 1383–1392

Aubrey WR and Yoxall CW (2001) Evaluation of the role of the neonatal nurse practitioner in resuscitation of preterm infants at birth. *Archives of Disease in Childhood*, 85 (2), 96–100

Australian Nursing and Midwifery Council (2004) *Nurse Practitioner Standards Project: Report to the Australian Nursing and Midwifery Council, ANMC*. Australian Nursing and Midwifery Council, Dickson, ACT, Australia

Baker RW, O'Sullivan JP, Hanley J and Coleman DV (1999) The characteristics of false negative cervical smears – implications for the UK cervical cancer screening programme. *J Clin Pathol*, 52, 358–362

Bankhead CR, Brett J, Bukach C, et al. (2003) The impact of screening on future health-promoting behaviours and health beliefs: a systematic review. *Health Technology Assessment* (Winchester, England), 7 (42), 1–92

Benedet JL, Matisic JP and Bertrand MA (2004) The quality of community colposcopic practice. *Obstetrics and Gynaecology*, 103 (1), 92–100

Bentley E, Cotton S, Cruickshank M, et al. (TOMBOLA Group) (2006) Refining the management of low-grade cervical abnormalities in the UK National Health Service and defining the potential for human papillomavirus testing: a commentary on emerging evidence. *Journal of Lower Genital Tract Disease*, 10 (1), Jan, 26–38

Berrington de Gonzalez A, Sweetland S and Green J (2004) Comparison of risk factors for squamous cell and adenocarcinomas of the cervix: a meta-analysis. *British Journal of Cancer*, 90 (9), 1787–1791

Bosze P (2006) Colposcopy used in a primary setting. *European Journal of Gynae Oncology*, 27 (1), 5–9

Brown D, Berran P, Kaplan KJ, Winter WE and Zahn C (2005) Special situations: abnormal cervical cytology during pregnancy. *Clinical Obstetrics and Gynaecology*, 48 (1), 178–185

Byrom J, Douce G, Jones PW, Tucker H, Millinship J and Dhar K (2006) Should punch biopsies be used when high grade disease is suspected at initial colposcopic assessment? A prospective study. *International Journal of Gynaecological Cancer*, 16 (1), Jan/Feb, 253–256

Byrom J, Dunn PD, Hughes GM, et al. (2003) Colposcopy information leaflets: what women want to know and when they want to receive this information. *Journal of Medical Screening*, 10 (3), 1431–1437

Castledine G (2003) The development of advanced nursing practice in the UK, in McGee P and Castledine G (eds), *Advanced Nursing Practice*, 2nd edition. Blackwell, Oxford

Chargui R, Damak T, Khomsi F, et al. (2006) Prognostic factors and clinicopathologic characteristics of invasive carcinoma of the uterine cervix. *American Journal of Obstetrics and Gynaecology*, 194 (1), 43–48

Cox JT (2005) Management of women with cervical cytology interpreted as ASC-US or as ASC-H. *Clinical Obstetrics and Gynaecology*, 48 (1), 160–177

Cruickshank ME, Anthony GB, Fitzmaurice A, et al. (2005) A randomized controlled trial to evaluate the effect of self-administered analgesia on women's experience of out-patient treatment at colposcopy. *BJOG*, 112, Dec, 1652–1658

Dainty L, Elkas JC, Rose GS and Zahn C (2005) Controversial topics in abnormal cervical cytology; 'See and Treat'. *Clinical Obstetrics and Gynaecology*, 48 (1), March, 193–201

Dalrymple JL, Gilbert WM, Leiserowitz GS, et al. (2005) Pregnancy-associated cervical cancer. *The Journal of Maternal Fetal and Neonatal Medicine*, 17 (4), 269–276

Dresang LT (2005) Colposcopy: an evidence-based update. *J Am Board Fam Pract*, 18, 383–392

Dunn TS, Killoran K and Wolf D (2004) Complications of outpatient LLETZ procedures. *Journal of Reproductive Medicine*, 49, 76–78

Farley J, McBroom JW and Zahn CM (2005) Current techniques for the evaluation of abnormal cervical cytology. *Clinical Obstetrics and Gynaecology*, 48 (1), March, 133–146

Ferris DG, Litaker M and ALTS Group (2005) Interobserver agreement for colposcopy quality control using digitized colposcopic images during the ALTS trial. *Journal of Lower Genital Tract Disease*, 9 (1), 29–35

Fickling D (2004) Australia recognises cancer risk for 'DES daughters'. *Lancet*, 363 (9426), 19 June, 2059

Freeman-Wang T, Walker P, Linehan J, Coffey C, Glasser B and Sherr L (2001) Anxiety levels in women attending colposcopy clinics for treatment for cervical intraepithelial neoplasia: a randomised trial of written and video information. *BJOG*, 108 (5), May, 482–484

Germann N, Haie-Meder C, Morice P, et al. (2005) Management and clinical outcomes of pregnant patients with invasive cervical cancer. *Annals of Oncology*, 16 (3), 397–402

Health and Social Care Information Centre Statistics (HSCIC) (2005) Cervical Screening Programme, England 2004–2005. *Health and Social Care Information Centre Bulletin*, 2005/09/HSCIC

Hill J, Bird HA, Harmer R, Wright V and Lawton C (1994) An evaluation of the effectiveness, safety and acceptability of a nurse practitioner in a rheumatology outpatient clinic. *British Journal of Rheumatology*, 33, 283–288

Houlard S, Perrotin F, Fourquet F, Marret H, Lansac J and Body G (2002) Risk factors for cervical stenosis after laser cone biopsy. *European Journal of Obstetrics, Gynecology, & Reproductive Biology*, 104 (2), 144–147

Howells REJ, Dunn PDJ, Isasi T, et al. (1999) Is the provision of information leaflets before colposcopy beneficial? *British Journal of Obstetrics and Gynaecology*, 106 (6), 528–534

Huff BC (2005) Can advanced practice clinicians perform loop electrosurgical excision procedures and cryotherapy? *American Society for Colposcopy and Cervical Pathology*, 9 (3), 143–144

Jolley S (2004) Quality in colposcopy. *Nursing Standard*, 18 (23), 39–44

Jolley S and Wright S (2006) A vital role for nurse colposcopists, in Jollet S (ed.) *Gynaecology: Changing Services for Changing Needs*. John Wiley, Chichester, UK, pp. 47–62

Legro-Janssen T, Schijf C (2005) What do women think about abnormal smear test results? A qualitative interview study. *Journal of Psychosomatic Obstetrics and Gynaecology*, 26 (2), June, 141–145.

Karnon J, Peters J, Platt J, Chilcott J, McGoogan E and Brewer N (2004) Liquid-based cytology in cervical screening: an updated rapid and systematic review and economic analysis. *Health Technology Assessment* (Winchester, England), 8 (20), May, iii, 1–78

Kleinberg MJ, Straughn JM Jr, Stringer JSA and Partridge EE (2003) A cost-effectiveness analysis of management strategies for cervical intraepithelial neoplasia grades 2 and 3. *American Journal of Obstetrics and Gynecology*, 188 (5), May, 1186–1188.

Krivak TC, Rose GS, McBroom JW, Carlson JW, Winter WE and Kost ER (2001) Cervical adenocarcinoma in situ: a systematic review of therapeutic options and predictors of persistent or recurrent disease. *Obstetrical and Gynaecological Survey*, 56 (9), 567–575

Kyrgiou M, Koliopoulos G, Martin-Hirsch P, Arbyn M, Prendiville W and Paraskevaidis E (2006) Obstetric outcomes after conservative treatment for intraepithelial or early invasive cervical lesions: systematic review and meta-analysis. *Lancet*, 367 (9509), 489–498

Lewis PL and Lashgari M (1994) A comparison of cold knife, CO_2 laser, and electrosurgical loop conization in the treatment of cervical intraepithelial neoplasia. *Journal of Gynecologic Surgery*, 10 (4), 229–234

Lindeque BG (2005) Management of cervical premalignant lesions. *Best Practice and Research Clinical Obstetrics and Gynaecology*, 19 (4), 545–561

Lindstrom AK, Hellberg D, Backstrom T and Stendahl U (2004) Diagnostic, endocrinological, behavioral, and DNA ploidy differences between squamous cell and adenomatous carcinoma of the cervix uteri. *Oncology Research*, 14 (7–8), 321–324

McPherson G, Horsburgh M and Tracy C (2005) A clinical audit of a nurse colposcopist. colposcopy: cytology: histology correlation. *Nursing Praxis in New Zealand*, 21 (3), Nov, 13–23

Marteau TM, Walker P, Giles J and Smail M P (1990) Anxieties in women undergoing colposcopy. *British Jnl Obstet Gynaecol*, 97, 859–861

Martin-Hirsch PL and Kitchener H (1999) Interventions for preventing blood loss during the treatment of cervical intraepithelial neoplasia. *Cochrane Database of Systematic Reviews*, 1999, Issue 1. Art. No.: CD001421. DOI: 10.1002/14651858.CD001421.

Martin-Hirsch PL, Paraskevaidis E and Kitchener H (1999) Surgery for cervical intraepithelial neoplasia. *Cochrane Database of Systematic Reviews*, Issue 2, Art No.: CD001318. DOI: 10.102/14651858.CD001318.

Massad S, Wright T, Cox JT, Twiggs L and Wilkinson E (2005) Managing abnormal cytology results in pregnancy. *Journal of Lower Genital Tract Disease*, 9 (3), 146–148

McCluggage WG (2003) Endocervical glandular lesions: controversial aspects and ancillary techniques. *J Clin Pathol*, 56, 164–173

Melnikow J, Nuovo J, Willan AR, Chan BKS and Howell LP (1998) Natural history of cervical squamous intraepithelial lesions: a meta-analysis. *Obstet Gynecol*, 92, 727–735

Mitchell H (1993) Improving consistency in cervical cytology reporting. *J Natl Cancer Inst*, 85 (19), 6 Oct, 1592–1596

Mitchell MF, Cantor SB, Ramanujam N, Tortolero-Luna G and Richards-Kortum R (1999) Fluorescence spectroscopy for diagnosis of squamous intraepithelial lesions of the cervix. *Obstetrics and Gynaecology*, 93 (3), 462–470

Montz FJ (2000) Management of high grade cervical intraepithelial neoplasia and low-grade squamous intraepithelial lesion and potential complications. *Clinical Obstetrics & Gynecology*, 43 (2), 394–409

Morris DL, McLean CH, Bishop SL and Harlow KC (1998) A comparison of the evaluation and treatment of cervical dysplasia by gynaecologists and nurse practitioners. *Nurse Practitioner*, 23 (4), April, 101–102

Moss SM, Gray A, Marteau T, Legood R, Henstock E and Maissi E (2004) Evaluation of HPV/LBC cervical screening pilot studies: http://www.cancerscreening.nhs.uk/cervical/evaluation-hpv-2006feb.pdf (accessed 15/6/07)

Mossa MA, Carter PG, Abdu S, Young M, Thomas V and Barton D (2005) A comparative study of two methods of large loop excision of the transformation zone. *BJOG*, 112 (4), April, 490–494

Muller CY and Smith HO (2005) Cervical neoplasia complicating pregnancy. *Obstet Gynaecol Clin N Amer*, 32, 533–546

National Council for the Professional Development of Nursing and Midwifery (NCPDNM) (2005) *A Preliminary Evaluation of the Role of Advanced Nurse Practitioner* (Sept). National Council for the Professional Development of Nursing and Midwifery, Dublin

National Statistics for Health and Social Care (2006) http://www.ic.nhs.uk/webfiles/publications/cervicscrneng2006/Cervical%20bulletin%202005–06.pdf (accessed 13/6/07)

Neale J, Pitts MK, Dunn PDJ, Hughes GM and Redman CWE (2003) An observational study of precolposcopy education sessions: what do women want to know? *Health Care for Women International*, 24, 468–475

NHMRC (2005) Screening to prevent Cervical Cancer: Guidelines for the Management of Asymptomatic Women with Screen Detected Abnormalities: http://www.nhmrc.gov.au/publications/synopses/wh39syn.htm (accessed 18/6/07)

NHSCSP (1999) Histopathology Reporting in Cervical Screening. NHSCSP Publication no. 10, April. NHSCSP, London

NHSCSP Luesley D and Leeson S (eds) (2004) *Colposcopy and Programme Management*. NHSCSP Publication no 20, April NHSCP, London: http://www.cancerscreening.nhs.uk/cervical/publications/nhscsp20.pdf (accessed 18/6/07)

NHSCSP (2006a) *Taking Samples for Cervical Screening*. NHSCSP Publication No 23: http://www.cancerscreening.nhs.uk/cervical/publications/nhscsp23.pdf (accessed 13/6/07)

NHSCSP (2006b) *Cervical Screening: the Facts*: http://www.cancerscreening.nhs.uk/cervical/publications/nhscsp-the-facts-english-2006.pdf (accessed 7/2/07)

NICE (2003) *Guidance on the Use of Liquid Based Cytology for Cervical Screening* (Technology Appraisal Guidance 69). NICE, London

Noller KL, Bettes B, Zinberg S, et al. (2003) Cervical cytology screening practices among obstetrician-gynecologists. *Obstet Gynecol*, 102, 259–265

Norstrom A, Jansson I and Andersson H (1997) Carcinoma of the uterine cervix in pregnancy. A study of the incidence and treatment in the western region of Sweden 1973 to 1992. *Acta Obstetricia et Gynecologica Scandinavica*, 76 (6), 583–589

Nursing and Midwifery Council (2004) *Consultation on a Framework for the Standard for Post-registration Nursing*. NMC, London

Olaniyan OB (2002) Validity of colposcopy in the diagnosis of early cervical neoplasia: a review. *Afr J Reprod Health*, 6, 59–69

Orbell S, Hagger M, Brown V and Tidy J (2004) Appraisal theory and emotional sequalae of first visit to colposcopy following an abnormal cervical screening result. *British Journal of Health Psychology*, 9, 533–555

Ostor AG (2000) Early invasive adenocarcinoma of the uterine cervix. *International Journal of Gynaecological Pathology*, 19 (1), 29–38

Palmer JR, Wise LA, Hatch EE, et al. (2006) Prenatal diethylstilbestrol exposure and risk of breast cancer. *Cancer Epidemiology, Biomarkers & Prevention*, 15 (8), Aug, 1509–1514

Posner T and Vessey M (1988) *Prevention of Cervical Cancer: the Patient's View*. King's Fund, London

Raab SS, Andrew-JaJa C, Condel JL and Dabbs DJ (2006) Improving Papanicolaou test quality and reducing medical errors by using Toyota production system methods. *American Journal of Obstetrics and Gynecology*, 194 (1), Jan, 57–64

Rieck GC, Bhaumik J, Beer HR and Leeson SC (2006) Repeating cytology at initial colposcopy does not improve detection of high-grade abnormalities: a retrospective cohort study of 6595 women. *Gynaecologic Oncology*, 101 (2), 228–233

Rostad KE (2002) The psychological impact of abnormal cytology and colposcopy. *British Journal of Obstetrics and Gynaecology*, 109, April, 364–368

Sadler L and Sykes P (2005) How little is known about cervical cancer in pregnancy? *Annals of Oncology*, 16 (3), 341–343

Saito T, Takehara M, Lee R, et al. (2004) Neoadjuvant chemotherapy with cisplatin, aclacinomycin A and mitomycin C for cervical adenocarcinoma – a preliminary study. *International Journal of Gynaecological Cancer*, 14 (3), 483–490

Scheungraber C, Kleekamp N and Schneider A (2004) Management of low-grade squamous intraepithelial lesions of the uterine cervix. *British Journal of Cancer*, 90 (5), March, 975–978

Schorge JO, Knowles LM and Lea JS (2004) Adenoma of the cervix. *Current Treatment Options in Oncology*, 5, 119–127

Sharples LD, Edmunds J, Bilton D, et al. (2002) A randomized, controlled trial of nurse practitioner versus doctor led outpatient care in a bronchiectasis clinic. *Thorax*, 57, 661–667

Sherman ME, Carreon JD and Schiffman M (2006) Performance of cytology and human papillomavirus testing in relation to the menstrual cycle. *British Journal of Cancer*, 94 (11), 1690–1696

Shipman SD and Bristow R (2001) Adenocarcinoma in situ and early invasive adenocarcinoma of the uterine cervix. *Current Opinion in Oncology*, 13 (5), 394–398

Smith T (2000) Colposcopy. *Nursing Standard*, 15 (4), 11 Oct, 47–52, 54, 55

Solomon D, Schiffman MH and Tarone R (2001) Comparison of three management strategies for patients with atypical squamous cells of undetermined significance: baseline results from a randomized trial. *J Natl Cancer Inst*, 93, 293–299

Solomon D, Stoler M, Jeronimo J, Khan M, Castle P and Schiffman M (2007) Endocervical curettage in women undergoing colposcopy for equivocal or low-grade cytologic abnormalities. *Obstetrics and Gynecology*, 110 (2, part 2), 288–295

Todd RW, Wilson S, Etherington I and Luesley D (2002) Effect of Nurse Colposcopists on a hospital-based service. *Hospital Medicine* (London), 63 (4), April, 218–223

VCCR Victorian Cervical Cytology Registry (2002) *Statistical Report 2002*: http://www.vccr.org/stats.html (accessed 18/6/07)

Zaino RJ (2002) Symposium part I: adenocarcinoma in situ, glandular dysplasia, and early invasive adenocarcinoma of the uterine cervix. *International Journal of Gynecological Pathology*, 21 (4), Oct, 314–326

Chapter 3

Surgery

'So it actually wasn't half as painful and half as difficult as I expected the operation to be.'

(Patient after a radical hysterectomy, Dipex CC10 transcript: http://www.dipex.org/EXEC (accessed 30/7/07))

Introduction

Treatment options in cervical cancer are principally determined by two factors: stage and tumour size. For early stage disease (i.e. the cancer is clinically localised to the cervix), and small tumours (less than 4 cm) surgical resection is the treatment of choice. However, as the disease progresses, negative surgical margins become increasingly difficult to achieve and surgical resection becomes technically more and more difficult. It is at this stage that chemo-radiotherapy provides a more attractive treatment option (see Chapter 4). In cases of recurrent or advanced disease, surgery is once again frequently utilised, either with palliative or curative intent.

This chapter focuses on the surgical management of cervical cancer, beginning with a review of the different surgical interventions and a discussion of their possible side effects. Pertinent nursing issues associated with these side effects are also examined. Lymph node dissection is an important part of the surgery for cervical cancer but is also associated with considerable morbidity. Lymph node dissection, sentinel lymph node biopsy and the management of lymphoedema are discussed. The chapter ends with a description of the surgical interventions for advanced disease and the nursing issues associated with pelvic exenteration.

Surgical management of cervical cancer

From a surgical perspective there are basically three categories of cervical cancer:

(1) non-invasive/micro-invasive cancer
(2) early stage disease (IB1)
(3) locally advanced/recurrent disease

The treatment options for each stage of disease are illustrated in Table 3.1 and the surgical options are discussed more fully below.

Table 3.1 Treatment algorithm for cervical cancer (Waggoner 2003)

Stage	Clinical features	Treatment
IA1	Invasion 3.0 mm or less	If patient desires fertility, conisation of cervix. If she does not, simple hysterectomy (abdominal or vaginal)
	With lymphovascular space invasion	Hysterectomy with or without pelvic lymphadenectomy
IA2	3.0–5.0 mm invasion, <7.0 mm lateral spread	Radical hysterectomy with pelvic lymphadenectomy Radiotherapy
IB1	Tumour 4 cm or less	Radical hysterectomy with pelvic lymphadenectomy plus chemotherapy for poor prognosis surgical-pathological factors*
IB2	Tumour bigger than 4 cm	Radical hysterectomy with pelvic lymphadenectomy plus chemotherapy for poor prognosis surgical-pathological factors* Chemoradiotherapy Chemotherapy plus adjuvant hysterectomy
IIA	Upper two thirds vaginal involvement	Radical hysterectomy with pelvic lymphadenectomy Chemoradiotherapy
IIB	With parametrial extension	Chemoradiotherapy
IIIA	Lower third vaginal involvement	Chemoradiotherapy
IVA	Lower extension within pelvis	Chemoradiotherapy Primary pelvic exenteration
IVB	Distant metastases	Palliative chemotherapy Chemoradiotherapy

*Pelvic lymph node metastases; large tumour; deep cervical stromal invasion; lymphovascular space invasion; positive vaginal or parametrial margins

Surgical management of non-invasive and micro-invasive cancer

A microinvasive carcinoma is one that invades to a depth of 5 mm or less, and shows 7 mm or less horizontal spread. Microinvasive squamous cell carcinoma has a very low risk of metastasis or recurrence (1% or less), and so can be treated conservatively by either cone biopsy or simple hysterectomy if less than 3 mm deep or the same procedure plus pelvic lymphadenectomy if between 3 and 5 mm deep, with the expectation of a cure (Garg et al. 2006).

Different cone biopsy strategies are discussed in Chapter 2. In the treatment of micro-invasive disease a cold knife cone biopsy will usually be chosen in preference to the loop electrosurgical excisional procedure because it allows better assessment of the surgical margins.

Surgical management of early stage disease (IB1)

Unlike bulky, late stage disease, which is generally treated with chemoradiotherapy, there is no standard treatment for early stage cervical cancer. Three management options can be proposed: surgery alone, combined radiation therapy plus surgery, and radiation therapy alone.

Radiotherapy is feasible in almost all patients and has a five-year survival rate of 78% to 91% (Landoni et al. 1997). Surgery has a five-year survival rate of 54 to 90%, mostly achieved with adjuvant therapy (Landoni et al. 1997). The choice between these management options depends on the experience and beliefs of the team treating the patients, the policy of the institution and the age and general health of the patient involved (Landoni et al. 1997, Morice and Castaigne 2005).

The surgical options for women with early stage disease are either radical hysterectomy or, more recently, the fertility-preserving radical trachelectomy, both of which are discussed below.

In order to minimise long-term post-operative complications, some surgeons are now suggesting that a simple hysterectomy or even cone dissection performed in conjunction with pelvic lymph node dissection may be adequate to treat some women with early stage cervical cancer (Covens et al. 2002, Querleu and Leblanc 2003, Selman et al. 2005). One major concern with this approach is that it leaves a risk of undetected parametrial disease.

Radical trachelectomy

The radical trachelectomy procedure is without question one of the most exciting new developments in the field of conservative surgery in gynecologic oncology in the last decade.

(Plante and Roy 2001)

It is estimated that 10–15% of cervical cancers are diagnosed in women who are still in their childbearing years (Van der Vange et al. 1995). For patients wishing to begin or complete a family a hysterectomy is obviously a devastating treatment option. For this reason a new surgical approach was developed by Daniel Dargent in the 1990s known as the radical trachelectomy. This is a fertility sparing surgical technique in which the cervix is removed but the uterus remains. It can only be performed in patients with very favourable prognostic factors (i.e. early-stage disease less than 2 cm in diameter).

The procedure begins with a laparoscopic pelvic lymphadenectomy. The nodes are sent for frozen section evaluation and if negative the surgeon proceeds to a trachelectomy. The trachelectomy specimen is also sent for frozen section analysis of the endocervical margin which needs to be clear of disease. If this is not the case then more endocervix is removed, or a complete vaginal radical hysterectomy is performed (Plante and Roy 2001).

To date, there have been many successful pregnancies following radical trachelectomies. Despite initial concerns about potential infertility problems related to the shortened cervix and possibly inadequate or hostile mucus production, most women seem able to become pregnant 'naturally' without assisted reproductive help. The main complication of pregnancy which has been reported is prematurity (Plante and Roy 2001). Bernardini et al. (2003) followed up a cohort of 39 women who wished to conceive post-trachelectomy. The result was twelve term pregnancies and another six in which the baby was premature. It has been proposed that a complete surgical closure of the cervix after conception may help to promote full term pregnancy.

Interestingly, in one series of trachelectomy patients there were five women with a history of infertility *prior* to their radical trachelectomy. Of these, three successfully managed to conceive after the procedure (Covens et al. 1999).

In general, radical trachelectomy has been associated with a low rate of disease recurrence. The cases in which recurrence has been reported serve to confirm that conservative surgery should not be performed in patients who have poor prognostic features. Patients with tumour size greater than 2 cm or with lymph node involvement are not candidates for this procedure and neither are women with a poor prognosis histological subtype (Morice and Castaigne 2005).

Hysterectomy

Until the introduction of the radical trachelectomy the principal treatment option for women with early stage cervical cancer was hysterectomy. Today hysterectomy is the most common major gynaecological operation in the developed world (Farquhar et al. 2005).

There are a number of different types of hysterectomy including:

(1) Subtotal or supracervical hysterectomy – the uterus is removed but the cervix is not.
(2) Total hysterectomy – removal of the uterus in its entirety, including the cervix.
(3) Radical hysterectomy – removal of the uterus, cervix, nearby lymph nodes, upper portion of the vagina and parametrium. Five classes of radical hysterectomy for cervical cancer have been described, each requiring progressively wider resections (Piver et al. 1974).

Post-hysterectomy complications

It is estimated that about half of women who have a hysterectomy will experience some side effects (Kim and Lee 2001, Walsgrove 2001). However, whilst much has been written about the physical, psychological and social sequelae of having a hysterectomy, interpretation of this literature requires caution. One of the key issues is that the vast majority of hysterectomies are carried out for benign conditions. Only 15% are performed for cancer

---

Box 3.1 Surgical approaches

As well as different types of hysterectomy there are also a number of different surgical approaches:

(1) Abdominal: an abdominal hysterectomy is generally conducted when there is a need for extensive exploration such as in the case of cancer. An abdominal hysterectomy can be performed with a vertical incision or a bikini line cut. The bikini line cut, directly above the pubic hairline, leaves a less obvious scar and results in a shorter recovery time (Reidel et al. 2003). Although an abdominal hysterectomy causes less damage to the urinary tract and blood vessels than other techniques, it is also associated with more pain, a lengthier hospital stay and longer recovery time.
(2) Vaginal: a vaginal hysterectomy involves making an incision in the upper portion of the vagina and removing the uterus through the vagina. Advantages include avoidance of the morbidity associated with abdominal incisions, decreased intra-operative blood loss, decreased post-operative morbidity, faster recovery and decreased expense (Davis et al. 2003). However, it is not used in situations in which extensive exploration of the abdomen is required.
(3) Laparoscopic: laparoscopic surgery involves making three or four small incisions in the abdomen. A type of endoscope called a laparoscope is inserted through one of the incisions into the abdominal cavity. The surgeon is then able to view the pelvic organs on a video screen and insert surgical instruments through the other incisions. Laparoscopic procedures result in shorter hospitalisation and recovery time than abdominal hysterectomy but require a skilled surgeon and are associated with greater operating time and higher costs. There has been understandable scepticism about incorporating laparascopic techniques into surgery for cancer because of reservations about inadequate assessment of the extent of disease. However, laparoscopic techniques have been used for radical hysterectomy with good results. Obviously, patient selection and surgical skill and experience are important factors (Querleu and Leblanc 2003).

Within the USA, 60–70% of all hysterectomies are abdominal, with only 30% vaginal and 10% laparoscopically assisted (Davis et al. 2003, Flory 2005).

> **Box 3.2 Early post-operative complications from a radical hysterectomy**
>
> (Hatch 1994)
>
> (1) blood loss (0.8l)
> (2) ureterovaginal fistula (1–2%)
> (3) pulmonary embolus (1–2%)
> (4) small bowel obstruction (1%)
> (5) febrile morbidity (25–50%)

– and this includes cancer of the uterus, ovaries and pelvis (Brown 2000, quoted in Walsgrove 2001). The indication for performing the hysterectomy is not always specified in the literature and therefore the degree to which it is applicable to cervical cancer is unclear.

Although some simple hysterectomies may be performed for early stage disease, for the most part it is the radical hysterectomy which is used in the treatment of cervical carcinoma. Because this is the most extensive type of hysterectomy, it is the one that is associated with the most complications. The main physical complications from a radical hysterectomy result from damage to the pelvic floor and its nerve supply. In order to prevent these toxicities, surgeons are constantly striving to improve their technique. 'Nerve sparing' approaches have been shown to significantly reduce the incidence of post-operative complications (Sakuragi et al. 2005, Todo et al. 2006). However, such strategies require prolonged operation time and are not considered standard therapy at this time.

Some of the early post-operative complications following a radical hysterectomy are listed in Box 3.2. The intermediate to long-term post-operative morbidities principally affect three systems: the genital system, urinary system and anorectal system. These are discussed in greater detail below.

Genital system

Hysterectomy can affect the genital system in two ways. It can impact reproductive and sexual function.

Reproductive function

Radical hysterectomy will render women of reproductive age infertile and may induce an early menopause. In order to preserve fertility some women will be eligible for a radical trachelectomy as described above. Where post-operative radiotherapy is planned ovarian transposition may also be undertaken. This involves moving the ovaries to the inferior pole of each kidney in order to escape the radiotherapy field. The procedure may be performed either at the time of hysterectomy or, on some occasions, laparoscopically as a separate operation. Ovarian transposition is usually only carried out for squamous cell cervical cancer because it is extremely rare for SCC to metastasise to the ovaries and therefore it is considered safe that they avoid the irradiation (Shimada et al. 2006).

Unfortunately, the procedure is not without complications. The blood flow can be disrupted during movement, rendering the ovaries dysfunctional. Furthermore, even when the ovaries have been moved they may still be exposed to scatter radiation. Ovarian transposition, fertility and menopause are discussed more fully in Chapter 7.

Sexual function

'I feel that your sexual identity and how you function in that is uppermost a part of your recovery process. I mean, you cannot separate one from the other. So if your cure ends up disrupting your sexual personhood, it's a terrible sentence to take.' (Woman following treatment for gynaecological cancer – Bruner and Boyd 1999.)

The physiological and psychosexual effects of the cervical cancer are inextricably linked, and the psychosexual aspects of the disease are discussed more fully in Chapter 6. Here we will briefly review the physical effects of radical hysterectomy on sexual function. It is a topic about which there is a fairly extensive literature but caution is required with interpretation of the research because many studies are associated with methodological problems (see Box 3.3).

The physiology of the sexual response is complex and not completely understood. However, radical hysterectomy is thought to affect sexual function and sensation in a number of ways. For example, it is believed to cause:

- altered mobility of the pelvic organs during coitus
- limitations in the expansion of the upper vagina during the arousal phase
- reduced mucus production (from removal of the cervix)
- reduced amount of sensitive tissue in the pelvic area
- removal of the uterus results in an absence of uterine contractions which are considered sexually pleasurable by some women
- removal of the cervix is thought to compromise sexual pleasure in many women
- removal of the ovaries induces early menopause and hormonal alterations
- disruption in blood circulation to the pelvis may impair an adequate lubrication-swelling response

---

Box 3.3 Methodological factors in the post-hysterectomy sexual function research

Although there appears to be a sizeable body of literature about the effects of hysterectomy on sexual function, many studies suffer from methodological deficits including:

(1) Retrospective versus prospective data collection: many of the studies are retrospective and may be affected by recall bias. Conversely, some of the prospective studies required data to be collected at stressful times such as pre-operatively and therefore may be influenced by patient anxiety.

(2) Timing of pre and post-operative assessments: it has been estimated that physical recovery from a hysterectomy may take six months and therefore the post-surgery assessment is best performed a considerable time post-operatively. The timing of assessments varies widely between studies.

(3) Sample size: many of the studies have small, non-random samples.

(4) Type of surgery: there is not always specification of or distinction between hysterectomy types (total versus subtotal) or surgical techniques (vaginal, abdominal, laparoscopic or combined).

(5) Hormonal status: it is not always clear whether concurrent oophrectomy was performed and whether or not hormone replacement therapy instigated.

(6) Measurement tools: Non-standardised or poorly-defined terms may be used – particularly in the assessment of sexual satisfaction. Furthermore there is often a failure to define what constitutes sexual activity (Meston and Bradford 2004)

(7) Other factors: sexual function is complex and affected by a large number of variables which have not always been adequately accounted for. These include:
  (a) age at hysterectomy
  (b) pre-operative menopausal status
  (c) presence of gynaecological problems preceding hysterectomy
  (d) pre-operative psychiatric morbidity
  (e) partner relationship/support (Meston and Bradford 2004)
      (Katz 2002, Maas and Kulie 2003, Meston and Bradford 2004, Flory et al. 2005)

• damage to the nerve supply of the upper vagina and uterus interferes with lubrication and orgasm
• formation of scar tissue in the upper vagina may prevent full ballooning of the vagina, limiting arousal

(Katz 2002, Flory 2005)

Pieterse et al. (2006) recently assessed post-radical hysterectomy morbidities in a cohort of 94 women compared with a control group. They found that the operation had a negative effect on sexual function not only when compared with the controls but also when compared with the sexual situation before the treatment. The changes or problems included less lubrication, a narrow and short vagina, senseless areas around the labia, dyspareunia, and sexual dissatisfaction.

Jensen et al. (2003) report similar findings. In this longitudinal study short-term sexual problems included difficulties with orgasm, dyspareunia, sexual dissatisfaction, distress because of reduced vaginal size during intercourse, inability to complete intercourse and dissatisfaction with appearance. These difficulties persisted from five weeks to six months after surgery. In the longer term, radical hysterectomy appeared to have a persistent negative effect on sexual interest and vaginal lubrication during the two years post-surgery.

Urinary dysfunction

The frequency of surgically-induced urinary tract morbidity varies in the literature, with clinically significant long-term bladder dysfunction occurring in 30–75% of patients (Benedetti-Panici et al. 2004). Fortunately, for the most part the changes are transient and if post-operative bladder care is adequate then vesical function often recovers spontaneously within six to twelve months (Benedetti-Panici et al. 2004, Jackson and Naik 2006). Nevertheless, long-term storage and voiding problems are reported in over 30% of cases, and at least 16% of women may be severely disabled by their symptoms (Naik et al. 2001). At the same time it should be remembered that a significant proportion of women who have not undergone a radical hysterectomy report regular urinary problems – in particular incontinence (O'Brien et al. 1991, Naik et al. 2001).

Causes of urinary dysfunction

This may be from direct trauma to the bladder at the time of surgery (Naik et al. 2001) or from ureteral injuries such as post-operative fistulas. The latter have become much less common than they once were, with ureterovaginal fistulas occurring in less than 1–2% of radical hysterectomy cases (Plante and Roy 2001). Today, by far the most important cause of urinary dysfunction after radical hysterectomy is from damage to the visceral autonomic nerve supply which is thought to occur during the dissection of the parametrium and the vaginal cuff (Jackson and Naik 2006).

It has been suggested that there are two phases in post-operative bladder dysfunction. Immediately post-operatively the bladder becomes small and hypertonic (Jackson and Naik 2006). Urinary retention can be a problem and is managed by catheterisation. In the longer term the bladder may become over-distended and hypotonic. It has been suggested that longer term complications are a particular risk if the bladder is poorly managed immediately post-operatively, although the data to support this are conflicting (Jackson and Naik 2006).

Incontinence is probably one of the most debilitating complications and can be a short or long-term problem (Jackson and Naik 2006). Naik et al. (2001) looked at the rate of urinary incontinence before and after radical hysterectomy. Regular incontinence *prior* to surgery was reported by 14.8% women . This number rose to 48.1% at six weeks post-surgery and dropped again to 29.6% three months after surgery. Although 31.2% of women still reported urinary incontinence at 12 months, it is of interest that only about half of these women sought medical advice about their incontinence. The study also indicates that for some women the incontinence recovered spontaneously.

Management of urinary incontinence is difficult and the most effective strategies focus on prevention. It is now widely accepted that the degree of urinary tract dysfunction is directly proportional to the radicality of the surgery (Benedetti-Panici et al. 2004). For example, Landoni et al. (2001) reported that Piver class II hysterectomies were as effective as Piver class III, but were associated with less morbidity with respect to bladder function.

At the moment the principal strategy for reducing the incidence of post-operative urinary dysfunction involves modifying the surgical technique appropriately. It is a trend which has been noted in other aspects of cervical cancer care, and means decreasing the radicality of surgery amongst low risk groups:

> It may be unnecessary to stick rigidly to the dogma of extensive radical surgery when modified treatment may be equally effective but less disabling. Such patients may be offered a range of therapeutic options based on a detailed knowledge of their individual fertility requirements and tumour characteristics.
>
> (Jackson and Naik 2006)

Bowel dysfunction

Anorectal complications may have an equally negative impact on quality of life for radical hysterectomy patients and yet there is a smaller amount of literature about these problems (Jackson and Naik 2006). After radical hysterectomy, women may experience acute and chronic bowel dysfunction characterised by constipation, difficulty with evacuation and loss of defacatory urge (Jackson and Naik 2006). The incidence of bowel dysfunction after hysterectomy is thought to be approximately 40% (Jackson and Naik 2006).

Nursing issues in the management of a patient undergoing a radical hysterectomy

Pre-operative preparation

In the 1980s and 1990s a number of studies indicated that there were shortcomings in women's perceptions of the information they received during their hospitalisation for hysterectomy. For example, Corney et al. (1992) talked to 105 women after surgery for gynaecological malignancies about their information requirements: 77 of the women had cancer of the cervix, 69 of whom had been treated by hysterectomy and 8 by pelvic exenteration. Even six months after surgery, 38% of women said they still felt anxious and 23% felt depressed.

The study does not specify the type of information the women had been given pre-operatively. However, a third of them reported needing to know more about the physical, psychological and sexual side effects of the surgery. Furthermore, a quarter of the partners stated that they would also have liked to receive more information on the illness and its treatment. Fears expressed by this group of women at the time of surgery, are shown in Table 3.2.

Since this study was published a number of papers have looked at different pre-operative educational interventions such as the provision of leaflets, booklets and videos (Scriven and Tucker 1997). Evaluation of some of the educational tools indicate that preoperative instruction can improve post-hysterectomy outcomes and alleviate anxiety (Williams et al. 1988, Bernhard 1993). However, although pre-operative teaching has been found to yield better immediate post-operative outcomes than no pre-operative instruction, the

Table 3.2 Some factors which frighten patients about hysterectomy (Corney et al. 1992)

Factor causing concern	Percentage of patients
None	10.8
Having cancer	48.4
Dying	6.5
Having an operation	4.3
Going into hospital	5.3
After-effects of surgery	4.3
Concerns with sexual problems	5.3
How family will cope	10.8
Fear of radiotherapy/other treatment	4.3

magnitude and consistency of benefits have not always been large and its effect on long-term outcomes is uncertain (Oetker-Black 2003).

In recent years different strategies for the provision of information and support have been explored, such as the Internet. Many hospitals have developed websites providing differing levels of information about the services they provide. Cancer-associated organisations such as BACUP have a longstanding reputation for providing good-quality data for cancer sufferers and their families, formerly by telephone and now on-line as well. Other hysterectomy specific websites such as Hystersisters (www.hystersisters.com) may also have a role in the provision of information to women (Bunde et al. 2006).

Post-operative care

Post-operatively radical hysterectomy patients return to the ward with intravenous hydration and a urinary catheter. Their abdominal wound will differ depending on the surgical approach and surgeon preference, but unless the operation has been performed laparascopically, it will be either vertical or transverse. Patients will frequently have a pelvic drain in situ. Regional policies vary regarding post-operative analgesia but most commonly this will be delivered via either an epidural or patient controlled analgesia (PCA).

As mentioned above, one significant post-operative risk is urinary retention and so women return to the ward with either a supra-pubic (SPC) or transurethral catheter (TUC) in situ. Regional practices vary regarding catheter management and are not always research based (Roberts and Naik 2006). Typically, a supra-pubic catheter will be clamped a few days after surgery so that the woman can try and void normally again. After each urination the catheter is unclamped and the remaining urine is measured (the 'residual volume'). Residual volumes need to reach a specified low value (e.g. less than 100 ml) in order for the catheter to be removed.

A recent study by Roberts and Naik (2006) compared supra-pubic catheterisation with intermittent self-catheterisation (ISC) post-operatively for radical hysterectomy. The ISC cohort returned from theatre with a transurethral catheter which was removed at day five after surgery. After this the woman voided normally, performing self-catheterisation after each void in order to assess the residual volume.

Self-catheterisation was found to be highly acceptable to the patients in this study, resulting in fewer disturbances at night, greater freedom to lead a normal life and less anxiety and embarrassment than an SPC.

Box 3.4 Abnormal post-operative pain following hysterectomy

There is a small group of patients who develop severe chronic post-operative suprapubic or groin pain which is not relieved by the usual analgesia strategies. These patients commonly complain of:

- numbness at and below the incision site
- pain and burning along the incision line
- referred pain elsewhere in the pelvic region or groin

Typically, they have been seeking help for their pain for some time. Their management began with narcotic medication and moved on to antidepressants and psychiatric counselling as standard analgesia failed.

Such pain may be caused by a number of factors including: contracture because of scar tissue, hernia, infection, abscess, suture granuloma or pelvic pathology. However, once these have been ruled out, a diagnosis of neuroma might be considered.

A neuroma is a damaged part of a peripheral nerve that forms after trauma. It can also form when a peripheral nerve becomes engulfed in scar tissue, (for example following surgery). If diagnosed promptly neuromas can be effectively managed with surgical excision.

Characteristics of a post-operative neuroma are:

(1) intractable and severe pain which lasts beyond six months post-operatively
(2) delayed onset of post-operative pain
(3) hyperaesthesia surrounding the incision
(4) immediate or delayed occurrence of areas of numbness
(5) referred pain into the groin or along a nerve's sensory distribution

(Ducic 2006)

Cervical cancer and the lymphatic system

The lymphatic system is part of the immune system and carries lymphocytes to respond to antigens and communicate responses to other parts of the body. It also carries excess fluid back to the venous bloodstream through a series of ducts or tubules. The thoracic duct drains the left arm, both legs and three quarters of the trunk. The right lymphatic duct drains the right arm and remaining quarter of the trunk. The amount of lymph generated by an average person ranges from two to four litres every day.

Lymph nodes are found at the articulations of large joints and in the mesentery system and neck. They act as filters for waste and help regulate protein content in the lymph fluid. Lymph node involvement is probably the most significant negative prognostic factor in cervical cancer.

Lymph node dissection accompanies most definitive surgery, with the exception of very early stage disease. However, it is only after the lymph node dissection has been performed that the presence or absence of nodal disease can be determined. Pelvic lymph node metastases are detected in less than 20% of women with stage IB cancer and less than 30% of women with stage IIA (Barranger et al. 2004). Thus, as many as four out of five patients are exposed to the risks of lymphadenectomy but will derive no benefit from it.

In recent years efforts have been made to identify women who have lymph node involvement pre-operatively in order to avoid unnecessary surgery on patients whose nodes are clear. This process of sentinel lymph node biopsy is described in Box 3.5.

Lymph node dissection is associated with two potential morbidities: lymphocele (lymphocyst) formation and lower limb lymphoedema, both of which are discussed below.

Box 3.5 Sentinel lymph node biopsy

Sentinel lymph node mapping has been investigated in several cancer types including breast cancer and melanoma. It was first tested in cervical cancer in 2000 and a number of studies have indicated that it may be effective in reducing the need for invasive surgery in this context (Singh 2004).

The sentinel node is defined as the first node in the lymphatic system that drains a tumour site (Barranger et al. 2004). The sentinel lymph node can thus be seen as a 'gatekeeper'. If this node contains metastatic cells then they may also have passed through and infected other lymph nodes. If, however, the node is clear, the assumption is made that other nodes in the chain are clear too. Thus, if the sentinel lymph node can be identified and biopsied pre-operatively a lymphadenectomy can be avoided in cases in which the nodes are negative. Furthermore, patients with nodal involvement may be better treated with radiation therapy alone. Thus, a positive lymph node biopsy may also result in avoiding surgery altogether (Morice and Castaigne 2005).

The SLNB procedure is relatively straightforward. On the day of surgery a blue dye and/or radiocolloid is injected into the cervix. The dye enters the lymphatic fluid and drains into the lymphatic vessels. If the dye enters a lymph node the node will take on a blue colour. Any blue lymph node is considered to be a sentinel node (there may be more than one). Radioactivity of the nodes may be measured to confirm this if a radioisotope has been used.

Sentinel lymph node biopsy may or may not be preceded by a procedure called lymphoscintigraphy. This involves the pre-operative injection of a radiocolloid dye into the cervix. Approximately 30 minutes after the injection a lymphoscintigram is performed. A lymphoscintigram is a nuclear imaging technique whereby the path of the radioactive dye can be traced.

Whilst it is probably true to say that the usefulness of this sentinel lymph node biopsy is yet to be quantified in cervical cancer patients, it is certainly feasible technically and holds the promise of reducing morbidity considerably.

Lymphocele (lymphocyst)

A lymphocele is a cystic mass that contains lymph from injured lymph vessels. It is a potential acute morbidity from surgical procedures in which large amounts of lymphatic tissue are excised. Unlike blood, lymph contains only a low concentration of clotting factors, so once injured a lymphatic vessel is prone to continue leaking.

Charkviani et al. (2000) reviewed their data on a large cohort of women who underwent a radical hysterectomy and found the incidence of lymphocyst formation post-hysterectomy to be about 4%, arising more frequently in patients less than 30 or older than 60 years old. In 18% of women the cysts were asymptomatic, requiring no further therapy; 44% of the cysts required some form of drainage.

Lower limb lymphoedema

Lymphoedema is a chronic and progressive condition resulting from an abnormality of, or damage to the lymphatic system. Any reduction in the capacity of the lymphatic system to drain fluid from the interstitium and return it to the blood circulation will cause fluid to build up in the skin and subcutaneous tissues of the affected part of the body.

(Badger et al. 2004b)

The term 'primary lymphoedema' refers to lymphoedema which develops without any recognised precipitating factor and is generally thought to be congenital in origin. Secondary lymphoedema is caused by injury to the lymphatic system which impairs lymph flow, for example as a result of paralysis, blockage or damage through trauma, surgery, radiotherapy, tumours or infection such as filariasis (Lacovara and Yoder 2006, Gary 2007).

Whilst commonly accepted, these explanations may be over-simplifications because not all cancer patients who are exposed to lymph node damage develop lymphoedema. Furthermore, it is a condition which can develop at any time – even many years after treatment, when there is no evidence of active disease (Williams 2004).

Lymphoedema is a progressive disorder and differs from other long-term chronic oedemas because of its duration – greater than three months (Dell and Doll 2006) and also because of the skin and tissue differences it causes (Honnor 2006). There are four main features of true lymphoedema:

- excess protein in the tissues
- excess oedema in the tissues
- chronic inflammation
- excess fibrosis

Acute lymphoedema is characterised by soft, pitting oedema that can be temporarily relieved by a number of measures which are discussed later in this chapter. However, if early identification and intervention is not initiated, it can progress to a chronic condition in which the skin reacts to the persistent oedema by producing cytokines and growth factors that promote fibrosis (Gary 2007). Elastin is replaced by collagen, leading to a permanent thickening and hardening of the tissues and an enlarged and deformed extremity which is much less responsive to treatment.

The study of lymphoedema in the cancer population is complicated by a real paucity of good quality data. Its aetiology is still imperfectly understood and whilst there are recognised management strategies which are commonly used and widely accepted, few of these have been tested in the context of large, multicentre randomised trials. Much of the lymphoedema research has focused on upper limb lymphoedema following treatment for breast cancer, with comparatively little about lower limb lymphoedema.

Incidence

It is difficult to ascertain the incidence of lymphoedema. Different studies employ different criteria to define the condition, making comparison problematic. Some studies are quite old and may refer to surgical and radiotherapy techniques which are now obsolete (Williams 2004). Others do not have long enough follow-up, which can be a problem as lymphoedema may develop quite late after definitive treatment (McCallin et al. 2005).

Werngren-Elgstrom and Lidman (1994) used interviews and limb volume measurements to assess the incidence of lower limb lymphoedema after treatment for cancer of the cervix and found that out of 54 women 22 developed measurable lower limb lymphoedema. Of the 54 patients 15 had a slight swelling (defined as a volume increase of more than 5%), three had moderate swelling (volume increase greater than 10%), and four had severe swelling (greater than 15% volume increase). Fifty-three of the women in this study had also received radiotherapy.

Matsuura et al. (2006) also looked at a cohort of 341 women treated for cervix cancer in their institution in Japan five years after treatment in order to assess post-operative morbidities. Here, 14% of women undergoing hysterectomy developed leg oedema. These patients did not receive radiotherapy, although another sub-group of women who did were assessed at the same time and had only a marginally higher incidence of lymphoedema at 15%.

In an Australian study of 743 women treated for gynaecological cancer, a diagnosis of lower limb lymphoedema was made in 18% of the total sample (Ryan et al. 2003a); 53% were diagnosed within three months of treatment, 18% within six months, 13% within twelve months and 16% in up to five years. The highest risk was amongst women with vulvar carcinoma who had had complete resection of their lymph nodes.

Symptoms

As well as limb enlargement, lymphoedema may be associated with a number of other symptoms. Ryan et al. (2003b) interviewed women about their experience of LLL. Initial changes described were in appearance (85%) or sensation (15%). Swelling, visible lumps, puffiness and reddened areas were seen. Changes in sensation included pain, hardness, heat, tenderness and pins and needles. The pain was described as 'heaviness', 'fullness', 'ache', 'tightness', 'sharp pain' or a 'throbbing sensation'.

Diagnosis

Lymphoedema can be diagnosed by ultrasound, duplex ultrasound, CT scan or MRI. Probably the 'gold standard' for diagnosis is the lymphoscintigram, which uses a radiolabelled protein to measure lymphatic function, lymph movement, lymph drainage, and response to lymphoedema treatment (Gary 2007).

Risk factors

It is not really understood why some people develop lymphoedema and others do not (Cole 2006). Data regarding the relevance of the number of lymph node removed is conflicting. Some authors suggest that it is the overall extent of the surgery rather than simply the number of nodes excised that is the significant factor (Larson et al. 1986).

In other cases, infection appears to trigger the lymphoedema – or perhaps its diagnosis. Certainly it is a condition characterised by recurrent attacks of infection/inflammation due to reduced local immunity (Mortimer 1995).

Trauma has also been implicated in the development of upper limb lymphoedema (ULL), and this may have a role in LLL. Venepuncture, injections and blood pressure measurements are generally contraindicated in a limb which has undergone lymph node dissection. The evidence base for this, however, appears to be mainly from case studies and anecdotes. One small audit by Cole (2006) found that of 14 women who underwent an axillary lymph node dissection and had a subsequent venepuncture in the affected arm, none developed ULL at 2 months follow-up.

Other reported triggers include cellulitis, a fall, an ascetic tap, sunburn, a mosquito bite, and air travel (Ryan 2003b, McCallin et al. 2005). Stasis, temperature extremes (being close to a radiotor or hot spa), and even overactivity can further compound the swelling (Ryan 2003b).

Lymphoedema grading

There are a number of grading systems for lymphoedema, one of which (the International Society of Lymphology) is illustrated in Table 3.3.

Although this is basically a three grade system, some practitioners also recognise a 'stage 0', referring to a latent or sub-clinical condition where swelling is not evident even though there is impaired lymph transport.

It can be seen that the grading system is not based on limb size alone, but also on the quality of the tissue. Often the most difficult limbs to treat are not the largest but those which have become solid. The presence of fibrotic tissue makes it difficult for fluid to drain and affected tissues become 'woody'. A vicious cycle is set up as the continued presence of fluid in these areas of hardened tissue provides an environment for further fibrosis and hence a stimulus for further thickening (Badger et al. 2004a).

Table 3.3 International Society of Lymphology grading system

Grade	Description
I	Early accumulation of fluid relatively high in protein content (e.g. in comparison with 'venous' oedema). Subsides with limb elevation.
II	Limb elevation alone rarely reduces the tissue swelling and pitting is manifest. Fibrosis of limb begins.
III	Encompasses lymphostatic elephantiasis where pitting is absent and trophic skin changes such as acanthosis, fat deposits and warty overgrowths develop.

Within each stage severity based on volume difference can be assessed as: minimal (<20% increase) in limb volume, moderate (20% to 40% increase) or severe (>40% increase). (http://www.u.arizona.edu/~witte/ISL.htm accessed 18/4/07)

Management

There is no cure for lymphoedema. However, a number of management strategies have been identified and are now commonly used in many countries throughout the world. Each is aimed at reducing the LLL and its associated discomfort. As mentioned above, the evidence base for these strategies is poor and much of the existing research involves women with ULL. The relevance of this to LLL is untested.

The basic principle behind lymphoedema management is decongestion of the compromised lymphatic pathways in order to reduce the size of the limb. This is achieved by encouraging the development of collateral drainage and stimulating the function of remaining patent routes (Mortimer 1995, Foldi 1998). Care can be seen as falling into two phases, 'treatment' and 'maintenance'. The former aims to reduce and control limb size and the latter to maintain any improvements to limb dimensions that have been made.

A number of different strategies are employed simultaneously and are sometimes referred to as complex decongestive physiotherapy (CDP). These strategies include:

(1) Manual lymphatic drainage

Gentle massage techniques are used to clear the trunk of oedema so that the flow from the affected limb can move into the healthy parts of the lymphatic system more easily (Dell and Doll 2006). Patients may also be taught to perform a simplified form of massage known as 'simple lymph drainage' (SLD) or 'self-administered massage' (SAM) (Badger et al. 2004b).

Pneumatic compression devices are marketed for use in lymphoedematous limbs but there is controversy as to their usefulness. While pneumatic compression therapy (PCT) has been demonstrated to reduce swelling, the way in which it does so and the possibility of the rapid displacement of fluid to elsewhere in the body have caused concern (Badger et al. 2004b). PCT is thought to assist with the reabsorption of water, but fails to mobilise protein molecules, which if left in situ may accelerate the process of fibrosis. Furthermore, guidelines regarding optimum pumping pressures, length and frequency of sessions, and treatment requirements are not always provided with the pumps (Gary 2007).

(2) Compression bandaging/fitted garments

Compression bandaging and hosiery is used after massage to encourage fluid to continue flowing through the new pathways and to deter it from going back into previously congested areas. It also provides a barrier against trauma (Dell and Doll 2006). There is a certain amount of debate as to whether bandages or compression hosiery are more effective at reducing oedema (Badger et al. 2004b). In practice, bandaging is often required to reduce swelling initially and is followed by the fitting of compression garments once the lymphoedema has been reduced (Linnitt 2005).

Compression garments are not always considered to be comfortable, aesthetically pleasing or very affordable. Of the 72% women who had compression garments prescribed in one study, 20% were unable to keep on wearing them Ryan (2003b).

(3) Special exercises

The role of exercise is not fully understood in the context of lymphoedema. Whilst on the one hand it is considered a helpful part of therapy, excessive exercise has also been mentioned as a potential trigger for the condition.

The rationale for exercise is that the pressure on the skin above the lymph channels afforded by compression garments in conjunction with active movement is thought to stimulate the muscles below the lymph channels to create a gentle, natural pumping mechanism. This is thought to direct the lymphatic flow into the trunk (Dell and Doll 2006).

(4) Meticulous skin care

The need for meticulous skin care is based on the observation that local infections appear to potentiate or exacerbate lymphoedema. This is thought to result from reduced function of the lymphatic system which leads to compromised immunity in the affected part of the body (Mortimer 1995). Recurrent infections in the skin (erysipelas), subcutaneous tissues (cellulitis), lymphatic vessels (lymphangitis) or lymph nodes (lymphadenitis) are observed in patients with lymphoedema and it is not unusual for patients to require admission to hospital for a course of intravenous antibiotics during an inflammatory episode (Badger et al. 2004c).

Each inflammatory episode is considered likely to damage the lymphatics still further and so prevention is clearly preferable to treatment (Badger et al. 2004b). Athlete's foot is not uncommon in patients with LLL and control of this may be useful in reducing outbreaks of cellulitis (Mortimer 2000).

In the light of this it seems logical to recommend good foot and skin care to women with lymphoedema. Long-term, low-dose, prophylactic antibiotics may also be prescribed for patients experiencing recurrent infections. Penicillin V is seen as the antibiotic of choice since streptococcus is thought to be the most common infecting organism (Badger et al. 2004c).

Efficacy of CPD

CPT studies have been generally clinical case reports of treatment that occurs in clinics, with small sample sizes, no blinding of therapists or patients to treatment and no control group.

(McCallin et al. 2005)

It has already been mentioned that the data supporting many of the interventions for lymphoedema is scanty. Overall, the results of CPD have been described as 'extremely variable', with efficacy rated from none to 'providing much relief' (Ryan 2003b).

Badger et al. (2004b) performed a Cochrane review of the literature in order to assess the effect of physical treatment programmes on both physical and psychological aspects of lymphoedema. Only three studies, involving a total of 150 patients were found to meet the inclusion criteria for the review (i.e. high level evidence through randomised controlled studies with at least six months' follow-up). Each of these three studies looked at different aspects of the CPT. The authors stated that there is currently not enough evidence to draw conclusions about the best physical therapy to use in the treatment of lymphoedema.

Other reviewers have reported similar findings. For example, McCallin et al. (2005) concluded: 'From this review it is evident that while CPD may be an effective treatment regimen for secondary lymphoedema, there is wide disagreement amongst researchers as to the optimal components and time frame for the intervention.'

Another factor which is important in the long-term control of lymphoedema but has also been poorly addressed in the literature is long-term compliance. Ongoing maintenance care is required to keep a lymphoedematous limb under control but in practice this can be time consuming and difficult to sustain.

Pharmacological interventions

The role of pharmacotherapy in the management of lymphoedema is unclear. A number of medications have been used with varying degrees of success. One group of drugs which has been investigated is the benzopyrones, the drug category which includes warfarin. These drugs are formed from a variety of naturally occurring substances such as plant extracts and were originally developed for use in vascular medicine (Badger et al. 2004c). They act by reducing vascular permeability and hence the amount of fluid forming in the subcutaneous tissues (Badger et al. 2004c). These drugs are also thought to increase macrophage activity, and encourage lysis of extracellular protein which in turn reduces the formation of fibrotic tissue in the lymphoedematous limb (Piller 1976, Hoult and Paya 1996).

However, notwithstanding claims for their efficacy, there have been concerns about potential toxicity. Warfarin used in the management of lymphoedema is prescribed at higher doses than that used for haematological and cardiac implications. Fears about liver toxicity when used in the management of LLL have resulted in its withdrawal for this indication in Australia (Badger et al. 2004c).

Badger et al. (2004c) performed another Cochrane review of the benzopyrone-related literature for the management of LLL. They concluded that whilst on an individual basis, patients may report an improvement in symptoms such as heaviness, tightness or aching when taking these preparations, this should be balanced against the lack of information about the long-term side effects of these drugs. Once again it was stated that it is not possible to draw any firm conclusions about the role of benzopyrones in lymphoedema from the current data.

Diuretics have also been used in the management of lymphoedema. Evidence of their efficacy is limited and they can cause significant damage through hyponatraemia and dehydration (Gary 2007). Furthermore, they may bring about an increase in the increased concentration of proteins in the interstitium, exacerbating inflammation and fibrosis.

Calcium channel blockers are contraindicated in the presence of lymphoedema because calcium is essential for smooth muscle contraction in the walls of the collecting vessels (Mortimer and Levick 2004). If smooth muscle contraction is decreased, it may decrease the flow of lymph and compromise the overall functioning of the lymphatic system (Gary 2007).

Prevention and education

The psychological and social sequelae of lymphoedema are considerable. The condition may necessitate changes in clothing and activities and may also have considerable economic implications. Some women describe it as 'worse than cancer' (Ryan 2003b).

Because of the gaps in our understanding of lower limb lymphoedema, guidance regarding prevention strategies is difficult to provide. Women are commonly advised to avoid injections and other types of trauma to the affected limb (Cole 2006). Similarly, they are advised to maintain good skin hygiene to that limb. However, on the whole, provision of lymphoedema-related information in general has been found to be poor.

This does not relate simply to lymphoedema prevention but also to its diagnosis and management. Ryan (2003b) found 34% of women had difficulty finding information about the condition. On initial presentation to health professionals with limb changes, 27% of patients were not informed about LLL or specialist care for the condition. Common reactions included statements like; ' it's nothing', 'it's sciatica', 'it will clear up'. Overall, 38% of women said the information they were given about LLL was inadequate and 13% of women said they had never heard of LLL at all.

The management of locally advanced/recurrent disease

Landoni et al. (1997) reported that among patients treated for locally advanced cervical cancer (IB–IIA), 25% will experience recurrence after therapy. For patients who have been pre-treated with radiotherapy and have reached their maximum radiotherapy dose, surgery is the standard treatment for recurrent cervical cancer in the pelvic cavity. Unfortunately, this will frequently be 'salvage' surgery, meaning surgery with a palliative approach in which cure is not feasible. The emphasis instead is on relieving symptoms and improving quality of life.

There is, however, a small sub-group of patients for whom radical surgery is contemplated with curative intent. The operation is known as pelvic exenteration and is only performed if there is no extra-pelvic disease. Traditionally, it is undertaken through a laparotomy, although a laparoscopic approach has also been used (Ferron et al. 2006).

The procedure was developed more than fifty years ago and entails en bloc resection of most of the pelvic viscera, including the reproductive, urinary and lower gastrointestinal organs. Whilst it is probably used most frequently for the treatment of recurrent cervical cancer, it is also used in the management of other pelvic tumours, including cancer of the uterus, vagina, vulva, colon and bladder.

Over time the operative technique has improved. The original operative mortality rate was 23%, compared with 10% more recently (Brunschwig 1948, Chi et al. 1999). The five-year survival rate after the operation ranges from 23% to 61% (Carter et al. 2004). Surgeons will only conduct the operation on women who have good prognostic indicators and therefore potential candidates are thoroughly investigated to confirm the absence of any metastatic disease.

The operation falls into two phases; the exenterative phase consisting of excision of the pelvic viscera and the reconstructive phase which involves the creation of a neovagina, reinforcement of the pelvic floor, and restoration of bowel continuity (Salom and Penalver 2003). The latter phase is of particular importance for the psychosocial wellbeing of the woman in that it avoids permanent colostomy. Studies of psychosexual health involving exenterative cases have indicated that the fewer the stomas required and the inclusion of a vaginal reconstruction at the time of resection correlates with improved quality of life (QOL) with minimal deterioration of body image (Turns 2001).

Suitable candidates for this surgery need to be of good performance status and without significant co-morbidity. Ideally the tumour will be mobile and not fixed to the pelvic side wall – a positron emission tomography (PET) scan will be performed to exclude extrapelvic or side wall disease. Complaints of lower back pain, unilateral leg oedema, sciatic leg pain and hydronephrosis may suggest pelvic sidewall and metastatic involvement, contraindicating this form of surgery.

Post-operative morbidity after pelvic exenteration

The consequences of this radical surgery affect not only the integrity of the body but also the emotional, functional, social and sexual aspects of individuals.

(Carter et al. 2004)

The procedure is, not surprisingly, associated with significant post-operative morbidity (see Table 3.4). Kakuda et al. 2003 reported that 45% of patients will require at least one re-admission to hospital and 32% require additional operative procedures. Potential problems include:

Table 3.4 Potential acute complications of pelvic exenteration (adapted from Ruth-Sahd and Zulkosky 1999)

Complication	Signs	Management
Upper gastrointestinal haemorrhage	Bright red effluent from NG tube or haematemesis Melaena from colostomy Hypovolaemic changes	Antacids Fluid replacement Prepare for endoscopy to identify bleeding point
Pelvic haemorrhage	Hypovolaemic changes Blood from drains/incisions	Fluid replacement May require surgery
Intraoperative myocardial infarction	Unstable haemodynamic condition Chest pain Abnormal cardiac enzymes	Monitor and assess vital signs as per institutional post-operative procedure
Pulmonary emboli	Dyspnoea, anxiety, chest pain, haemoptysis, tachycardia	Oxygen, anticoagulants and bedrest
Iliac artery thrombosis	Sudden onset of diffuse abdominal pain	May require surgery
Conduit infarction	Ileal conduit pale in colour and may be painful	Monitor May require surgery
Urinary retention	Decreased urinary output	Monitor Conduit skin opening may need to be enlarged by surgeon
Colostomy retraction	Colostomy slips back into the abdominal cavity and is not visible on the skin surface	Monitor May require surgery
Peristomal hernia	The area around the stoma bulges and is painful	Monitor May require surgery
Small bowel obstruction	Abdominal pain, cramps, nausea and vomiting, abdominal distention, high pitched bowel sounds, decreased output from colostomy	Insert NG tube for decompression May require laparotomy
Prolonged ileus	Absent or decreased bowel sounds, abdominal distention, vomiting and cramps	NG tube for decompression NBM IV fluids May require laparotomy
Perineal hernia	Bulging perineal area Increased pressure and pain in the perineal area	May require surgery
Intra-abdominal abscess	Fever, abdominal tenderness, possible offensive drainage from incisions	Antibiotics and may require surgical or radiologically guided drainage
Necrotising fasciitis	Increased pain, tenderness and drainage around incision or ostomy areas, elevated white blood cell count, fever, subcutaneous emphysema	Will require surgical debridement
Conduit-related obstruction due to renal calculi	Excruciating intermittent flank pain, radiating across the abdomen, chills, fever, haematuria	Will require opiates for pain relief May require surgery for removal of calculi
Urinary fistulae	Faecal contents in ileal conduit drainage bag	Will require surgery

---

Box 3.6 Creation of a neovagina

The creation of a neovagina can be performed during the initial pelvic exenteration surgery or as a separate operation at a later date. In the former situation, myocutaneous grafts are used from the gracilis and rectus abdominis muscles (Pawlick et al. 2006). These flaps have the added benefit of providing extra tissue to cover the pelvis – in fact the formation of a neovagina has been associated with decreased post-operative morbidity through filling the potential space left following the operation (Pawlick et al. 2006).

Gleeson et al. (1994) evaluated the outcome of 14 patients who underwent vaginal recon-struction. Most patients wanted to resume intercourse post-surgery and those who did not wanted a normal anatomy. Results were disappointing, with a high incidence of complications (necrosis, fistula). Only one of the five previously sexually active survivors had resumed inter-course. Compromised vaginal depth with dyspareunia, vaginal discharge and vulvar pain were obstacles to normal sexual function.

---

(1) gastro-intestinal: intestinal obstruction, enteroperitoneal fistula, perineal and peristo-mal hernias
(2) urological: urinary conduit leak, stricture and calculi
(3) pelvic: fistulae and wound breakdown
(4) infective: the incidence of wound abscesses remains high and an interventional radiolo-gist is often required to drain pelvic collections which do not resolve with antibiotics alone

The radicality of the procedure is not the only factor which is likely to contribute to post-operative morbidity. Other factors include delayed wound-healing as a result of a previously irradiated surgical field, long operative time, blood loss and intestinal contami-nation. Some patients have poor pre-operative nutritional status because of the disease process and may require post-operative total parenteral nutrition. Routinely, patients are admitted to intensive care for 48 to 72 hours post-procedure.

Five-year survival after pelvic exenteration for gynaecological malignancies is approxi-mately 40% (Salom and Penalver 2003). Negative prognostic factors for the procedure are:

- large pelvic recurrences
- pelvic and para-aortic lymph node involvement
- positive margin status
- short time to recurrence
- non-squamous cell carcinoma

(Salom and Penalver 2003, Pawlick et al. 2006)

Preparing patients for this operation is difficult, mainly because the extensiveness of the procedure is almost incomprehensible to them (Ruth-Sahd and Zulkosky 1999). Patients return to the intensive care unit with an endotracheal and nasogastric tube in situ. They also frequently have two abdominal incisions, two abdominal drains, a colostomy and an ileal conduit (Ruth-Sahd and Zulkosky 1999). They may have a neo-vagina formed either during the initial surgery or in a separate operation later on. The muscle required for this is obtained from the thighs and so surgical scars will also be present on the medial aspect of each one. Alternatively, skin and muscle from the abdominal wall may be used – a transverse rectus abdominis musculocutaneous or TRAM flap.

Whilst many studies have concentrated on the physical morbidity of this surgery, its psychological sequelae are just as significant.

Dempsey et al. (1975) interviewed sixteen patients who had undergone pelvic exenteration for gynaecological cancer. The post-operative period appeared to be a difficult time for all, and most were totally amnesic for two or three days post-surgery. Immediate post-operative complaints included fatigue, irritation from the nasogastric tube, insomnia and pain. All patients had been concerned about dealing with a stoma, but by three months were comfortable with it. Most women reported that their sexual activity had been compromised by the surgery, although none felt it had had a negative effect on their marriage. The conclusion of the authors was that despite the magnitude of the surgery, quality of life post-exenteration is satisfactory. These conclusions are confirmed by other research indicating that although patients demonstrated high levels of anxiety post-operatively and also scored low on sexual functioning scales, there was nevertheless a reasonable level of adjustment in major life areas (Anderson and Hacker 1983).

Good psychological and social recovery is assisted by a thorough pre-operative psychiatric assessment (Turns 2001). Furthermore, pre-operative involvement by the whole team is important, including the stoma therapist, sexual counsellors and nursing staff. Involvement of the patient's family, and in particular her partner, is very valuable.

Conclusion

Surgery has an important role in the management of both early stage and advanced cervical cancer. It is a dynamic area with the ongoing refinement of fertility-preserving and nerve sparing techniques. However, surgery can also be associated with significant morbidity. This is a challenge for cervical cancer patients. Although modern therapies offer a real chance of cure this is not without a cost, this being the ongoing management of treatment-related toxicity.

Frequently asked questions

(1) I am having a radical hysterectomy. How long will I be in hospital for?
   This will vary according to which surgeon performs the operation and whether or not you experience any post-operative complications. However, most women will be in hospital for five to eight days after the surgery.
(2) When can I have sex again after a radical hysterectomy?
   Once again, different surgeons have different guidelines, but somewhere in the region of six weeks is usually recommended.
(3) When can I drive again after radical hysterectomy?
   Your surgeon will guide you and will probably advise not before four weeks following the operation.
(4) When can I start to lift things and return to work after a radical hysterectomy?
   Most surgeons will advise that you do not lift or return to work for six weeks following the operation.
(5) How can I avoid lower limb lymphoedema following my operation?
   It is difficult to avoid this complication as it appears to be related to the extent of your surgery. However, early detection is very important for effective management, so be aware of any changes in limb size or sensation and seek advice from a lymphoedema specialist. The use of support stockings post-operatively may help.

Resources

National Lymphedema Network: http://www.lymphnet.org
British Lymphology Society: http://www.lymphoedema.org/bls/
The Lymphoedema Association of Australia: www.lymphoedema.org.au
Lymphoedema Support Network: www.lymphoedema.org/lsn/
UK Lymph: www.uklymph.com/
BACUP: http://www.cancerbackup.org.uk/Home
Jo's Trust: http://www.jotrust.co.uk/
Trachelectomy: http://www.trachelectomy.co.uk/
The Cancer Council: http://www.cancercouncil.com.au/

References

Andersen BL and Hacker MF (1983) Psychosexual adjustment following pelvic exenteration. *Obstet Gynaecol*, 61, 331–338

Badger C, Preston N, Seers K and Mortimer P (2004a) Benzopyrones for reducing and controlling lymphoedema of the limbs. *Cochrane Database of Systematic Review*. Issue 2. Art. No.: CD003140. DOI: 10.1002/14651858.CD003140.pub2

Badger C, Preston N, Seers K and Mortimer P (2004b) Physical therapies for reducing and controlling lymphoedema of the limbs. *Cochrane Database of Systematic Reviews*. Issue 4. Art. No.: CD003141. DOI: 10.1002/14651858.CD003141.pub2

Badger C, Preston N, Seers K and Mortimer P (2004c) Antibiotics/anti-inflammatory for reducing acute inflammatory episodes in lymphoedema of the limbs. *Cochrane Database of Systematic Reviews*. Issue 2. Art. No.: CD003143. DOI: 10.1002/14651858.CD003143.pub2

Barranger E, Cortez A, Commo F, et al. (2004) Histopathological validation of the sentinel node concept in cervical cancer. *Anna Oncol*, 15 (6), June, 870–874

Benedetti-Panici P, Zullo MA, Plotti F, Manci N, Muzii L and Angioli R (2004) Long-term bladder function in patients with locally advanced cervical carcinoma treated with neoadjuvant chemotherapy and type 3–4 radical hysterectomy. *Cancer*, 100 (10), 2110–2117

Bergmark K, Avall-Lundqvist E, Dickman P, Henningsohn L and Steineck G (2002) Patient rating of distressful symptoms after treatment for early cervical cancer. *Acta Obstet Gynecol Scand*, 81, 443–450

Bernardini M, Barrett J, Seaward G and Covens A (2003) Pregnancy outcomes in patients after radical trachelectomy. *Am J Obstet Gynaecol*, 189 (5), Nov, 1378–1382

Bernhard LA (1993) Sexual counseling of women having gynecologic surgical procedures. *AWHONNS Clinical Issues in Perinatal & Womens Health Nursing*, 4 (2), 250–257

Brown K (2000) *Management Guidelines for Women's Health Nurse Practitioners*. FA Davis, Philadelphia PA

Bruner DW and Boyd CP (1999) Assessing women's sexuality after cancer therapy: checking assumptions with focus group technique. *Cancer Nursing*, 22 (6), 438–447

Brunschwig A (1948) Complete excision of pelvic viscera for advanced carcinoma. *Cancer*, 1, 177–183

Bunde M, Suls J, Martin R and Barnett K (2006) Hystersisters online: social support and social comparison among hysterectomy patients on the Internet. *Annals of Behavioral Medicine*, 31 (3), 271–278

Burghardt E, Baltzer J, Tulusan AH and Haas J (1992) Results of surgical treatment of 1028 cervical cancers studied with volumetry. *Cancer*, 70, 648–655

Butler-Manuel SA, Buttery LDK, Ahern RP, Polak JM and Baton DPJ (2000) Pelvic nerve plexus trauma at radical hysterectomy and simple hysterectomy: the nerve content of the uterine supporting ligaments. *Cancer*, 89, 384–841

Carter J, Dennis SC, Abu-Rustum N, Brown CL, McCreath W and Barakat RR (2004) Brief report; total pelvic exenteration – a retrospective clinical needs assessment. *Psycho-oncology*, 1, 125–131

Charkviani L, Kekelidze N and Charkviani T (2000) Management of lymphocysts after cervical carcinoma surgery. *European Journal of Gynaecological Oncology*, 21 (5), 487–480

Chi DS, Gemignani ML, Curtin JP and Hoskins WJ (1999) Long-term experience in the surgical management of cancer of the uterine cervix. *Semin Surg Oncol*, 17, 161–167

Choi SH, Kim SH, Choi HJ, Park BK and Lee HJ (2004) Preoperative magnetic resonance imaging staging of uterine cervical carcinoma: results of prospective study. *J Comput Assist Tomogr*, 28 (5), Sept/Oct, 620–627

Cole T (2006) Risks and benefits of needle use in patients after axillary node surgery. *British Journal of Nursing*, 15 (18), 969–979

Corney R, Everett H, Howells A and Crowther M (1992) The care of patients undergoing surgery for gynaecological cancer: the need for information, emotional support and counseling. *Journal of Advanced Nursing*, 17, 667–671

Covens A, Rosen B and Murphy J (2002) How important is removal of the parametrium at surgery for carcinoma of the cervix? *Gynaecol Oncol*, 84, 145–149

Covens A, Shaw P, Murphy J, et al. (1999) Is radical trachelectomy a safe alternative to a radical hysterectomy for patients with stage IA–B carcinoma of the cervix? *Cancer*, 86, 2273–2279

Davis G, O'Boyle AL, Towers G, Seymour S and Russell S (2003) Selecting the most appropriate technique for vaginal hysterectomy. *Journal of Pelvic Medicine and Surgery*, 9 (3), May/June, 133–144

Dell DD and Doll CC (2006) Caring for a patient with lymphoedema. *Nursing*, 36 (6), 49–51

Dempsey MG, Buchsbaum HJ and Morrison J (1975) Psychosocial adjustment to pelvic exenteration. *Gynaecol Oncol*, 3, 325–374

Ducic I, Moxley M and Al-Attar A (2006) Algorithm for treatment of post-operative incisional groin pain after caesarian delivery or hysterectomy. *Obstet Gynaecol*, 108 (1), 27–31

Farquhar C, Sadler L, Harvey SA and Stewart AW (2005) The association of hysterectomy and menopause: a prospective cohort study. *BJOG*, 112 (7), July, 956–962

Ferron G, Querleu D, Martel P, Letourneur B and Soulie M (2006) Laparoscopy-assisted vaginal pelvic exenteration. *Gynecologic Oncology*, 100 (3), 551–555

Flory N (2005) Psychosocial effects of hysterectomy – literature review. *Journal of Psychosomatic Research*, 59, 117–129

Foldi E (1998) The treatment of lymphoedema. *Cancer*, 83 (12, Suppl American), 2833–2834

Frumovitz M, Coleman RL, Gayed IW, et al. (2006) Usefulness of preoperative lymphoscintigraphy in patients who undergo radical hysterectomy and pelvic lymphadenectomy for cervical cancer. *American Journal of Obstetrics & Gynecology*, 194 (4), 1186–1195

Garg K, Rabban J, Chen L and Zaloudek C (2006) Microinvasive carcinoma of the cervix. *Pathol Case Review*, 11 (3), May/June, 121–129

Gary D (2007) Lymphoedema diagnosis and management. *Journal of the American Academy of Nurse Practitioners*, 19 (2), 72–78

Gleeson N, Baile W, Roberts WS, et al. (1994) Surgical and psychosexual outcome following vaginal reconstruction with pelvic exenteration. *Eur J Gynaecol Oncol*, 2, 89–95

Grigsby P and Herzog TJ (2001) Current management of patients with invasive cervical carcinoma. *Clin Obstet Gynaecol*, 44 (3), Sept, 531–537

Hatch KD (1994) Cervical cancer, in Berek JS and Hacker NF (eds) *Practical Gynecologic Oncology*. Williams and Wilkins, Philadelphia (2nd edn), pp. 243–283

Heller PB, Malfetano JH, Bundy BN, et al. (1990) Clinical-pathologic study of stage IIB, III, and IVA carcinoma of the cervix: extended diagnostic evaluation for para-aortic node metastasis. A Gynecologic Oncology Group study. *Gynecol Oncol*, 38, 425–430

Honnor A (2006) The staging of lymphoedema and accompanying symptoms. *British Journal of Community Nursing*, 11 (10), S6–S8

Hoult JR and Paya M (1996) Pharmacological and biochemical actions of simple coumarins: natural products with therapeutic potential. *General Pharmacology*, 27 (4), 713–722

Jackson KS and Naik R (2006) Pelvic floor dysfunction and radical hysterectomy. *Int J Gynaecol Cancer*, 16 (1), Jan/Feb, 354–363

Jensen PT, Groenvold M, Klee MC, Thranov I, Petersen MA and Machin D (2003) Early stage cervical carcinoma, radical hysterectomy and sexual function. *Cancer*, 100 (1), 97–106

Kakuda JT, Lamont JP, Chu DZ and Paz IB (2003) The role of pelvic exenteration in the management of recurrent rectal cancer, *Am J Surg*, 186, 660–664

Katz A (2002) Sexuality after hysterectomy, *JOGNN*, 31 (3), May/June, 256–262

Kim KH and Lee KA (2001) Symptom experience in women after hysterectomy. *JOGNN*, 30 (5), Sept/Oct, 472–480

Lacovara JE and Yoder LH (2006) Secondary lymphoedema in the cancer patient. *Medsurg Nursing*, 15 (5), 302–306

Landoni F, Maneo A, Colombo A, et al. (1997) Randomised study of radical surgery versus radiotherapy for stage IB–IIA cervical cancer. *Lancet*, 350 (9077), 23 Aug, 535–540

Landoni F, Maneo A, Cormio G, Perego P, Milani R and Caruso O (2001) Class II versus Class III radical hysterectomy in stage IB–IIA cervical cancer: a prospective randomised study. *Gynaecol Oncol*, 80, 3–12

Larson D, Weinstein M, Goldberg I, et al. (1986) Edema of the arm as a function of the extent of axilliary surgery in patients with stage I–II carcinoma of the breast treated with primary radiotherapy. *Int J Radiat Oncol Biol Phys*, 12 (9), 1575–1582

Linnitt N (2005) Case study detailing treatment of bilateral lower limb lymphoedema. *Wound Care*, June, S28–S31

Maas CP and der Kulie MM (2003) The effect of hysterectomy on sexual functioning, in Weijenborg PT (ed.) *Annual Review of Sex Research*, 14, 83–113

Matsuura Y, Kawagoe T, Toki N, Tanaka M and Kashimura M (2006) Long-standing complications after treatment for cancer of the uterine cervix – clinical significance of medical examination at five years after treatment. *Int J Gynaecol Cancer*, 16 (1), 294–297

McCallin M, Johnston J and Bassett S (2005) How effective are physiotherapy techniques to treat established secondary lymphoedema following surgery for cancer? A critical analysis of the literature. *NZ Journal of Physiotherapy*, 33 (3), 101–112

Meston CM and Bradford A (2004) A brief review of the factors influencing sexuality after hysterectomy. *Sexual and Relationship Therapy*, 19 (1), 5–12

Moore DH (2006) Cervical Cancer. *Obstet Gynaecol*, 107 (5), May, 1152–1161

Morice P and Castaigne D (2005) Advances in the surgical management of invasive cervical cancer. *Curr Opin Obstet Gynaecol*, 17 (1), Feb, 5–12

Mortimer P (1995) Managing lymphoedema. *Clinical and Experimental Dermatology*, 20, 98–106

Mortimer P (2000) Swollen lower limb – 2: lymphoedema. *BMJ*, 320, 1527–1529

Mortimer PS and Levick JR (2004) Chronic peripheral oedema: the critical role of the lymphatic system. *Clinical Medicine*, 4 (5), 448–453

Naik R, Mayne C, Nwabinelli J, et al. (2001) Prevalence and management of (non-fistulous) urinary incontinence in women following radical hysterectomy for early stage cervical cancer. *Eur J Gynaecol Oncol*, 22, 26–30

O'Brien J, Austin M, Sethi P and O'Boyle P (1991) Urinary incontinence: prevalence, need for treatment and effectiveness of intervention by nurse. *BMJ*, 303, 1308

Oetker-Black SL, Jones S, Estok P, Ryan M, Gale N and Parker C (2003) Preoperative teaching and hysterectomy outcomes. *AORN*, 77 (6), June, 1215–1231

Pawlick TM, Skibber JM and Rodriguez-Bigas MA (2006) Pelvic exenteration for advanced pelvic malignancies. *Annals of Surgical Oncology*, 13 (5), 612–623

Pieterse QD, Maas CP, Kuile MM, et al. (2006) An observational, longitudinal study to evaluate miction, defaecation, and sexual function after radical hysterectomy with pelvic lymphadenectomy for early stage cervical cancer. *International Journal of Gynaecological Cancer*, 16 (3), 1119–1129

Piller NB (1976) Conservative treatment of acute and chronic lymphoedema with benzo-pyrones. *Lymphology*, 9 (4), 132–137

Piver MS, Rutledge F and Smith JP (1974) Five classes of extended hysterectomy for women with cervical cancer. *Obstet Gynaecol*, 44, 265–272

Plante M and Roy M (2001) New approaches in the surgical management of early stage cervical cancer. *Curr Opin Obstet Gynecol*, 13 (1), 41–46

Querleu D and Leblanc E (2003) Laparoscopic surgery for gynaecologcial oncology. *Curr Opin Obstet Gynaecol*, 15 (4), 309–314

Reidel MA, Knaebel HP, Seiler CM, et al. (2003) Postsurgical pain outcome of vertical and transverse abdominal incision: design of a randomized, controlled equivalence trial. *BMC Surgery*, 3, 9 (http://www.biomedcentral.com/1471-2482/3/9 accessed 2/7/07)

Roberts K and Naik R (2006) Catheterization options following radical surgery for cervical cancer. *British Journal of Nursing*, 15 (19), 1038–1044

Rojas-Espaillant LA and Rose PG (2005) Management of locally advanced cervical cancer. *Curr Opin Oncol*, 17 (5), September, 485–492

Rose P (2001) Type II radical hysterectomy: evaluating its role in cervical cancer. *Gynecol Oncol*, 80, 1–2

Ruth-Sahd LA and Zulkosky KD (1999) Cervical cancer: caring for patients undergoing total pelvic exenteration. *Critical Care Nurse*, 19 (1), Feb, 46–57

Ryan M, Stainton C, Slaytor EK, Jaconelli C, Watts S and MacKenzie P (2003a) Aetiology and prevalence of lower limb lymphoedema following treatment for gynaecological cancer. *Australia and New Zealand Journal of Obstetrics and Gynaecology*, 43, 148–151

Ryan M, Stainton MC, Jaconelli C, Watts S, MacKenzie P and Mansberg T (2003b) The experience of lower limb lymphoedema for women after treatment for gynaecologic cancer. *Oncology Nursing Forum*, 30 (3), 417–423

Sakuragi N, Todo Y, Kudo M, Yamamoto R and Sato T (2005) A systematic, nerve-sparing radical hysterectomy technique in invasive cervical cancer for preserving post-surgical bladder function. *International Journal of Gynaecological Cancer*, 15 (2), 389–397

Salom EM and Penalver MA (2003) Pelvic exenteration and reconstruction. *Cancer J*, 9, 415–424

Scriven A and Tucker C (1997) The quality and management of written information presented to women undergoing hysterectomy. *Journal of Clinical Nursing*, 6 (2), 107–113

Selman TJ, Luesley DM, Murphy DJ and Mann CH (2005) Is radical hysterectomy for early stage cervical cancer an outdated operation? *BJOG*, 112, 363–365

Shimada M, Kigawa J, Nishimura R, et al. (2006) Ovarian metastasis in carcinoma of the uterine cervix. *Gynecologic Oncology*, 101 (2), May, 234–237

Singh N and Arif S (2004) Histopathologic parameters of prognosis in cervical cancer – a review. *Int J Gynaecol Cancer*, 14 (5), Sept/Oct, 741–750

Soutter WP, Hanoch J, D'Arcy T, Dina R, McIndoe GA and DeSouza NM (2004) Pretreatment tumour volume measurement on high-resolution magnetic resonance imaging as a predictor of survival in cervical cancer. *BJOG*, 111 (7), 741–747

Spencer C and Fang H (2005) Cervical cancer, in Lancaster T and Nattress K (eds), *Gynaecological Cancer Care: a Guide to Practice*. Ausmed Publications, Melbourne. pp. 63–77

Todo Y, Kuwabara M and Watari H (2006) Urodynamic study on postsurgical bladder function in cervical cancer treated with systematic nerve-sparing radical hysterectomy. *Int J Gynaecol Cancer*, 16 (1), Jan/Feb, 369–375

Turns D (2001) Psychosocial issues: pelvic exenterative surgery. *Journal Surg Oncology*, 76, 224–236

Van der Vange N, Weverling G, Ketting B, et al. (1995) The prognosis of cervical cancer associated with pregnancy: a matched cohort study. *Obstet Gynecol*, 85, 1022–1026

Waggoner SE (2003) Cervical cancer. *Lancet*, 361, 2217–2225

Walsgrove H (2001) Hysterectomy. *Nursing Standard*, 15 (29), April 4, 47–55

Werngren-Elgstrom M and Lidman D (1994) Lymphoedema of the lower extremities after surgery and radiotherapy for cancer of the cervix. *Scandanavian Journal of Plastic and Reconstructive Surgery*, 28, 289–293

Williams AF (2004) Understanding and managing lymphoedema in people with advanced cancer. *Journal of Community Nursing*, 18 (11), 30–40

Williams PD, Valerrama DM, Gloria MD, et al. (1988) Effects of preparation for mastectomy/hysterectomy on women's post-operative self-care behaviors. *International Journal of Nursing Studies*, 25 (3), 191–206

Chapter 4

Radiotherapy

'Few therapeutic modalities in medicine induce more misunderstanding, fear and anxiety than the use of radiation in cancer treatment.'
(Rotman et al. 1977, p. 744, quoted by Wells 2003, p. 39)

Introduction

Whilst surgery is recognised as the optimal treatment for early stage cervical cancer, radiotherapy is the treatment of choice for more advanced disease (large stage IB tumours and beyond). In recent years significant improvements have been made to radiotherapy as a primary treatment through the addition of concurrent chemotherapy. Radiotherapy may also be used in conjunction with surgery, although in general this is avoided because of the increased toxicity which arises from using the two modalities together. Nevertheless, adjuvant radiotherapy may be employed post-surgery where there are positive surgical margins or other poor prognostic factors. Radiotherapy also remains a common salvage therapy for disease which recurs after surgery, and has an important role in the palliation of symptoms associated with advanced disease.

In this chapter we will review the indications for radiotherapy, different radiotherapy treatment modalities, radiotherapy and chemoradiotherapy toxicities and the nursing management of patients undergoing radiotherapy and chemoradiotherapy.

The great debate: surgery versus radiotherapy

The management of stage IA cervical cancer (microscopic invasive disease) has been shown to be effective with simple hysterectomy, giving greater than 95% five-year survival (Cannistra 1996). However, unfortunately, many patients present with more advanced disease than this.

For patients with bulky lesions (stage IIB and above) surgery is not really a good treatment option (Dargent et al. 2005). It becomes technically too difficult and the likelihood of achieving negative surgical margins is very small (Grigsby and Herzog 2001). In this situation radiotherapy – or more specifically chemoradiotherapy – is the treatment of choice.

Whilst in some cases it is very clear whether to proceed with surgery or with radiotherapy, there are also intermediate situations in which the optimal treatment modality is debatable. For example, patients with IB or IIA disease could reasonably be treated either surgically or with radiotherapy. In this situation it is believed that both strategies are equally effective, resulting in a five-year survival rate of 80% to 90% (Eifel et al. 1997). The equivalence of the two techniques is basically supported by one seminal study by Landoni et al. (1997).

Box 4.1 Radiotherapy versus surgery

Advantages of surgery over radiotherapy

The advantage of surgery over radiotherapy is that radical hysterectomy allows the gonadal function of at least one ovary to be saved, thereby avoiding the effects of early menopause in younger women. It allows the status of the lymph nodes – the most important variable associated with survival – to be assessed accurately. It limits the radiation associated shortening and fibrosis of the vagina, (although radical hysterectomy is also associated with a degree of vaginal shortening). Furthermore, pelvic relapses can be successfully cured by radiotherapy, whereas salvage surgery after primary irradiation carries a high rate of failures and severe morbidity (Landoni et al. 1997).

Advantages of radiotherapy over surgery

Radiotherapy has some distinct logistical advantages over surgery in certain situations. For example, it is easier to deliver in patients who are obese, are elderly, or have severe illness – major contraindications to the surgical approach. It also avoids the risks of anaesthesia and the laparotomy scar, and iatrogenic mortality is rare (Landoni et al. 1997).

Landoni et al. (1997) performed a phase III trial in which patients with stages IB and IIA cervical cancer were randomised to receive either external irradiation and brachytherapy or a radical hysterectomy and lymph node dissection. The final results demonstrated that the overall survival rate was 83% for each group. Disease-free survival rates were also similar for the two groups at five years: 74% for surgery and 74% for irradiation. Of note is the fact that more than 60% of the patients who were initially treated with a radical hysterectomy and lymph node dissection also received post-operative pelvic irradiation in this study.

Surgery plus adjuvant radiotherapy

As well as controversy about the selection of surgical versus non-surgical cases, controversy also exists regarding the indications for combining the two treatment modalities. What are the indications for adjuvant radiotherapy after radical surgery?

Depending on the institutional selection criteria, as many as 50% of surgical patients may also be submitted to adjuvant radiotherapy (Dargent et al. 2005). Adjuvant radiotherapy is thought to reduce recurrence rates by treating subclinical disease – that is the 'invisible' metastases that develop in the pelvic tissue left *in situ*.

Situations in which post-operative radiotherapy may be considered are where there are:

- only small tumour-free margins
- positive lymph nodes
- unsuspected higher disease stage after surgery
- large tumour diameter
- vascular or lymphovascular space involvement
- inadequate primary surgery (simple hysterectomy without lymphadenectomy in stages IB and higher)
- deep stromal invasion
- spread to the pelvic cellular tissue

(Dargent et al. 2005, Munstedt et al. 2005)

Although improvements in the management of cervix cancer have reduced the incidence of many of the most severe treatment-related complications over the past 20 years, the highest complication rate remains following the combination of surgery and adjuvant radiotherapy. The morbidity due to radiotherapy given after pelvic dissection is twice that

---

Box 4.2 Some radiation effects on cells

(1) Free radicals damage DNA so that the cell is unable to divide properly at the next mitosis.
(2) Radiation triggers immediate cell death (apoptosis).
(3) Radiation influences the genes controlling the cell cycle (e.g. p53, RB gene).
(4) Radiation damages the cell membrane causing signals to be transmitted to the nucleus which influence cell behaviour.

(From Munroe (2003) in Faithfull and Wells, pp. 19)

---

of radiotherapy given without (Landoni et al. 1997). This particularly applies to long-term (delayed in onset) complications such as oedema of the lower limbs, urethral stenosis, rectal and bladder fistulas and bowel morbidity (Munstedt et al. 2005).

How does radiotherapy work?

Therapeutic radiation for the treatment of patients with cancer is usually produced by a machine called a linear accelerator. Linear accelerators create electromagnetic waves which interact with the atoms of tissues, causing them to give up their energy. The radiation produced is similar to X-rays but much more penetrating. Radiation may also be emitted from the nuclei of radioactive elements such as cobalt 60. This is known as gamma radiation.

Radiotherapy brings about structural damage to the nucleus and the cytoplasm of the cell. While both types of damage are important, it is the nuclear damage to the DNA which has the critical effect in causing radiation-induced cell death and in rendering malignant cells unable to divide. The effects of radiation on cells are summarised in Box 4.2.

Radiation effects on a tumour may not be immediately apparent. Some cancer cells will not show any obvious evidence of damage until they attempt to divide, and only then will they die. This can be observed clinically by looking at the response of a bulky carcinoma of the cervix immediately after completion of a course of definitive radiotherapy. CT scanning may well indicate residual tumour is present but re-examination on later follow-up will generally show complete resolution of the disease (Ahamed and Jhingran 2004).

Methods of radiotherapy administration

Radiotherapy for cervical cancer is delivered in two ways: Intra-cavity Brachytherapy (ICBT) and External Beam Radiotherapy (EBRT). Most women will begin with EBRT and finish with ICBT, which is administered 10–14 days after the last dose of EBRT.

A number of studies have shown that the combination of EBRT and ICBT is more effective than EBRT alone. For example, Longsdon and Eifel (1999) reported the pelvic failure rate to be 45% with EBRT alone versus 24% in stage IIIB patients receiving both EBRT and ICBT. Coia et al. (1990) similarly observed a significant increase in the pelvic failure rate (by 31%) when ICBT was not included in treatment protocols for stages I, II and III cervical carcinoma

External beam radiotherapy (EBRT)

External beam radiotherapy aims to reduce tumour size, (preferably to 4 cm or less). It is aimed at both primary and locoregional disease sites (particularly the regional lymph nodes).

Intra-cavity Brachytherapy (ICBT)

Brachytherapy involves the insertion of a radioactive source into the vagina and cervix. It is a treatment modality which has been around since shortly after the discovery of radium – indeed, little has changed in the technique in the last 40 years (Ahamed and Jhingran 2004). It has been shown to provide a good chance of cure even in cases of advanced cervical cancer, with five-year survival rates of 85% to 90% for stage IB disease (Barillot et al. 1997), 50% to 80% for stage IIB and 25% to 50% for stage III cancer (Coia et al.1990).

Brachytherapy may be administered at a high dose rate (HDR) or low dose rate (LDR). Low dose brachytherapy (LDB) is the traditional approach used in cervical cancer and is defined as a dose rate of less than 2 Gy/hr (traditionally 0.6–0.8 Gy/hr). It requires a hospital admission for 72–96 hours, during which time the patient is confined to a single room on bedrest and the radiotherapy is administered using a remote afterloading device (see Box 4.3). The treatment is typically administered over 36–40 hours, or less if given in two LDR fractions.

LDB is physically and psychologically demanding on cervical cancer patients and also presents a challenge to nursing staff (see Box 4.4). In part this is because of the physical isolation patients have to endure and in part because they are effectively immobilised by the radiation applicators. It is imperative that these applicators remain in the correct position so that the radiotherapy is delivered to the right place. For this reason the applicators are stitched in place and the patient is generally nursed 'flat' (the head of the bed should not be tilted by more than 30°). Clearly, this makes activities of daily living difficult. Eating can be a particular problem and many patients find 'finger food' the easiest to manage until mobile again (Gosselin and Waring 2001).

Elimination may also be difficult. Most patients will be catheterised, which makes urination easier. Some centres also institute a low residue diet and administer constipating medications in order to arrest bowel movements during the treatment period. If a patient does feel they are going to have a bowel movement the radiation physician needs to be informed so that the radioactive sources and applicator can be removed (Gosselin and Waring 2001). If linen changes are necessary the patient will be 'log-rolled' in order that the radioactive sources are not displaced.

Box 4.3 Remote afterloading devices and radiation safety

The principles of radiation safety are simple:

- minimise time of exposure
- maximise distance from sources of radiation
- use appropriate shielding

(Crownover et al. 1999)

Any potential exposure to radiotherapy is hazardous. The risk of exposure can be minimised through the use of remote afterloading devices. The radioactive source is attached to a cable and housed within a computer-controlled robotic machine which is known as an afterloader. When treatment is delivered, the radioactive source is pushed from the remote afterloader through tubing which is connected to the radiation applicator within the cervix. The Selectron machine and the Gammamed are examples of remote afterloading devices.

With high dose brachytherapy the patient is only 'hot' whilst in the treatment room and so this should not pose a threat to nursing staff, provided that they do not enter the room during treatment. In patients receiving LDB, the afterloading device reduces the risk of radiation exposure to theoretically negligible levels.

General nurses caring for these patients should wear a film badge or something similar to monitor their radiation exposure. Nursing staff assignments should be rotated to reduce cumulative exposure to any individual, and ideally it is recommended that pregnant staff are excluded from caring for LDB patients (Crownover et al. 1999).

Perineal discomfort may be a problem for patients undergoing LDB. Appropriate (generally opiate) analgesia should be administered and patient-controlled analgesia is often employed. The combination of prolonged immobility plus a higher risk of thromboembolic complications because of their cancer diagnosis means that anti-embolism measures such as the administration of subcutaneous heparin and compression hosiery should be instituted.

Although low dose brachytherapy is still widely utilised, it is clearly a discomforting procedure and for this reason high-dose brachytherapy has become increasingly popular over the last two decades. Several studies indicate treatment results equivalent to those of low-dose rate therapy, except maybe in stage III disease (Petereit et al. 1999, Kapp et al. 1998 from Ahamed and Jhingran 2004). The principal advantage of HDB over the LDB is that it can be administered on an out-patient basis. Both types of brachytherapy are associated with similar medium and long-term toxicities.

HDR brachytherapy refers to a dose rate of greater than 12 Gy/hr. The patient undergoes a number of ICBT applications, commonly ranging from three to six, usually at weekly intervals, depending on the treatment protocol and stage of disease (Ahamed and Jhingran 2004). Each HDB treatment takes five to ten minutes and the patient generally spends a total of 15–30 minutes in the radiation treatment room.

Radiotherapy simulation and planning

EBRT planning

As with any therapeutic agent, the dose of radiotherapy must be calculated and tailored for each patient. Once the total dose is established then it is broken down into a number of small treatments known as 'fractions'.

The radiation dose and the specific area to which it should be delivered is determined during a planning visit. The dosage calculation and design of treatment fields is based on a combination of computed tomography (CT) imaging and a computerised dose calculation system which allows three-dimensional planning. Patients undergo scanning in the treatment position, using a machine called a simulator. This allows identification of the volume of abnormal tumour tissue to be irradiated (the gross tumour volume (GTV)). Because there is uncertainty regarding the extent of microscopic tumour extension along tissue planes, and there will also be organ movements, an extra margin of tissue is added to the GTV. This more generous volume is known as the clinical target volume (CTV) and is the area which is irradiated. It will also include the regional lymph nodes (Ahamed and Jhingran 2004).

Additional measures to localise the position of the tumour include the insertion of gold seeds around its periphery. This occurs during the staging exploration under anaesthetic (EUA) in cases where advanced disease is detected. Some centres also insert a tampon into the vagina during planning in order to establish the position of the cervix. The EBRT treatment area is then defined by tattoos or marks to the skin which some patients dislike as it can make them feel 'branded' (Wells 2003).

Clearly, because the focus of radiotherapy planning is on absolute technical accuracy, this can result in something of a dehumanising experience for the patient (Wells 2003, p. 43). Interestingly, there is little published research exploring the experience of radiotherapy planning for the patient (Wells 2003). What is known is that many patients find the whole radiotherapy environment anxiety provoking – the size of the machines, the noises they make and the very concept of therapy using radiation.

ICBT planning

Patients receiving brachytherapy will invariably be catheterised and will also require the insertion of a rectal tube during planning. These help to identify the location of the bowel and bladder so that the radiotherapy dosage to these areas can be minimised.

A computerised tomography (CT) or magnetic resonance imaging (MRI) scan can also be obtained to accurately determine the residual tumour to be treated, although the applicators have to be CT/MRI compatible.

A variety of different applicators can be used for the insertion of radioactive implants into the woman's cervix. Some involve sutures to the skin, whilst other methods (principally those used for HDR brachytherapy) can avoid this by utilising specially designed undergarments. Placement of applicators may require a general anaesthetic or can sometimes be performed under local. Once the applicator has been inserted the woman is required to remain on strict bedrest.

The prescription dose for brachytherapy to the cervix is determined through identification of a hypothetical point 'A', which represents an area 2 cm above the cervical os and

---

Box 4.4   Low dose brachytherapy – the patient experience

> I said it's barbaric, I'll tell you. I know it sounds awful but I did, honestly, it's how I felt. I think it's like star wars. I said how do you expect me to lay all that time.
>
> (patient comment in Warnock, 2005).

It is perhaps a little surprising that there is only a small amount of nursing research looking at the management of the patient undergoing low dose brachytherapy. It is a procedure requiring skilled nursing intervention and it might be expected that there would be a larger body of literature on the patients' experience of the procedure and their perceived needs.

What we do learn from the available literature is that there is a high level of anxiety amongst women receiving intracavity brachytherapy (Andersen et al. 1984, Brandt 1991). We also learn that nurses are not necessarily fulfilling their potential in alleviating this anxiety. Andersen and Adamsen (2001) performed an interesting study in which they continuously videoed five patients receiving intracavity brachytherapy for anal or gynaecological cancer. They found that nurses spent only 27% of the available time with the patients. The majority of their communication was focused around physical care. It is of note that the patients had no expectations of receiving psychological support from the nurses.

More recently Warnock (2005) published a study building on a smaller, qualitative trial of ten women performed by Velji and Fitch (2001). Thirty-two women who were undergoing LDB participated and were questioned before, during and after treatment. Nursing staff also completed two-hourly checklists during treatment, assessing how they felt the participants were faring.

In anticipation of their forthcoming therapy the pre-treatment comments of most women were negative. There was apprehension regarding a number of issues including treatment length, being alone, lying still and pain.

Most patients did indeed experience a degree of pain during therapy and fourteen required analgesia with a strong opioid such as morphine. In a third of cases nurses underestimated the level of pain experienced by the patient. Other problems reported during treatment were:

- lying still
- backache
- length of treatment
- pain/discomfort on applicator removal
- difficulty eating
- nausea
- abdominal wind
- being alone

Some patients described coping mechanisms which they found to be helpful during treatment such as distraction (e.g. watching TV, listening to music) or positive thinking. They also described aspects of nursing care that they perceived as useful. These included being turned regularly, analgesia and sedative administration, back massages and occasional nursing visits to reduce loneliness.

2 cm on either side of the uterine axis along the plane of the uterus. This is thought to signify the region of maximum radiation tolerance (Ahamed and Jhingran 2004). In recent years sophisticated, computer-aided planning techniques have been developed whereby the radiation dose is applied more accurately to the residual tumour volume, making point A less relevant. Despite this, the dose to point A is still recorded for the purposes of data comparison.

Radiotherapy treatment factors

To provide effective treatment with radiotherapy a number of conditions must be satisfied:

(1) Dosage
   Clearly, the dose that can be administered is limited by the radiation tolerance of the surrounding normal tissues. To eliminate microscopic lymph node disease the classic treatment is to give the whole pelvis external beam X-ray therapy to a dose of 45–50.4 Gy in 25 to 28 daily fractions of 1.8 Gy each. Although this will not prevent relapse in 100% of patients, it will in most and the chance of long-term toxicities is less than 5% (Ahamed and Jhingran 2004).
   The addition of ICRT to radiotherapy regimens allows provision of a higher dose to the target area. Most authorities consider the optimal dosage to point A to be approximately 80 or 85 Gy, depending on the tumour size (although often tumour control can be achieved with smaller doses).
(2) Length of treatment time
   When a tumour is damaged by radiation, cells that are not dividing enter the cell cycle to replace the cells that have been destroyed. This process is known as repopulation. In some cases it may result in the tumour growing even more quickly than before treatment began.
   Treatment delays can allow time for sufficient repopulation to occur to reduce tumour control (Fyles et al. 1992). It has been estimated that the reduction in pelvic control and survival resulting from such delays is approximately 1% per day for each additional day beyond the optimal treatment time (Perez et al. 1995). Today, most authorities would consider a treatment duration of 55 days or less to be acceptable for cervical cancer (Lehman and Thomas 2001).
(3) Fractionation
   The rationale behind the fractionation of radiotherapy is to allow repair of non-malignant tissue. By breaking the treatment up into a number of fractions a higher total dose can be administered because the normal cells have time to repair themselves. Conversely, malignant cells lack this capacity for repair. The tissues which make up the bladder, rectum and skin can repair most of the damage caused by a fraction of radia-tion before the next fraction of treatment – indeed, it has been estimated that half the sublethal DNA damage will be repaired after 30 to 90 minutes (Adamson 2003). Certainly, most normal tissues will have repaired themselves within six hours.
(4) Anaemia
   Anaemia is a powerful prognostic factor in patients with cervical cancer and there is a considerable body of evidence to suggest that patients experiencing significant anaemia during their course of treatment have a worse outcome (Loizzi et al. 2003). Grogan et al. (1999) found that the poorest survival rates were amongst patients whose haemoglobin was less than 120 g/l at presentation/throughout therapy, or those whose initially high haemoglobin fell during the course of treatment. It is assumed that this is because of impaired oxygen delivery to the tumour tissue.
   For this reason, attempts are made to achieve and maintain haemoglobin levels between 11 and 13 g/dL during radiation treatment (Fyles et al. 2000). There are two ways of manipulating haemoglobin levels: either through the use of blood transfusion

or by administering erythropoietin (EPO), the cytokine responsible for stimulating red blood cell production.

Transfusion, whilst generally effective at maintaining good haemoglobin levels, is not without its problems. Sometimes there is a scarcity of transfusion products and there are also transfusion-related risks. These risks include acute and chronic transfusion reactions, viral infections and the possibility of increased tumour recurrence due to transfusion induced immunosuppression. Moreover, blood transfusions can only increase the haemoglobin level for a limited time, meaning that multiple transfusions may be required throughout an average treatment programme (Loizzi et al. 2003).

The role of EPO in maintaining haemoglobin levels during radiotherapy is not fully understood. A recent Gynaecology Oncology Group (GOG) trial of patients with stage IIB to IVA cervical cancer randomised patients to receive chemotherapy/radiotherapy (CT/RT) versus CT/RT plus EPO (40,000 units SC weekly). Out of the planned 406 patients, 109 were accrued, but the study was closed prematurely because of sponsor concerns regarding thromboembolic events – even though the incidence of such events was not found to be statistically higher than amongst non-EPO users. This unfortunately means that the role of EPO in this context has yet to be determined (Thomas et al. 2006)

Optimising radiotherapy treatment

Chemoradiotherapy (CRT)

Whilst radiotherapy is unarguably an effective treatment modality for the management of cervical cancer, over the years a number of endeavours have been made to improve and refine the technique. By far the most important of these involves the addition of concurrent chemotherapy. This has also been found to be helpful in the management of squamous cell carcinoma of the anus, oesophagus, bladder, lung, head and neck (Lehman and Thomas 2001).

During the 1990s a number of clinical trials were instigated in order to assess the value of chemoradiotherapy in cervical cancer. Prior to this, studies had failed to demonstrate any benefit to administering chemotherapy *prior to* or *following* radiotherapy. However, the new studies examined the value of administering chemotherapy *concurrently* with radiotherapy. The results of five of them led to an unusual step by the US National Cancer Institute. In 1999 a clinical alert was released to practising oncologists urging that 'strong consideration should be given to the incorporation of concurrent cisplatin-based chemotherapy with radiotherapy in women who require radiotherapy for the treatment of cervix cancer' (National Cancer Institute 1999, in Lehman and Thomas 2001).

The five trials on which this recommendation was made differed in their inclusion criteria, chemotherapy schedules and radiotherapy prescriptions (see Table 5.2 on p. 104). However, a total of 1800 women were involved and the results demonstrated a significant absolute improvement in survival when patients with locally advanced cervical cancer were treated with concomitant chemoradiation (Keys et al. 1999, Morris et al. 1999, Rose et al. 1999, Whitney et al. 1999, Peters et al. 2000).

The results of a sixth trial conducted by the National Cancer Institute of Canada were released shortly after this announcement was made and interestingly this failed to corroborate the results of the other five trials. Closer analysis of the trial methodology suggests that this was possibly because of differences in staging techniques. The Canadian study did not use surgical staging but CT scans to identify and exclude patients with para-aortic nodal metastasis, a method which has been shown to be less accurate (Pearcey et al. 2002).

More recently Greene et al. (2005) performed a systematic review of the literature looking at chemoradiotherapy. It was concluded that it improves response and survival, particularly amongst patients with stage I and II disease. It is associated with a notable reduction in distant metastases and a benefit can be observed regardless of the chemo-therapy agent used. In summary, a potential survival benefit of 12% was attributed to CRT. Greene concluded:

> Concomitant chemoradiation appears to improve overall survival and progression-free survival in locally advanced cervical cancer. It also appears to reduce local and distant recurrence, suggesting concomitant chemotherapy may afford radiosensitisation and systemic cytotoxic effects. Some acute toxicity is increased, but the long-term side effects are still not clear.

As an update of and extension to Greene's review, two of the co-authors, Vale and Tierney (2006), have conducted a meta-analysis using individual patient data. Their analysis includes 15 trials with a combined patient cohort of 4254 women. They found a 24% reduction in the risk of death and an 8% improvement in five-year survival with chemoradiation.

An important question to be answered with CRT treatment is whether or not it results in a greater level of toxicity than RT alone (Greene et al. 2005, Vale and Tierney 2006). Not only is there the issue of the additional chemotherapy-related toxicity, but also of whether radiotherapy-associated toxicities such as bowel toxicity are exacerbated by the addition of chemotherapy.

Addressing these factors, Kirwan et al. (2003) performed a Cochrane-type review of chemoradiation toxicities based on 4580 patients. Looking at acute toxicity there was no significant increase in grade 1 and 2 gastrointestinal, genito-urinary or dermatological toxicity. However, grade 3 and 4 haematological toxicities were persistently more common in the CRT arm with a two-fold increase in white blood count toxicity and a three-fold increase in platelet toxicity. One death in the CRT group was attributable to neutropenic sepsis. There was no significant difference in haemoglobin level although a trend towards more anaemia was noted in CRT group.

Most non-haematological grade 3 and 4 toxicities were more common in the CRT group and gastrointestinal toxicities were twice as common. There were no differences in either neurological or skin toxicity at any grade. Of the twelve toxic deaths reported, ten were in the CRT group.

Data on long-term toxicity was much less available, reported in only eight trials, seven of which indicated that there was no statistical difference between the two treatment groups. It has been suggested that this may simply be the result of under-reporting of late events (Kirwan et al. 2003).

Intensity modulated radiotherapy

In recent years a new radiotherapy technique has been developed which is known as intensity-modulated radiotherapy (IMRT). Rather than having a single, large radiation beam pass through the body, IMRT allows the beam to be broken into thousands of tiny, pencil-thin beams, each with a different intensity, which enter the body from many more angles. IMRT aims to protect surrounding tissues (especially bladder and bowel) from high doses of radiation, thus reducing some radiation-associated toxicities (Ahamed and Jhingran 2004).

Image guided radiotherapy

Changes in treatment planning over recent years mean the delivery of radiation can be more accurate. These improvements utilise CT, PET, ultrasound and MRI scanning in conjunction with specialised computer software. The result is an improved therapeutic ratio, permitting biologically higher doses with a greater degree of accuracy.

> **Box 4.5 Informational needs for patients undergoing radiotherapy**
>
> A number of studies would seem to indicate that patients' informational needs are not being met prior to radiation therapy, and that the information that is supplied is not always appropriate (Coulter et al. 1999). The type of information that patients appear to want is that which focuses on the principles of radiotherapy and the side effects of their treatment (Fieler et al. 1996). Furthermore, sensory information about what they can expect to feel has been found to be useful (Porock 1995, Christman and Cain 2003). For example, for a patient receiving EBRT it may be helpful to know that:
>
> - the treatment table is hard and narrow
> - the gantry will rotate around them
> - the bed may be moved up and down
> - there may be a buzzing or ticking sound from the machine during treatment
> - they will be alone in a dimmed room but closely watched either through a CCTV system or window and intercom
>
> (Wells 2003)
>
> Traditionally, leaflets, booklets and videos have been utilised to prepare patients for radiation therapy, although ensuring that the information is up to date and is in the correct languages is sometimes difficult with this kind of material. More recently, the provision of computerised information has been explored (Jones et al. 1999). To a certain extent the optimal modality of information provision is likely to be a matter of individual choice, and the importance of basic communication with a knowledgeable health professional should not be under-estimated. Jones et al. (1999) found that 80% of patients preferred a ten-minute consultation with a specialist nurse or radiographer to computer or booklet information.
>
> Adequate information provision is particularly important for patients undergoing brachytherapy – especially low dose brachytherapy. It has been suggested that basic preparation should include details about the length of time required for the procedure, the instruments that will be used and the anticipated schedule of events (Gosselin and Waring 2001). Patients will also require information about nutrition, bowel and bladder management, pain management, fatigue and radiation safety.

Treatment-related toxicities

As with any cytotoxic therapy, the success of radiotherapy lies with delivering the optimal dose to the diseased tissue and sparing the surrounding healthy tissue. Radiotherapy affecting the adjoining normal structures results in treatment-related toxicities.

The extent of radiation damage to normal tissues depends on several factors, including the radiation dose, the target organ, the volume of tissue irradiated, and the division rate of the irradiated cells (Ahamed and Jhingran 2004). It is estimated that approximately 12% of radiotherapy patients will experience major complications as a result of their treatment (Landoni et al. 1977). Radiotherapy-related toxicities can be subdivided into two categories: early and late effects.

Early or acute effects are generally of short duration and resolve with medical management, whereas late complications of radiotherapy lead to damage which may permanently impair quality of life (Ahamed and Jhingran 2004, Greene et al. 2005). In part this is related to the type of tissue involved. Early toxicities are manifest in those cells which are rapidly dividing such as the skin, mucosa and bone marrow. Slowly dividing tissues, such as the spinal cord and kidney, tend to show no immediate response to radiotherapy, with damage only becoming apparent in the ensuing months and years. Unlike acute damage, this damage may never be completely repaired (Adamson 2003).

Definitions of acute toxicities vary between studies, some classifying them as toxicities occurring during treatment and up to 42 days after completion of therapy, others using

60 days and others 90 (Kirwan et al. 2003). They include small bowel enteritis (crampy abdominal pain), cystitis (frequency, urgency, and haematuria), and radiodermatitis (erythema and dry and moist desquamation). Because a typical plan for pelvic irradiation also treats significant amounts of bone marrow, bone marrow suppression may also be a problem. This is an issue of increasing concern, given that most cases of cervix cancer are treated with concurrent chemotherapy and some patients will develop distant metastasis that will require chemotherapy later on (Ahamed and Jhingran 2004).

The aetiology of late toxicities is not fully understood and appears to be complex, involving a combination of cellular, vascular and cytokine changes (Small and Kachnic 2005). Late toxicites can occur months or even years after the termination of treatment. Denton et al. (2000) performed a national audit of the outcomes of women treated with radiotherapy for cervix cancer in the UK and found the rate of late severe complications at five years to be 8%. Four of the 91 patients who developed complications died as a result of their morbidity. The team encountered many difficulties related to the retrospective nature of their review and the poor clinical documentation of toxicities.

Even when toxicity data is collected prospectively, available radiation toxicity scales are not always sensitive enough to accurately reflect the true level of morbidity. Studies have estimated the incidence of serious late effects to be between 1 and 19%. Examples of late effects include organ stricture, fistula, necrosis and ulceration, connective tissue fibrosis, enteritis, and secondary malignancies (Ahamed and Jhingran 2004).

Acute radiotherapy toxicities

Fatigue

'In patients with cancer, fatigue is a pervasive, discouraging and debilitating symptom that can adversely affect daily functioning, quality of life, health and personal well-being . . . the fatigue experienced by patients with cancer differs from the ordinary fatigue of day-to-day living in that it tends to be more severe, more distressing, prolonged and unrelieved by ordinary measures such as sleep and rest.'

(Magnan and Mood 2003)

Fatigue is a radiation side effect which has been well addressed in the nursing literature and which significantly impacts quality of life. Reports of an association between radiation and fatigue appear as early as the nineteenth century in the literature. Fatigue has been described as 'a subjective experience of unusual, excessive or overwhelming tiredness that results in a decreased desire or capacity for mental or physical activity' (Mock et al. 2003). It constitutes both an acute and a long-term toxicity of radiotherapy treatment.

Most of us have our own perceptions of fatigue from personal experience, but the feelings described by cancer patients appear to be incomparable with 'normal' feelings of fatigue. Piper et al. (1987) reported cancer fatigue to be more distressing to patients than pain. Fatigue is now considered to be the most prevalent symptom of patients with cancer, affecting 70–95% of those receiving treatment with chemotherapy, radiotherapy or biotherapy (Mock 2003). It is also a significant survivorship issue and can lead to a marked reduction in normal functioning. However, many patients consider it to be an inevitable consequence of cancer and therefore fail to discuss it with their health care providers (Donovan and Ward 2005).

Magnan and Mood (2003) looked at the incidence of fatigue amongst a sample of 384 gynaecology oncology patients (6% of whom had cervix cancer). They found the time of onset varied widely. On average it was near the middle of the second week, although a substantial proportion of women (20%) reported it started on the first day of radiotherapy. Ahlberg et al. (2005) in a study of women with uterine cancer found fatigue to be cumulative over the course of treatment and other studies have indicated it is worst during the last week of treatment. It can persist for months or even years after treatment has ended (Ahlberg et al. 2005).

The mechanism of radiation induced fatigue is not completely understood. It may result from the release of metabolites during cellular destruction, or it could be related to the increased requirements of the body for cellular repair. The individual patient's experience of fatigue is likely to be influenced by a number of factors, including haemoglobin level, health state, global symptom distress, cachexia, anorexia and mood disturbance (Magnan and Mood 2003, Faithfull 2003a). Starting radiotherapy in a good state of health is associated with a delayed onset of fatigue and lower levels of fatigue distress (Magnan and Mood 2003).

Management of fatigue

Whilst the literature exploring the concept of fatigue and its prevalence is widespread, solutions to the problem tend to be a little more difficult to find. However, a number of interventions have been recommended, such as:

- assess pre-treatment levels of fatigue (it may be related to prior therapy or disease) and maintain ongoing assessments excluding possible physiological causes such as anaemia or treatable psychological morbidity
- encourage patients with fatigue to maintain a diary of daily activity – it helps with planning activities
- forewarn patients of the possibility of fatigue – many patients are surprised by its severity
- suggest a combination of self-care strategies, e.g. goal setting, prioritising activities; rest helps some patients but makes others feel worse
- exercise – if able, suggest patients undertake some form of activity such as a 30-minute brisk walk three times a week
- optimise sleep quality
- teach relaxation strategies
- promote use of massage and healing touch
- manage insomnia or hypersomnia with consistent naps/no late afternoon naps
- advise to avoid caffeine
- educate regarding good nutrition
                    (Faithfull 2003a, Donovan and Ward 2005, Madden and Newton 2006)

Of these, it is only really the role of exercise that is supported by a good body of evidence (Stricker et al. 2004). Whilst the benefits of exercise seem to be clear, the clinical issue is how to develop appropriate exercise programmes. Any such intervention needs to be tailored to an individual's specific disease and treatment characteristics and will preferably be home-based (Stricker et al. 2004).

Bowel toxicity

'About a week after starting the treatment I just started off with violent diarrhoea. In fact one day I was just in the kitchen and without any warning I just couldn't even get out in the hallway, it just come [sic] away from me.'

(Abayomi et al. 2005)

Bearing in mind the anatomical position of the cervix, it is not surprising that it is the intestinal sequelae which are amongst the most common acute and chronic side effects in patients undergoing radiation therapy (Perez et al. 1999).

Acute radiation enteritis (ARE) refers to inflammation of the lining of the small intestine as a result of radiotherapy. It is also sometimes called radiation colitis. Radiation proctitis refers to irritation of the rectum. Either or both may occur at any stage during the treatment period, resulting in diarrhoea which disappears on completion/within three months of treatment. Acute lower gastrointestinal tract toxicities may sometimes progress beyond three months post-therapy, becoming a chronic toxicity.

It is estimated that as many as 70% of patients undergoing pelvic radiotherapy experience ARE (Resbeut et al. 1997). Furthermore, approximately 20% of these patients will require

---

Box 4.6 Pharmacological management of radiation-induced diarrhoea

Codeine phosphate, loperamide: antidiarrhoeals which decrease gastric motility but can also cause dizziness and constipation.

Cholestyramine, colestipol hydrochloride: drugs that bind with bile acids. May be beneficial but generally considered unpalatable (Chary and Thompson 1984).

Sucralfate: forms a protective coating on the gastrointestinal mucosa (Henriksson et al. 1992) may have a role in the management of acute and chronic radiation-induced bowel toxicity.

Aspirin: anti-inflammatory drugs. Mixed data on whether or not effective (Faithfull 2003b). Would not be considered standard practice.

Octreotide: Somatostatin analogue. Multiple antidiarrhoeal actions including suppression of gastric acid secretion, reduction in motility and pancreatic exocrine function, increases water absorption along with electrolytes and nutrients (Solomon and Cherny 2006).

---

their radiotherapy to be interrupted, potentially compromising its overall efficacy (Faithfull 2003b). Diarrhoea may be associated with discomforting and embarrassing abdominal cramping and bloatedness, and proctitis may be so severe that it becomes haemorrhagic.

Radiotherapy is thought to cause a shortening and flattening of the villi so that there is a smaller surface area in the bowel for the absorption of fluid. The consequent malabsorption of bile salts, vitamin B12 and lactose contributes to the severity of gastrointestinal symptoms (Faithfull 2003b).

Management strategies generally begin with pharmacological interventions. A range of anti-diarrhoeal medications are available (see Box 4.6). These may be combined with other measures such as dietary manipulations.

A number of studies have attempted to assess the usefulness of different diets in ameliorating the gastrointestinal effects of radiotherapy. Because of the changes to the gastrointestinal tract described above, low fat and low lactose diets have both been found to have a beneficial effect on diarrhoea frequency and quality of life (Bye et al. 1992). Elemental diets have also been tested. These diets reduce food into its component parts which are then administered as supplements. It is a fairly radical approach to dietary therapy, sometimes employed with chronic gut disorders such as Crohn's disease. Compliance has been found to be low and calorie intake insufficient when used for patients undergoing pelvic radiotherapy (McGough et al. 2006).

Glutamine plays an important role in the support of mucosal growth and function and animal studies demonstrate that it protects both the upper and lower gastrointestinal tract from the effects of chemotherapy, radiotherapy and other causes of injury (Jensen et al. 1994). Kozelsky et al. (2003) conducted a phase III, randomised, double-blind study to determine the role of oral glutamine in the prevention of acute diarrhoea in patients undergoing pelvic radiation therapy but were unable to demonstrate any efficacy. However, the study group did not rule out the possibility that future trials might demonstrate a benefit for glutamine using a different dose, schedule, or formulation.

There is no clinical data to support the use of a low fibre diet for patients undergoing radiotherapy, which could lead to problems with constipation (Faithfull 2003b).

Skin: radiation-induced dermatitis

At one time, the level of radiation-induced skin reaction was used as a dose-determining parameter. Today, despite improvements resulting from the utilisation of linear accelerators, to some degree radiation skin reactions are inevitable – especially where there are skin folds (Wells and MacBride 2003).

Normal skin regeneration arises from the basal layer which lies between the dermis and the epidermis. Cells formed in the basal layer migrate upwards and are shed from the skin surface in the process of cell desquamation. Repopulation of the entire epidermis takes approximately four weeks (Wells and MacBride 2003).

Basal cell loss begins at doses of 20 to 25 Gy with low-grade damage (erythema or dry desquamation). Maximal skin depletion (moist desquamation/skin necrosis) arises when doses reach 50 Gy or above. For this reason most skin reactions will become apparent in the second and third weeks of radical treatment, peaking at the end, or within a week of its completion (Wells and MacBride 2003). The majority of acute skin reactions will have healed within four weeks of ceasing therapy (Rezvani et al. 1991).

As well as affecting the basal layer, radiation can also damage other structures within the skin causing:

(1) Dryness due to sweat and sebaceous gland destruction.
(2) Loss of elasticity due to skin atrophy and fibrosis.
(3) Erythema: transient erythema may occur within 24 hours of the first dose and is caused by dilation of the capillaries and increased vascular permeability. Erythema beyond this period is caused by erythrocyte and leukocyte extravasation within the dermis. Another common skin reaction is increased pigmentation caused by increased production of melanocytes – the body's attempt at protecting the basal layer from further damage (Wickline 2004).
(4) Hyperpigmentation, flaky and pruritic skin: usually seen after two to four weeks of treatment.
(5) Temporary (usually) hair loss: generally occurs after about three weeks of therapy (Wickline 2004).
(6) Telangiectasia: spidery red lines across the skin surface from fibrosis of the blood vessels.

Risks factors for skin toxicity may be either patient or treatment related (Wells and MacBride 2003). Patient factors include moist areas or skin folds within the radiation field, poor general health and skin condition and poor nutritional status. Treatment factors include high radiation dose and application of skin boluses.

Interventions

'Recommendations regarding the prevention and management of radiation dermatitis are diverse and rarely evidence-based.'

(Wickline 2003)

Dermatological interventions can be classified into two categories: preventative and therapeutic. Preventative measures include skin hygiene recommendations and application of topical agents. Once moist desquamation has occurred the situation changes and there is effectively an open wound – analogous to a second degree burn. Whilst some topical substances may still be recommended in this context, moist desquamation may be more appropriately managed by application of an appropriate dressing.

Skin hygiene

Patients are commonly advised to avoid use of products such as soap and talcum powder during therapy, although the data for this is equivocal. In the past it has been claimed that skin reactions could be induced or exacerbated by the application of perfumed products or substances containing metal which may be associated with 'radiation scatter'. This theoretical possibility has been questioned in the light of modern radiotherapy techniques (Lavery 1995) but in the absence of further data to guide practice, many centres chose to adhere to these recommendations.

Roy et al. (2001) randomised a group of breast cancer patients between washing their treatment area with soap or not washing it at all during therapy and found that there was no difference in treatment-related reactions. Similarly, Westbury et al. (2000) randomised patients receiving cranial irradiation between washing and not washing their hair during treatment and found no difference in toxicity between the two groups.

It is very difficult to find any good literature on the issue of vaginal douching during radiotherapy (White and Faithfull 2006). However, looking at the general literature on the subject, douching is not recommended and may carry negative health risks (Cottrell 2006).

Topical products

A number of topical preparations have been advocated as beneficial in either preventing or treating radiation reactions. For example, sucralfate is thought to stimulate cell growth by increasing the amounts of prostaglandin E and epidermal growth factor. It also has an anti-inflammatory effect (Wickline 2004). There is some limited data supporting its use as a topical agent in the prevention of radiation reactions.

A number of 'natural' therapies have also been put forward for the prevention (and sometimes management) of skin reactions, including aloe vera, almond oil, chamomile and vitamin C. There is currently no strong data regarding the efficacy of any of these products (Wickline 2004).

To treat radiation reactions a number of creams are commonly used in the clinical setting. For mild reactions moisturising agents such as aqueous cream are often recommended. With more severe reactions products such as hydrocortisone 1% may be useful, although they may also mask infection and should only be used with caution (Wells and MacBride 2003). There is no evidence to illustrate that steroid creams reduce progression to moist desquamation (Lavery 1995), and once again the data on their general efficacy appears to be mixed (Wells and MacBride 2003).

Gentian violet has traditionally been used for the management of radiation skin effects because of its antibacterial and antifungal properties, although by modern day wound-healing standards its tissue irritating effects make it an unlikely candidate for radiation-induced wounds. Gentian violet also stains clothing and skin (Mak et al. 2005). Furthermore, it has been found to be carcinogenic in some animal studies and for this reason has been withdrawn from clinical use in the UK (Lavery 1995).

Dressings

The optimal dressing to apply to ulcerated areas of radiation dermatitis is problematic. Since the 1960s a large body of data has advocated a warm, moist environment for the promotion of epithelialisation and wound-healing (Winter 1962, Alvarez 1983). The rationale for applying antiseptics to wounds in order to prevent infection has been questioned and is now believed to be ineffective – indeed detrimental – because it damages healthy, granulating tissue (Wilson et al. 2005). The use of transparent, hydrocolloid and hydrogel dressings promotes a warm, moist environment which is conducive to healing and thus may have a role in the treatment of radiation-induced dermatitis.

The College of Radiographers (2001) recommend the use of hydrocolloid dressings with light to moderately-exuding wounds and alignate sheets where there is heavy exudate. This will form a hydrophilic gel on contact with the wound, promoting the necessary moist environment. Simple (dry) dressings are not advocated because of the trauma resulting from changing them. Some centres employ the use of products used in the management of burns (e.g. silver-containing creams such as Flamazine) instead of hydrocolloid dressings.

In conclusion, a review of the literature on the management of radiotherapy skin reactions ultimately leaves more questions than it answers. This is particularly true of pelvic radiotherapy. The practicalities of applying dressings to difficult anatomical areas such as the groin has not been widely addressed. Furthermore these dressings will need to be removed prior to each radiotherapy treatment in order to avoid a bolus dose of radiation to the skin. This goes against the principle of hydrocolloid dressings which should preferably remain in situ for several days in order to promote optimal healing.

However, endeavours have been made to produce guidelines incorporating 'best practice' recommendations where research is deficient (National Health Service Scotland Quality Improvement Statement 2004). On the basis of the existing literature, a number of guarded statements have been made in order to guide practice:

- Patients can wash their perineum safely with mild, unperfumed soap and warm water during therapy. Friction to the area should be avoided by using a patting motion when drying and wearing loose clothing.
- Simple moisturiser can be used but perfumed skin products are probably best avoided because of a theoretical risk of causing or worsening skin toxicity.
- Talc may block sweat glands and hair follicles, resulting in worse reactions.
- Biafine, chamomile cream, almond ointment, topical vitamin C, gentian violet are not proven effective and should not be used.
- Transparent, hydrocolloid and hydrogel dressings can be beneficial, although the research supporting them only involved small sample sizes.
- Hydrogel dressings are the most pleasing dressings to patients because they are non-adherent, allow for atraumatic removal and are soothing when applied.
- Aloe vera has not been shown to provide major benefit, although one study reported it prolongs the time to skin damage at higher doses of RT. It appears to be a fairly benign product and probably does no harm (Wickline 2004)
- Sucralfate and corticosteroid creams are the most promising agents in prevention and treatment of radiation dermatitis (sucralfate cream is not currently commercially available in the UK).

(Wells and McBride 2003, Wickline 2004)

Urologenital complications

The close proximity of the bladder and urethral tissues to the cervix renders irradiation to these areas virtually unavoidable during pelvic radiotherapy. The incidence of acute bladder toxicity varies from 23% to 80% (Faithfull 2003c) and is the most common radiotherapy associated side effect in some series (Yalman et al. 2002).

Acute radiation induced cystitis results from damage to the rapidly dividing cells in the bladder mucosa. This causes inflammation, oedema, lymphocytic infiltration and degeneration of the epithelium. The sensitivity of the bladder lining increases, leading to pain and instability of the bladder muscles, reduced bladder capacity, increased frequency and dysuria. Further damage may lead to ulceration, submucosal petechiae, loss of protein into the urine and occasionally haematuria.

Radiation damage to the bladder occurs at doses of approximately 15 to 30 Gy, and therefore acute bladder symptoms tend to arise two or three weeks into treatment when these levels of radiation have been reached (Woodhouse 1990). On the whole it persists only for a short period of time, although occasionally acute radiation cystitis may become prolonged and develop into a late reaction, as discussed in the following section (Denton et al. 2003).

Pharmacological interventions are sometimes helpful, employing agents to alkalinise the urine, anticholinergic drugs and non-steroidal anti-inflammatories. A good fluid intake is also advocated and some centres recommend patients drink cranberry juice. Cranberries contain a substance that can prevent bacteria from sticking to the walls of the bladder and there is some evidence to suggest that regular consumption of cranberry juice may be helpful in preventing urinary tract infections (Jepson and Craig 2007).

Also significantly affected by both external beam radiotherapy and brachytherapy are the female reproductive organs. The ovaries have a very low radiation tolerance and therefore a premature menopause is inevitable if the ovaries have not been transposed prior to commencing radiotherapy. Ovarian transposition, fertility and menopause are discussed more fully in Chapter 7.

The vagina can also be the site of considerable toxicity. The acute toxicities are discomforting and include vaginal and vulval mucositis, pain and ulceration (Denton and Maher 2003). However, it is probably true to say that it is the chronic vaginal effects that have the most enduring impact on patient quality of life, as discussed in the following section.

Late radiotherapy toxicities

There remains a surprising dearth of literature regarding the long-term effects of radiotherapy, despite repeated calls in the literature for more information on the subject.

Late stage complications may appear at any time from a few months to 20 years or more after the completion of radiotherapy (Shibata et al. 1982 in Yamashita et al. 2006) and may not have any obvious correlation with acute toxicities (Kirwan et al. 2003).

The underlying pathology of late adverse effects is quite different from that seen with acute reactions. Whereas on the whole acute radiation injuries result from damage to the epithelial cells of the organ involved, late toxicities tend to arise from damage to deeper tissues and supporting structures such as blood vessels. These cells have a slow turnover rate; thus, although they sustain radiation damage at the time of treatment it is not expressed until cell division is attempted some time later.

Some of the late radiation-induced toxicities from pelvic radiotherapy are discussed below.

Vaginal stenosis

Vaginal stenosis is a narrowing of the vagina and occurs commonly post-pelvic radiotherapy – particularly brachytherapy. As with the other long-term radiation toxicities, it is associated with fibrosis, resulting in loss of elasticity and sensation in the vagina, vaginal shortening and telangiectasia (Denton and Maher 2003). In the worst cases the entire vagina is obliterated, making vaginal examination and sexual intercourse impossible (Brand et al. 2006).

Other radiotherapy-induced vaginal changes include:

- vaginal dryness
- atrophic vaginitis
- vaginal/vulval ulceration or necrosis
- shortened vaginal canal
- dyspareunia
- post-coital bleeding

(Denton and Maher 2003)

The incidence of vaginal stenosis amongst patients undergoing pelvic radiotherapy is unknown with widely divergent estimates reported in the literature (1.2% to 88% (Hartman and Diddle 1972, Eltabbakh et al. 1997). In some series it is the commonest late effect post-cervical radiotherapy (Yalman et al. 2002), yet in others it is barely mentioned. This disparity can partly be explained by patient population factors and partly by methodological differences. For example, the frequency of stenosis tends to be higher in prospective studies in which patients are specifically asked about it. Studies dependent on retrospective analysis of clinical notes are less likely to pick it up as a problem and consequently its incidence is likely to be underestimated (Brand et al. 2006).

Other factors which may influence incidence of vaginal stenosis include:

- dose and technique of RT
- effects of combined cancer treatments prior to and concurrent with RT
- stage of disease
- age (a statistically significant increase in the incidence of stenosis has been found with age greater than 50

- menopausal status
- sexual activity

(Brand et al. 2006, White and Faithfull 2006)

The average length of time it takes to develop vaginal stenosis also varies widely between studies. Brand et al. (2006) found it to begin a median of 7.5 months after completion of treatment, whereas other studies have cited much earlier development – as early as three months (Hartman and Diddle 1972).

The mainstay of therapy rests with prevention. This is principally achieved through regular vaginal dilation which serves to break down any developing adhesions. One way of achieving this is through regular sexual intercourse, although intercourse alone may not be adequate as the sole means of prophylaxis. In one study, 57% of women developed stenosis one year after completing brachytherapy despite the fact that they were sexually active (Decruze et al. 1999). Most commentators now agree that the best prevention strategy is to prescribe vaginal dilators to women undergoing pelvic irradiation, although this has never been tested in the context of a randomised, controlled study. It is generally considered that such a trial would be unethical because the benefits of vaginal dilation appear to be clear (Decruze et al. 1999, Denton and Maher 2003).

Although there is overall agreement regarding the appropriateness of vaginal dilation, the optimal regimen to use remains the subject of some debate. Recent questionnaire studies in Australia and the UK show that there is no clear consensus on such issues as:

- when to commence vaginal dilation
- how frequently to perform it
- how long women should insert dilators for each time
- how long vaginal dilation should be continued

(Lancaster 2004, White and Faithfull 2006)

Another problem with the prescription of vaginal dilators is that of compliance. This has been found to be low in a number of studies. Several factors have been postulated which might have a negative effect on compliance. These include:

- inadequate information regarding the importance of vaginal dilatation
- anxiety
- fear of damaging vagina or spreading cancer
- modesty
- association with masturbation

(Lancaster 2004)

Many centres employ specialist nurses to teach patients about this delicate aspect of their care and it has been suggested that such an approach is helpful in improving uptake (Lancaster 2004).

Other methods of managing vaginal stenosis were recently evaluated in a Cochrane review by Denton and Maher (2003). These include the application of ointments (e.g. topical oestrogens, benzydamine) and the utilisation of novel therapies such as hyperbaric oxygen. Whilst data exists suggesting a role for such strategies, the general conclusion of the authors was that the quantity and quality of research evidence was not adequate to support their widespread implementation.

Chronic radiation cystitis

Delayed radiation toxicity of the bladder develops in a small but significant proportion of the treated population, with frequencies quoted in the region of 5% to 10% depending on the series, grading system and the method of calculation that have been used (Denton et al. 2003). The period of time after completion of radiotherapy at which late bladder toxicity occurs is extremely variable, ranging from a minimum of three months to three years or more (Denton et al. 2003).

Radiation associated damage to the bladder wall and vasculature results in the bladder submucosa becoming increasingly hypovascular, hypocellular and hypoxic. Ongoing fibrosis leads to reduced bladder capacity and telangiectasia. On cystoscopy these changes are characterised by patchy, bleeding ulcers and fistula formation is a further risk.

The clinical manifestations of late radiation cystitis are urinary frequency, urgency, dysuria, haematuria, sphincter dysfunction and reduced bladder capacity. A vicious cycle of bleeding, clot retention and obstructive uropathy may arise, eventually culminating in sepsis and renal failure (Denton et al. 2003).

Management strategies can be either surgical or pharmacological. Surgical management begins with diathermy to the bleeding points and ends with ileal diversion. However, because radiation-damaged tissues have a reduced capacity to replace normal collagen and cellular loss, they have a tendency to break down after surgery. For this reason surgical intervention is often not recommended on heavily irradiated tissue.

Non-surgical intervention may incorporate intravesical instillation of agents (e.g. alum or formalin) or may employ systemic therapies. Some agents are thought to enhance the integrity of the bladder either by correcting the epithelial breakdown or reducing vascular fragility (e.g. D-glucosamine, oestrogens) (Denton et al. 2003). Other treatments aim to reverse the radiation changes (e.g. superoxide dismutase, pentoxyfilline, hyperbaric oxygen – see also Box 4.7). Unfortunately, the data supporting each treatment strategy is poor. In a recent Cochrane review of the evidence on the management of late bladder toxicities it was concluded that the clinical trials to date did not include large enough numbers to draw any useful conclusions for practice and that there is a need for further studies (Denton et al. 2003).

Box 4.7 Hyperbaric oxygen

Hyperbaric oxygen therapy (HBOT) is a treatment modality occasionally employed for delayed radiation injuries. It involves high dose oxygen delivery to the patient in an environment in which the atmospheric pressure is two to three times that at sea level. This causes transient increases in tissue oxygen concentration resulting in fibroblast proliferation, collagen synthesis and vascular capillary formation. HBOT is thought to improve tissue quality, promote healing and prevent breakdown of irradiated tissue fields (Bennett et al. 2005). Typically, treatments involve pressurisation for periods between 60 and 120 minutes once or twice a day for a total of 30 to 60 sessions.

Although serious adverse events are rare, HBOT cannot be regarded as an entirely benign intervention (Bennett et al. 2005) and is potentially associated with a number of side effects including damage to the ears, sinuses and lungs, temporary worsening of short sightedness, claustrophobia and oxygen poisoning. In a recent Cochrane review HBOT was shown to have potential efficacy in the treatment of late radiation induced tissue injury to the head, neck and bowel, but it was felt that there was insufficient data confirming its use in other tissues (Bennett et al. 2005).

There have been several studies looking at the efficacy of employing HBOT for the repair of tissue injury following pelvic radiotherapy. For example, Neheman et al. (2005) found it to be an effective treatment option for patients with radiation induced haemorrhagic cystitis. They found that the procedure was well tolerated even in patients debilitated by advanced cancer and blood loss.

Fink et al. (2006) looked at the effect of HBOT on 14 patients who had received pelvic radiotherapy for cervical cancer at a centre in Australia. Patients were suffering from a range of long-term toxicities, including radiation cystitis, proctitis, vaginitis and vaginal vault ulceration. Ten patients healed or showed an improvement of more than 50%, resulting in an overall success rate of 71%. Fink et al. (2006) concluded that 'HBOT should be considered for patients with delayed radiation injuries not responding to other treatments.'

Chronic radiation enteritis (CRE)

Chronic radiation enteritis generally becomes manifest 6–12 months after completion of treatment, although it may also appear much later. The incidence of CRE reported in medical literature varies from 5% to 15% (Waddell et al. 1999). Incomplete repair of the gut mucosa, coupled with hyperplasia of the blood vessels, results in a thin, friable mucosal epithelium. Over time the gut walls become increasingly fibrotic leading to strictures, ulceration and necrosis. Microscopically marked changes are observed in the submucosa of the intestine characterised by atypical fibroblasts and collagen proliferation, alterations in the endothelial layer and occlusive vasculitis (Gavazzi et al. 2006). Diagnosis may be complicated by the fact that there is no real, definitive test for CRE.

Patients generally present with abdominal pain, the pattern of which can vary. Altered bowel function is also common and may be accompanied by tenesmus, bleeding and rectal strictures. Late bowel ulceration is often focal in nature, resulting in loss of specific sections of bowel, leading to perforation or fistula formation (Khoo 2003a) (see also Box 4.8).

Risk factors for CRE include:

- high total radiation dose: retrospective studies indicate severe complications occur in 5–15% patients treated with 40–45 Gray in five weeks
- high dose per fraction
- large volume of intestine irradiated
- previous abdominal surgery
- malnutrition
- diabetes mellitus
- hypertension
- vasculitis

(Bye et al. 1992, Abayomi et al. 2005, Gavazzi et al. 2006).

Management of CRE

There is a disappointingly meagre literature on the subject of management despite the fact that post-radiotherapy bowel toxicity is a significant problem (Andreyev 2005). Avoidance is the best strategy, but this is difficult if comprehensive pelvic treatment is to be ensured. Some centres treat patients in a prone position with a 'belly board' in order to keep the bowel out of the radiation field. The board has a hole where the bowel lies so that the

---

Box 4.8 CRE and bowel perforation

In extreme cases, CRE may result in perforation and/or obstruction of the bowel. The cause of the perforation is not fully understood but could be the result of a hot spot (high dose) in the irradiated bowel. Yamashita et al. (2006) looked at this issue in a retrospective study in Japan involving 95 Japanese women with cervical cancer. Of these women, 7% were diagnosed with small bowel perforation.

The time from radiotherapy to sigmoid perforation has been cited as 13 months (range, 3–98 months) and from the onset of gastrointestinal symptoms to perforation 90 days (Ramirez et al. 2001). Other studies have reported cases of acute perforation with a latency period of 14 years (Sher and Bauer 1990, Rao et al. 1996).

The presenting complaints of patients with bowel perforation following radiotherapy can be varied and unpredictable. The majority of patients will show no evidence of acute peritonitis on physical examination (Ramirez 2001). Whilst abdominal pain was seen in all of Yamashita's patients, only 14% of them described it as severe. Yamashita et al. (2006) concluded that a high degree of suspicion remains a priority in the care of irradiated patients who present with abdominal pain given the atypical presentation of perforation in this group.

Box 4.9 Smoking and radiation toxicity

Eifel et al. (2002) examined the records of 3489 patients treated with radiation therapy for stage I or II carcinoma of the cervix, in order to gain information about late complications. Major late complications were defined as any problems occurring or persisting for more than three months after treatment which required hospitalisation, transfusion, an operation, or caused severe symptoms including death.

Interestingly, heavy smoking was found to be the strongest predictor of overall complications. The most striking influence of smoking was on small bowel complications; even women who smoked less than one pack per day had a significantly increased risk. The risk was dose-related, with the incidence of small bowel complications increasing by more than five-fold for the heaviest smokers. Heavy smokers also had significantly increased risks of bladder and rectal complications. The increased incidence of gastrointestinal complications amongst smokers could suggest a synergistic effect of smoking and radiation on normal tissue which seems to be independent of other conditions (Eifel et al. 2002).

---

abdominal organs can 'fall through' by gravity. Other centres treat patients with a full bladder which similarly 'pushes' the bowel out of the way.

Surgery may be necessary in cases of CRE where there is identifiable mechanical obstruction, although often surgeons are reluctant to operate on these patients because of the irradiated tissue. Where proctitis or anal discomfort is a problem, steroid suppositories may be prescribed along with topical anaesthetics and regular systemic analgaesia. Rectal anti-inflammatories, sucralfate and metronidazole may also have a role, and selective laser treatment, electrocautery and silver nitrate or formalin rectal installations have been used for persistent bleeding (Khoo 2003b). Parenteral nutrition may be required in cases where nutritional intake is compromised (Gavazzi et al. 2006).

Pelvic fractures

Osteoradionecrosis may occur in any bone which is irradiated beyond its tolerance. Large doses of radiation lead to a reduced number of bone cells, resulting in enlarged, empty bone spaces or lacunae, together with fatty degeneration and hypocellularity of the bone. Radiation may also affect the bone microvasculature, decreasing its blood supply and thus causing hypoxia. These effects are exacerbated by other factors such as osteoporosis and steroid use (Khoo 2003b).

Pelvic radiotherapy appears to increase the risk of bone fractures. Baxter (2005) looked at 6428 women with anal, cervical or rectal cancer who had received pelvic radiotherapy. The incidence of pelvic fractures was 11% for those in the irradiated group versus 7% in the non-irradiated group. Many of the fractures were thought to be pelvic insufficiency fractures – hairline fractures resulting from radiation-induced weakening of pelvic bone, occurring because the pelvis was unable to support body weight (Small and Kachnic 2005).

Another study of post-menopausal women who received radiation therapy for advanced cervical cancer indicated the pelvic insufficiency fracture rate was 17% (Ogino et al. 2003). Insufficiency fractures can be asymptomatic or associated with pain. The majority of symptoms improve with conservative measures (Small and Kachnic 2005).

Second malignancies

Whereas the incidence of radiation-induced second malignancies is fairly well documented in diseases like lymphoma, information about second malignancies following pelvic radiotherapy is a little more difficult to come by. One Scottish study (Macara et al. 1998) did find an increased risk of malignancy amongst a cohort of women who had received pelvic irradiation, but interestingly this was not within the irradiated field. Instead, they found a significant increase in lung and pleural cancers, indicating that women treated for cervical cancer in the West of Scotland are at more risk of a subsequent cancer due to causes other than the late effects of radiotherapy.

Nevertheless, there is a theoretical risk of other malignancies as a long-term toxicity due to radiation (and chemotherapy) damage. Patients undergoing brachytherapy for prostate cancer, for example, have been shown to have a slightly higher incidence of bladder and colorectal cancers (Liauw et al. 2006).

Radiotherapy and quality of life

'It has stopped me going out. I've got a friend who usually picks me up and takes me shopping but I don't go anywhere . . . I've got a sister who lives around the corner. I don't go there as well . . . I haven't seen her for months and she only lives around the corner.'

(Frances, aged 54, in Abayoumi 2005)

The impact of a symptom on the patient's quality of life is significantly influenced by their individual perception of that symptom. Thus, the level of distress caused by a symptom depends on the individual experience of that symptom and the patient's beliefs about what it means. 'Symptom distress . . . represents an intricate interaction of physical, social and emotional forces and not merely a level of symptom severity' (Faithfull 2003d, p.100).

Fellowes et al. (2001) found that it was insufficient to wait for women to volunteer information about symptoms and side effects after treatment. It appears that patients need to be asked directly about specific symptoms because they themselves feel unclear about what 'counts' as a side effect and whether or not it is worth mentioning.

The impact of radiation therapy on quality of life and general functioning is different in the 'acute' and 'chronic' phases of treatment. Nail et al. (1986) looked at some of the acute effects in a sample of women with gynaecological cancers undergoing radiotherapy. The study examined the level of toxicity, quality of life and functional disruption caused by the treatment. Health related quality of life was thought to be worst during the treatment period, with high scores for diarrhoea, fatigue, nausea and anorexia. The severity of these symptoms was greatest during the third and last treatment weeks. Functional disruption (e.g. sleeping, mobility, eating) was greatest during the last week of treatment but progressively fell by three months follow-up.

The impact of long-term toxicities on quality of life is an even greater problem and is an important survivorship issue for many women who have undergone successful treatment for cervix cancer. Long-term bowel toxicity appears to be particularly debilitating. It has been suggested that as many as one in five women experience faecal incontinence after radiotherapy which affects their quality of life (Andreyev 2005).

Abayomi et al. (2005) performed a small, qualitative study exploring the impact of radiation-induced enteritis on quality of life amongst a cohort of women with cervical cancer. Not surprisingly, acute enteritis had a negative impact on quality of life during the treatment period. However, in the longer term, chronic enteritis was equally incapacitating, affecting women some 6 to 24 months after termination of treatment. Of the ten women interviewed a number described varying degrees of social withdrawal because of this: 'Well it's affected it dramatically because I don't see anyone and then if I am sitting here on me own and I hear the door I don't answer it, if I feel bad I won't answer it. I pretend I'm not in' (Julia, aged 41).

Bye et al. (2000) also assessed the influence of long-term toxicities three to four years after treatment amongst a cohort of women who had been treated for carcinoma of the endometrium and cervix. Once again, bowel toxicity was a significant problem for a large number of women – although it was not necessarily associated with increased emotional distress or a deterioration in their health related quality of life. It was only amongst the women who complained of *substantial* diarrhoea that impaired social functioning and reduced quality of life was an issue.

The other side effect that was reported in approximately 20% of women was pain in the lower back, hips and thighs. This was possibly related to radiation damage to the pelvic bones although it is also, as pointed out by the authors, a common complaint amongst the general population. In conclusion, when compared with the general population, the radiotherapy patients had more diarrhoea but less fatigue, less pain and similar social functioning. It was concluded that in general the health-related QOL of women after radiotherapy did not differ substantially from that of the normal population (Bye et al. 2000).

To conclude, there appears to be some divergence in the literature regarding the long-term QOL of women who have had treatment for cervix cancer. Some studies report high levels of psychological distress and others contradict this and report generally favourable adaptation after treatment (Bye et al. 2000). To some degree these differences can be explained by methodological and population differences. They could also be the result of 'response shift' – a redefinition of QOL values as a result of time and experiences.

Conclusion

It can be seen that radiotherapy is an essential component in the treatment of many women with cervical cancer. It is a therapy which has been dramatically improved in recent decades by the addition of concurrent chemotherapy, and it is one in which innovations continue to be made. However, improvements in survival are not without a cost. In this case the principal cost is the toxicities – particularly the long-term toxicities – which continue to impact women long after their cancer has been eradicated. The control and management of such toxicities provides the challenge for future decades of radiotherapy treatment.

Frequently asked questions

(1) Can I have sex during radiotherapy?
    Yes, but it is important to avoid pregnancy and infection during cancer treatment.
(2) Am I still 'radioactive' after I go home during my EBRT? Will I pass radiotherapy to my family?
    No, you are not radioactive and pose no risk to family and friends.
(3) Should I douche during radiotherapy?
    The role of douching is unclear at this time but it is not generally recommended (Cottrell 2006).
(4) Will I lose my hair?
    It is possible that you may lose your pubic hair during treatment but this will usually (although not always) grow back.
(5) Should I eat a special diet during treatment?
    A diet low in fat and lactose (milk products) is recommended. Bland foods are generally preferred whilst nauseated or experiencing diarrhoea.

Resources

Cancer Research UK: http://www.cancerhelp.org.uk/help/default.asp?page=2778
International Gynaecologic Cancer Society: http://www.igcs.com.au/pil/CervicalCancer.htm
Cancer Bacup: http://www.cancerbackup.org.uk/Cancertype/Cervix/Treatment/Radiotherapy

References

Abayomi J, Kirwan J, Hackett A and Bagnall G (2005) A study to investigate women's experiences of radiation enteritis following radiotherapy for cervical cancer. *J Hum Nutr Diet*, 18 (5), 353–363

Adamson D (2003) The radiobiological basis of radiation side effects, in Faithfull S and Wells M (eds) *Supportive Care in Radiotherapy*. Churchill Livingstone, Edinburgh, UK. pp. 71–95

Ahamed A and Jhingran A (2004) New radiation techniques in gynaecological cancer, *Int J Gynaecolog Cancer*, 14 (4), 569–579

Ahlberg K, Ekman T and Gaston-Johansson F (2005) Fatigue, psychological distress, coping resources, and functional status during radiotherapy for uterine cancer. *Oncology Nursing Forum*, 32 (3), 633–640

Alvarez OM, Mertz PM and Eaglestein WH (1983) The effect of occlusive dressings on collagen synthesis and re-epithelialization in superficial wounds. *J Surg Res*, 35, 142–148

Andersen B, Karlsson J, Andersen B and Tewfik H (1984) Anxiety and cancer treatment: response to stressful radiotherapy. *Health Psychology*, 3 (6), 535–551

Andersen C and Adamsen L (2001) Continuous video recording: a new clinical research tool for studying the nursing care of cancer patients. *Journal of Advanced Nursing*, 35 (2), 257–267

Andreyev J (2005) Gastrointestinal complications of pelvic radiotherapy: are they of any importance? *Gut*, 54, 1051–1054

Barillot I, Horiot JC, Pigneux J, et al. (1997) Carcinoma of the intact uterine cervix treated with radiotherapy alone: a French cooperative study: update and multivariate analysis of prognostics factors. *Int J Radiat Oncol Biol Phys*, 38, 969–978

Baxter N, Habermann EB, Tepper JE, et al. (2005) Risk of pelvic fractures in older women following pelvic irradiation. *JAMA*, 294 (20), 2587–2593

Bennett MH, Feldmeier J, Hampson N, Smee R and Milross C (2005) Hyperbaric oxygen therapy for late radiation tissue injury. *Cochrane Database of Systematic Reviews*, (3), CD005005

Brand AH, Bull CA and Cakir B (2006) Vaginal stenosis in patients treated with radiotherapy for carcinoma of the cervix. *Int J Gynaecol Cancer*, 16, 288–293

Brandt B (1991) Informational needs and selected variables in patients receiving brachytherapy. *Oncology Nursing Forum*, 18 (7), 1221–1229

Bye A, Kassa S, Ose T, Sundfør K and Tropé C (1992) The influence of low fat, low lactose diets on diarrhoea during pelvic radiotherapy. *Clin Nutr*, 11, 147–153

Bye A, Trope C, Loge JH, Hjermstad M and Kaasa S (2000) Health related quality of life and occurrence of intestinal side effects after pelvic radiotherapy. *Acta Oncologica*, 39 (2), 173–180

Cannistra SA and Niloff JM (1996) Cancer of the uterine cervix. *The New England Journal of Medicine*, 334 (16), 1030–1038

Chary S and Thompson D (1984) A clinical trial evaluating cholestyramine to prevent diarrhoea in patients maintained on low fat diets during pelvic radiation therapy. *International Journal of Radiation Oncology, Biology, Physics*, 10, 1885–1890

Christman NJ and Cain LB (2003) The effects of concrete, objective information and relaxation on maintaining usual activity during radiation therapy. *Oncology Nursing Forum*, 31 (2), E39–E45

Coia L, Won M, Lanciano R, Marcial VA, Martz K and Hanks G (1990) The patterns of care outcome study for cancer of the uterine cervix: results of the second national practice survey. *Cancer*, 66, 2451–2456

College of Radiographers (2001) *Summary of Intervention for Acute, Radiotherapy-induced Skin Reactions in Cancer Patients: a Clinical Guideline*. College of Radiographers, London

Cottrell BH (2006) Discussing the health risks of douching. *AWHONN Lifelines*, 10 (2), 130–136

Coulter A, Entwistle V and Gilbert D (1999) Sharing decisions with patients: is the information good enough? *British Medical Journal*, 318, 318–322

Crownover RL, Wilkinson DA and Weinhous MS (19990 The radiobiology and physics of brachytherapy. *Hematology – Oncology Clinics of North America*, 13 (3), June, 477–487

Dargent D, Lamblin G, Romenstaing P, Montbarbon X, Mathevet P and Benchaib M (2005) Effect of radiotherapy on pelvic lymph node metastasis in cervical cancer stages IB2–IVA: a retrospective analysis of two comparative series, 15 (3), May/June, 468–474

Datta NR (2005) From 'points' to 'profiles', in Intracavity brachytherapy of cervical cancer. *Curr Opin Obstet Gynaecol*, 17 (1), 35–40

Decruze SB, Guthrie D and Magnani R (1999) Prevention of vaginal stenosis in patients following vaginal brachytherapy. *Clinical Oncology (Royal College of Radiologists)*, 11 (1), 46–48

Denton A, Bond S, Matthews S, et al. (2000) National audit of the management and outcomes of carcinoma of the cervix treated with radiotherapy in 1993. *Clinical Oncology*, 12, 347–353

Denton AS and Maher EJ (2003) Interventions for the physical aspects of sexual dysfunction in women following pelvic radiotherapy. *Cochrane Database of Systematic Reviews 2003*, Issue 1. Art no: CD003750. DOI:10.1002/14651858.CD003750

Denton AS, Clarke NW and Maher E J (2003) Non-surgical interventions for late radiation cystitis in patients who have received radical radiotherapy to the pelvis. *Cochrane Systematic Review*, Volume 4

Donovan HS and Ward S (2005) Representations of fatigue in women receiving chemotherapy for gynaecologic cancers. *Oncology Nursing Forum*, 32 (1), 113–116

Eifel P, Jhingran A, Bodurka DC, Levenback C and Thames H (2002) Correlation of smoking history with major complications of pelvic radiation therapy for cervical cancer. *Journal of Clinical Oncology*, 20 (17), Sept, 3651–3657

Eifel PJ, Berek JS and Thigpen JT (1997) Gynecologic Cancers. Section 2. Cancer of the cervix, vagina, vulva, in DeVita VT, Jr, Hellman S and Rosenberg SA (eds). *Cancer: Principles & Practice of Oncology*, fifth edition. Lippincott-Raven, Philadelphia. pp. 1427–1478

Einhorn N, Trope C, Ridderheim M, Boman K, Sorbe B and Cavallin-Stahl E (2003) A systematic overview of radiation therapy effects in cervical cancer. *Acta Oncologica*, 42 (5/6), 546–556

Eltabbakh GH, Piver MS, Hempling RE, et al. (1997) Excellent long term survival and absence of vaginal recurrences in 332 patients with low risk stage I endometrial adenocarcinoma treated with hysterectomy and vaginal brachytherapy without formal lymph node sampling: report of a prospective trial. *Int Jnl Radiath Oncol Biol Phys*, 38, 373–380

Faithfull S (2003a) Fatigue and radiotherapy, in Faithfull S and Wells M (eds) *Supportive Care in Radiotherapy*. Churchill Livingstone, Edinburgh. pp. 118–134

Faithfull S (2003b) Gastrointestinal effects of radiotherapy, in Faithfull S and Wells M (eds) *Supportive Care in Radiotherapy*. Churchill Livingstone, Edinburgh. pp. 247–267

Faithfull S (2003c) Urinary symptoms and radiotherapy, in Faithfull S and Wells M (eds) *Supportive Care in Radiotherapy*. Churchill Livingstone, Edinburgh. pp. 227–246

Faithfull S (2003d) Assessing the impact of radiotherapy, in Faithfull S and Wells M (eds) *Supportive Care in Radiotherapy*. Churchill Livingstone, Edinburgh. pp. 96–113

Faithfull S and Wells M (eds) (2003) *Supportive Care in Radiotherapy*. Churchill Livingstone, Edinburgh

Fellowes D, Fallowfield L, Saunders C, et al. (2001) Tolerability of hormone therapies for breast cancer; how informative are documented symptom profiles in medical notes for 'well-tolerated' treatments? *Breast Cancer Research Treatment*, 66, 73–81

Fieler VK, Wlasowicz GS, Mitchell ML, et al. (1996) Information preferences of patients undergoing radiation therapy. *Oncology Nursing Forum*, 23 (10), 1603–1608

Fink D, Chetty N, Lehm JP, Marsden DE and Hacker NF (2006) Hyperbaric oxygen therapy for delayed radiation injuries in gynaecological cancers. *Int J Gynaecol Cancer*, 16 (2), Mar/Apr, 638–642

Fyles A, Keane TJ, Barton M and Simm J (1992) The effect of treatment duration in the local control of cervix cancer. *Radiother Oncol*, 25, 273–279

Fyles AW, Milosevic M, Pintilie M, Syed A and Hill RP (2000) Anemia, hypoxia and transfusion in patients with cervix cancer: a review. *Radiotherapy & Oncology*, 57 (1), 13–19

Gavazzi C, Bhoori S, LoVullo S, Cozzi G and Mariani L (2006) Role of home parenteral nutrition in chronic radiation enteritis. *American Journal of Gastroenterology*, 101 (2), 374–379

Gosselin TK and Waring JS (2001) Nursing management of patients receiving brachytherapy for gynaecologic malignancies. *Clinical Journal of Oncology Nursing*, 5 (2), 59–63

Greene J, Kirwan J, Tierney J, et al. (2005) Concomitant chemotherapy and radiotherapy. *Cochrane Review*, 3

Grigsby P and Herzog J (2001) Current management of patients with invasive cervical carcinoma. *Clin Obstet Gynaecol*, 44 (3), 531–537

Grogan M, Thomas GM, Melamed I, et al. (1999) The importance of hemoglobin levels during radiotherapy for carcinoma of the cervix. *Cancer*, 86, 1528–1536

Hanks GE, Herring DF and Kramer S (1983) Patterns of care outcome studies: results of the National Practice in Cancer of the Cervix. *Cancer*, 51, 959–967

Hartman P and Diddle AW (1972) Vaginal stenosis following irradiation therapy for carcinoma of the cervix uteri. *Cancer*, 30, 426–429

Henriksson R, Franzen I and Littbrand B (1992) Effects of sucralfate on acute and late bowel discomfort following radiotherapy of pelvic cancer. *Journal of Clinical Oncology*, 10, 969–975

Jain G, Scolapio J, Wasserman E and Floch M (2002) Chronic radiation enteritis: a ten year follow-up. *Journal of Clinical Gastroenterology*, 35 (3), Sept, 214–217

Jensen JC, Schaefer R, Nwokedi E, et al. (1994) Prevention of chronic radiation enteropathy by dietary glutamine. *Ann Surg Oncol*, 1, 157–163

Jepson RG and Craig JC (2007) Cranberries for preventing urinary tract infections. *Cochrane Database of Systematic Reviews*. Issue 3. Art. No.: CD001321. DOI: 10.1002/14651858.CD001321. pub4

Jones R, Pearson J, McGregor S, et al. (1999) Randomised trial of personalised computer-based information for cancer patients. *BMJ*, 319, 1241–1247

Kapp KS, Stuecklschweiger GF, Kapp DS, et al. (1998) Prognostic factors in patients with carcinoma of the uterine cervix treated with external beam irradiation and IR-192 high-dose-rate brachytherapy. *Int J Radiat Oncol Biol Phys*, 42, 531–540

Keys HM, Bundy BN, Stehman FB, et al. (1999) Cisplatin, radiation, and adjuvant hysterectomy compared with radiation and adjuvant hysterectomy for bulky stage IB cervical carcinoma. *N Engl J Med*, 340, 1154–1161

Khoo V (2003a) Other Late Effects, in Faithfull S and Wells M (eds) *Supportive Care in Radiotherapy*. Churchill Livingstone, Edinburgh. pp. 348–371

Khoo V (2003b) Late toxicity: bone problems, in Faithfull S and Wells M (eds) *Supportive Care in Radiotherapy*. Churchill Livingstone, Edinburgh. pp. 337–347

Kirwan JM, Symonds P, Green JA, Tierney J, Collingwood M and Williams CJ (2003) A systematic review of acute and late toxicity of concomitant chemoradiation for cervical cancer. *Radiotherapy and Oncology*, 68, 217–226

Kozelsky TF, Meyers GE, Sloan JA, et al. (2003) Phase III double-blind study of glutamine versus placebo for the prevention of acute diarrhoea in patients receiving pelvic radiation therapy. *Journal of Clinical Oncology*, 21 (9), May, 1669–1674

Lancaster L (2004) Preventing vaginal stenosis after brachytherapy for gynaecological cancer: an overview of Australian practices. *European Journal of Oncology Nursing*, 8 (1), March, 30–39

Landoni F, Maneo A, Colombo A, et al. (1997) Randomised study of radical surgery versus radiotherapy for stage IB–IIA cervical cancer. *Lancet*, 350 (9077), 23 August, 535–540

Landoni F, Maneo A, Cormio G, et al. (2001) Class II versus class III radical hysterectomy in stage IB–IIA cervical cancer: a prospective randomized study. *Gynecol Oncol*, 80, 3–12

Lavery BA (1995) Skin care during radiotherapy; a survey of UK practice. *Clinical Oncology* (Royal College of Radiologists), 7, 187–187

Lehman M and Thomas G (2001) Is concurrent chemotherapy and radiotherapy the new standard of care for locally advanced cervix cancer. *Int J Gynaecol Cancer*, 11 (2), March/April, 87–99

Liauw SL, Sylvester JE, Morris CG, Blasko JC and Grimm PD (2006) Second malignancies after prostate brachytherapy: incidence of bladder and colorectal cancers in patients with 15 years of potential follow-up. *International Journal of Radiation Oncology, Biology, Physics*, 66 (3), 669–673

Logsdon MD and Eifel PJ (1999) FIGO IIIB Squamous cell carcinoma of the cervix; an analysis of prognostic factors emphasizing the balance between external beam and intracavitary radiation therapy. *Int J Radiat Oncol Biol Phys*, 43, 763–775

Loizzi V, Cormio G, Loverro G, Selvaggi L, Disaia PJ and Cappucini F (2003) Chemoradiation: a new approach for the treatment of cervical cancer. *Int J Gynaecol Cancer*, 13 (5), 580–586

Macara LM, Lamont D and Symonds RP (1998) Second malignancies in cervical cancer patients in the west of Scotland. *Scottish Medical Journal*, 43 (1), 16–18

McGough C, Baldwin C, Norman A, et al. (2006) Is supplementation with elemental diet feasible in patients undergoing pelvic radiotherapy? *Clinical Nutrition*, 25 (1), 109–116

Madden J and Newton S (2006) Why am I so tired all the time? Understanding cancer-related fatigue. *Clinical Journal of Oncology Nursing*, 10 (5), 659–661

Magnan MA and Mood DW (2003) The effects of health state, haemoglobin, global symptom distress, mood disturbance and treatment site on fatigue onset, duration and distress in patients receiving radiation therapy. *Oncology Nursing Forum*, 30 (2), E33–E39

Mak SS, Zee CY, Molassiotis A, et al. (2005) A comparison of wound treatments in nasopharyngeal cancer patients receiving radiation therapy. *Cancer Nursing*, 28 (6), 436–545

Mock V (2003) Clinical excellence through evidence-based practice: fatigue management as a model. *Oncology Nursing Forum*, 30 (5), 787–796

Mock V, Atkinson A, Barsevick A, et al. (2003) Clinical practice guidelines in oncology: cancer-related fatigue. Version 1. *Journal of the National Comprehensive Cancer Network*, 1, 308–331

Morris M, Eifel PJ, Lu J, et al. (1999) Pelvic radiation with concurrent chemotherapy compared with pelvic and para-aortic radiation for high-risk cervical cancer. *N Engl J Med*, 340, 1137–43

Munstedt K, Johnson P, Bohlmann MK, Zygmunt M, Von Georgi R and Vahrson H (2005) Adjuvant radiotherapy in carcinomas of the uterine cervix: the prognostic value of haemoglobin levels. *Int J Gynaecol Cancer*, 15 (2), 285–291

Munroe AJ (2003) Challenges in radiotherapy today, in Faithfull S and Wells M (eds) *Supportive Care in Radiotherapy*. Churchill Livingstone, Edinburgh. pp. 17–38

Nail LM, King KB and Johnson JE (1986) Coping with radiation treatment for gynecologic cancer: mood and disruption in usual function. *J Psychosom Obstet Gynaecol*, 5, 271–281

National Cancer Institute (NCI) Common Terminology Criteria: http://ctep.cancer.gov/forms/CTCAEv3.pdf (accessed 18/6/2008)

National Cancer Institute (NCI) (1999) *Concurrent Chemoradiation for Cervical Cancer*. Clinical announcement. February. National Cancer Institute, Bethesda MD

National Cancer Institute (NCI) (2006) http://www.cancer.gov/cancertopics/pdq/treatment/cervical/HealthProfessional/page4

National Health Service Scotland Quality Improvement Statement (NHSQIS) (2004) *Skincare of Patients Receiving Radiotherapy. Best Practice Statement NHS Scotland*: www.nhshealthquality.org (accessed 20/7/07)

Neheman A, Nativ O, Moskovitz B, Melamed Y and Stein A (2005) Hyperbaric oxygen therapy for radiation-induced haemorrhagic cystitis. *BJU*, 96 (1), 107–109

Ogino I, Okamoto N, Yoshimi O, Kitamura T and Nakayama H (2003) Pelvic insufficiency fractures in postmenopausal woman with advanced cervical cancer treated by radiotherapy. *Radiother Oncol*, 68, 61–67

Pearcey R, Brundage M, Drouin P, et al. (2002) Phase III trial comparing radical radiotherapy with and without cisplatin chemotherapy in patients with advanced squamous cell cancer of the cervix. *J Clin Oncol*, 20, 966–972

Perez CA, Grigsby PW, Castro Vita H and Lockett MA (1995) Carcinoma of the uterine cervix. I. Impact of prolongation of treatment time and timing of brachytherapy on outcome of radiation therapy. *International Journal of Radiation Oncology, Biology, Physics*, 32, 1275–1288

Perez CA, Grigsby PW, Lockett MA, et al. (1999) Radiation therapy morbidity in carcinoma of the uterine cervix: dosimetric and clinical correlation. *Int J Radiat Oncol Biol Phys*, 44, 855–866

Petereit DG, Sarkaria JN, Potter DM, et al. (1999) High-dose-rate versus low-dose-rate brachytherapy in the treatment of cervical cancer: analysis of tumor recurrence – the University of Wisconsin experience. *Int J Radiat Oncol Biol Phys*, 45, 1267–1274

Peters WA, Liu PY, Barrett RJ, et al. (2000) Concurrent chemotherapy and pelvic radiation therapy compared with pelvic radiation therapy alone as adjuvant therapy after radical surgery in high-risk early-stage cancer of the cervix. *J Clin Oncol*, 18, 1606–1613

Piper B, Lindsey A and Dodd M (1987) Fatigue mechanisms in cancer patients: developing nursing theory. *Oncology Nursing Forum*, 14 (6), 17–23

Porock D (1995) The effect of preparatory patient education on the anxiety and satisfaction of cancer patients receiving radiotherapy. *Cancer Nursing*, 18 (3), 206–214

Ramirez PT, Levenback C, Burke TW, Eifel P, Wolf JK and Gershenson DM (2001) Sigmoid perforation following radiation therapy in patients with cervical cancer. *Gynecol Oncol*, 82, 150–155

Rao SP, Anderson V, Shlasko E, Miller ST, Choi K and Rabinowitz S (1996) Intestinal perforation 14 years after abdominal irradiation and chemotherapy for Wilms' tumor. *J Pediatr Hematol Oncol*, 18, 187–190

Resbeut M, Marteau P, Cowen D, et al. (1997) A randomised double blind placebo controlled multicenter study of mesalazine for the prevention of acute radiation enteritis. *Radiother Oncol*, 44, 59–63

Rezvani M, Alcock CJ, Fowler JF, et al. (1991) Normal tissue reactions in the British Institute of Radiology study of three fractions per week versus five fractions per week in the treatment of carcinoma of the laryngo-pharynx by radiotherapy. *British Journal of Radiology*, 64, 1122–1133

Rose PG, Bundy BN, Watkins EB, et al. (1999) Concurrent cisplatin-based radiotherapy and chemotherapy for locally advanced cervical cancer. *N Engl J Med*, 340, 1144–1153

Rotman M, Rogow L, Delean G, et al. (1977) Supportive therapy in radiation oncology. *Cancer*, 39, 744–750

Roy L, Fortin A and Larochelle M (2001) The impact of skin washing with water and soap during breast irradiation: a randomized study. *Radiotherapy and Oncology*, 58, 333–339

Sher ME and Bauer J (1990) Radiation-induced enteropathy. *Am J Gastroenterol*, 85, 121–128

Shibata HR, Freeman CR and Roman TN (1982) Gastrointestinal complications after radiotherapy for carcinoma of the uterine cervix. *Can J Surg*, 25, 64–66

Slevin M, Nichols SE, Downer SM, et al. (1996) Emotional support for cancer patient: what do patients really want? *British Journal of Cancer*, 74 (8), 1275–1279

Small W and Kachnic L (2005) 'Postradiotherapy pelvic fractures: cause for concern or opportunity for future research?' *JAMA*, 294 (20), Nov 23/30, 2635–2637

Solomon R and Cherny NI (2006) Constipation and diarrhoea in patients with cancer. *Palliative and Supportive Care*, 12 (5), 355–364

Stricker CT, Drake D, Hoyer KA and Mock V (2004) Evidence-based practice for fatigue management in adults with cancer: exercise as an intervention. *Oncology Nursing Forum*, 31 (5), 963–976

Thomas GM, Ali S, Patel M, Abulafia O and Lucci JA (2006) A GOG phase III trial to evaluate maintaining haemoglobin (HGB) >/= 120G/L with erythropoietin (EPO) during chemoradiation (CT/RT) for cervical cancer. *International Journal of Gynaecological Cancer*, 16, (Suppl 3), 603–604

Vale CL and Tierney JF (2006) Concomitant chemoradiation for cervical cancer: a meta-analysis using individual patient data from randomized, controlled trials. *International Journal of Gynaecological Cancer*, 16, (Suppl 3), 603

Velji K and Fitch M (2001) The experience of women receiving brachytherapy for gynaecologic cancer. *Oncology Nursing Forum*, 28 (4), 743–751

Waddell BE, Rodriguez-Bigas MA, Lee RJ, et al. (1999) Prevention of chronic radiation enteritis. *J Am Coll Surg*, 189 (6), 611–624

Warnock C (2005) Patients' experiences of intracavity brachytherapy treatment for gynaecologic cancer. *European Journal of Oncology Nursing*, 9, 44–55

Wells M (2003) The treatment trajectory, in Faithfull S and Wells M (eds) *Supportive Care in Radiotherapy*. Churchill Livingstone, Edinburgh. pp. 39–59

Wells M and MacBride S (2003) Radiation Skin Reactions, in Faithfull S and Wells M (eds) *Supportive Care in Radiotherapy*. Churchill Livingstone, Edinburgh. pp. 135–159

Westbury C, Hines F, Hawkes E, Ashley S and Brada M (2000) Advice on hair and scalp care during cranial radiotherapy: a prospective, randomized trial. *Radiotherapy and Oncology*, 54, 109–116

White ID and Faithfull S (2006) Vaginal dilation associated with pelvic radiotherapy; a UK survey of current practice. *Int J Gynaecol Cancer*, 16, 1140–1146

Whitney CW, Sause W, Bundy BN, et al. (1999) Randomized comparison of fluorouracil plus cisplatin versus hydroxyurea as an adjunct to radiation therapy in stage IIB–IVA carcinoma of the cervix with negative para-aortic lymph nodes: a Gynecologic Oncology Group and Southwest Oncology Group study. *J Clin Oncol*, 17, 1339–1348

Wickline MM (2004) Prevention and treatment of acute radiation dermatitis: a literature review. *Oncology Nursing Forum*, 31 (2), 237–247

Wilson J, Mills J, Prather I and Dimitrijevich S (2005) A toxicity index of skin and wound cleansers used on *in vitro* fibroblasts and keratinocytes. *Adv Skin Wound Care*, 18 (7), 373–378

Winter GD (1962) Formation of scab and the rate of epithelialization of superficial wounds in the skin of the young domestic pig. *Nature*, 193, 293–294

Woodhouse C (1990) Injuries to the bladder, in Galland R and Spencer J (eds) *Radiation Enteritis*. Edward Arnold, London. pp. 162–167

Yalman D, Arican A, Ozsaran Z, et al. (2002) Evaluation of morbidity after external radiotherapy and intracavitary brachytherapy in 771 patients with carcinoma of the uterine cervix or endometrium. *European Journal of Gynaecological Oncology*, 23 (1), 58–62

Yamashita H, Nakagawa K, Tago M, et al. (2006) Small bowel perforation without tumour recurrence after radiotherapy for cervical carcinoma: report of seven cases. *Australas J Ageing*, 32 (2), 235–242

Chapter 5

Chemotherapy

'Chemotherapy and radiotherapy will make the ancient method of drilling holes in a patient's head to permit the escape of demons look relatively advanced.'

(Jr Krebs)

http://www.cybernation.com/victory/quotations/subjects/quotes_medicine.html

Introduction

In the treatment of cervical cancer, chemotherapy is principally reserved for two situations. First, as already described in Chapter 4, it can be used as an adjunct to radiotherapy, significantly improving its efficacy. Second, it may be employed as a treatment for progressive or recurrent disease which is unresponsive to surgery or radiotherapy.

A number of chemotherapy agents have been shown to have a role in the treatment of advanced cervical cancer, although unfortunately their efficacy is generally limited. The most active drug has been found to be cisplatin, for which the response rates are a disappointing 20% to 30% when administered as a single agent (Cannistra and Niloff 1996). Some of the other chemotherapy agents which are also used in the treatment of cervical cancer are listed in Table 5.1.

This chapter explores the role of chemotherapy in the management of cancer of the cervix. It begins with a discussion of the standard indications for chemotherapy, followed by a review of some of the literature, looking at experimental approaches such as neoadjuvant and intra-arterial chemotherapy. Some of the chemotherapy-related nursing issues are examined, focusing on care of the neutropenic patient and management of chemotherapy induced nausea and vomiting. Finally, the potential toxicities associated with cisplatin – the main chemotherapy agent used in cervical cancer – are outlined.

Chemotherapy as a radiosensitiser

The addition of concomitant chemotherapy to external beam radiotherapy is one of the major innovations in the management of advanced cervical cancer in recent decades (see Chapter 4). The survival benefit in early trials was such that it prompted the National Cancer Institute to issue a clinical alert recommending strong consideration to the incorporation of concurrent cisplatin-based chemotherapy with radiotherapy.

At one time it was assumed that the efficacy of combined chemoradiotherapy resulted from radiotherapy controlling the local disease and the chemotherapy controlling subclinical metastases outside the radiation field. However, it is now thought that the relationship between the two modalities is far more complex than this, with chemotherapy and radiotherapy acting synergistically, increasing the sensitivity of the tumour to radiation therapy.

Table 5.1 Some cytotoxic drugs active against squamous cell carcinoma of the cervix (response rates >/= 15%) (with permission Rein and Kurbacher 2001)

Drug	Patients (n)	Response rate (%)
Alkylating agents		
Cyclophosphamide	251	15
Ifosphamide	157	22
Melphalan	20	20
Heavy metal complexes		
Cisplatin	815	23
Carboplatin	175	15
Antibiotics		
Doxorubicin	266	17
Antimetabolites		
5 FU	142	20
Methotrexate	96	18
Plant alkaloids		
Vincristine	55	18
Vindesine	21	24
Vinorelbine	35	40
New agents		
Paclitaxel	52	17
Docetaxel	14	14
Topotecan	43	19
Irinotecan	142	20
Gemcitabine	45	11

A number of factors have been postulated to explain the clinical benefit of chemoradiotherapy. These include:

- the simultaneous activity of drug and radiation in different phases of the cell cycle and against different tumour cell sub-populations
- decreased tumour cell repopulation following fractionated radiation
- increased tumour cell recruitment from G_0 phase into a therapy-responsive cell cycle phase
- inhibition of the repair of sublethal radiation damage
- increased direct cytotoxicity

(Rose and Eifel 2001, Loizzi et al. 2003)

Which chemotherapy agents are the best radiosensitisers?

Cisplatin has consistently been found to be the most active radiosensitiser in the management of cervical cancer. In the past, clinicians have experimented with a variety of drug

Table 5.2 Chemotherapy regimens used for radiosensitising in cervix cancer
The regimens below were those used in the five studies which originally prompted the NCI
announcement to employ chemosensitising radiotherapy (Lehman and Thomas 2001)

Trial	Number of patients	Regimen
Keys et al.	369	XRT + cisplatin 40 mg/m^2 weekly × 6 weeks
Whitney et al.	368	XRT + cisplatin 50 mg/m^2 d 1, 29 plus 5 FU infusion 1 g/m^2 d 1–5, 30–33
Rose et al.	526	XRT + cisplatin 40 mg/m^2 weekly × 6 w Or XRT + cisplatin 50 mg/m^2 d 1 and 29 plus 5 FU infusion 1 g/m^2 d 1–4, 29–33 plus Hydroxyurea 2 g/m^2 (orally) 2×/wk for 6 wks
Morris et al.	386	XRT + cisplatin 75 mg/m^2 d 1 plus 5 FU infusion 1 g/m^2 d 1–5 (×3q3w)
Peters et al.	243	XRT + cisplatin 70 mg/m^2 plus 5 FU infusion 1 g/m^2 inf d 1–5 (×4q3w)

dosages and regimens, including once every three to four weeks, weekly, daily or by continuous infusion (see Table 5.2). However, the general consensus today is that weekly administration of cisplatin at 40 mg/m^2 during radiotherapy offers adequate radiosensitisation with minimal toxicity.

Some studies have also attempted to increase the effectiveness of cisplatin by adding other agents. For example, 5FU has shown synergy with cisplatin when used in animal models and has subsequently been used in a number of clinical studies (see Table 5.2). Its mode of action is again unclear but it is thought to interfere with the repair of radiation induced lesions (Loizzi et al. 2003). Hydroxyurea has also been added as a chemosensitiser in a number of studies, although more recent data from systematic reviews does not support its widespread use in this setting (Symonds et al. 2003, 2004).

Chemotherapy for recurrent or advanced disease

'The optimal treatment for patients with metastatic or recurrent cervical cancer is still undefined and chemotherapy is used with palliation intent.'

(Tambaro et al. 2004)

Cervical cancer is generally considered to be a chemorefractory disease, and therefore chemotherapy is only adopted when radiotherapy and surgery have been unsuccessful. Unfortunately, the fact that chemotherapy is only employed in pre-treated patients further compromises its efficacy. Both radical surgery and irradiation are known to destroy local vascularisation, reducing the efficacy of drugs administered systemically. Furthermore, as the tumour cells become increasingly hypoxic, they are exposed to intensive genetic stress which is also thought to bring about chemoresistance (Rein and Kurbacher 2001).

As well as compromising its efficacy, pre-treatment can also lead to increased toxicity for a number of reasons. These include limited bone marrow function because of prior radiotherapy and possible renal dysfunction, for example secondary to uretal obstruction.

Nevertheless, recurrent or resistant disease remains an accepted indication for chemotherapy, and once again it is cisplatin which is the most active agent in this setting. It is generally administered at doses ranging from 50–100 mg/m and is given every three weeks. Higher doses may result in an improved response but not necessarily improved survival

---

Box 5.1 Clinical considerations for administering radiosensitising chemotherapy

(1) Is it essential to give the chemotherapy on the day of radiotherapy? Is the preceding/following day acceptable if, for example, the linear accelerator breaks?
It is generally acknowledged that chemotherapy should be given on the day of radiotherapy. If the linear accelerator breaks down the radiotherapist may try to schedule two fractions the following day to catch up. In this case they may recommend not to treat with chemotherapy that day – discuss with your radiotherapy team.

(2) If given on the day of radiotherapy, does it matter whether it is given before or after the radiation?
The optimal timing of chemotherapy administration relative to the radiotherapy treatment time is still not clear. In some animal studies administration of cisplatin even as little as six hours after radiotherapy was found to confer only a small benefit beyond radiotherapy alone (Kallman et al. 1992). The general consensus is that chemotherapy should always be given prior to radiotherapy.

(3) Why isn't chemotherapy given with brachytherapy?
In the five seminal trials which supported the original NCI recommendations to use chemoradiotherapy (Keys et al. 1999, Morris et al. 1999, Rose et al. 1999, Whitney et al. 1999, Peters et al. 2000) chemotherapy was not used simultaneously with brachytherapy. With low dose brachytherapy there would be concerns about neutropenia and sepsis if chemotherapy was given concurrently.

(4) What is the optimal regimen of radiosensitising chemotherapy?
A number of different chemotherapy regimens have been used to date, but currently many centres administer 40 mg/m^2 of cisplatin a week during external beam radiotherapy (5–6 cycles).

(5) Is it necessary to administer electrolytes such as magnesium and calcium with the cisplatin pre-hydration?
Cisplatin is a drug associated with significant renal toxicity, as discussed later in this chapter. For this reason a standard regimen of pre-hydration is employed when using the drug. Electrolyte disturbances may also occur when using cisplatin and therefore some institutions administer calcium and magnesium supplements with the pre-hydration.

---

and are obviously associated with greater toxicity (Tambaro et al. 2004). Whilst it might be postulated that carboplatin would offer a good alternative to cisplatin in certain patients, the preliminary results with this drug are disappointing (Tambaro et al. 2004).

Other drugs with single agent activity which have been developed over recent decades include ifosfamide, paclitaxel, topotecan, irinotecan and gemcitabine. In particular, the topoisomerase I poisons irinotecan and topotecan have been found to be active even in patients failing platinum based chemotherapy (Eisenhauer and Vermorken 1996).

A variety of different two- to four-drug combination regimens have also been studied in clinical trials over the last two decades. Platinum has been combined with ifosfamide, bleomycin, 5-FU, mitomycin C and vinca alkaloids sometimes producing response rates exceeding those seen with single-agent protocols. However, most of the data related to combination chemotherapy are generated in small, non-randomised trials, thus substantially limiting their clinical utility (Rein and Kurbacher 2001).

Clearly, the decision of whether or not to administer chemotherapy involves careful assessment of the patient's clinical status. Whilst in some instances chemotherapy will bring about a symptomatic improvement, this needs to be balanced against potential toxicity.

No randomised study to date has compared the efficacy of cisplatin with best supportive care; thus, its impact on survival is unclear (Tambaro et al. 2004). Furthermore, so is its effect on quality of life. One small study does indicate that cisplatin based chemotherapy may achieve a palliation of pain in 67% of patients (Chambers et al. 1994) but this is an isolated trial and further research would be desirable. Unfortunately, large-scale research projects are extremely difficult in palliative care because of both small sample sizes and ethical factors. There is, however, some research suggesting that palliative chemotherapy offers a quality of life benefit in certain other cancers such as non-small cell lung cancer (Medley and Cullen 2002).

Eralp et al. (2003) endeavoured to identify the impact of various prognostic factors on survival in a population of patients with recurrent carcinoma of the cervix in order to help identify subgroups most likely to benefit from therapy.

Poor prognostic factors were found to be:

• presentation with advanced disease at initial diagnosis
• a progression-free interval of less than eight months
• a recurrence within a previously irradiated field

It was concluded that most patients with relapsed cervical cancer do not benefit from highly responsive multidrug regimens or dose-intense combinations: 'A careful prognostic judgement on case-by-case basis may not only assist in choosing the best therapeutic option, but also may help circumvent ethical issues that may arise from employing toxic regimens without a substantial survival benefit' (Eralp et al. 2003).

Neoadjuvant chemotherapy

Unfortunately, adjuvant chemotherapy (i.e., chemotherapy administered after definitive therapy such as surgery) has not been found to be helpful in the management of cervical cancer. However, another approach which has generated considerable interest is the use of neoadjuvant chemotherapy – that is chemotherapy which is administered *prior* to radiotherapy or surgery. Of course the obvious and worrying risk with this is that it involves delaying the initiation of definitive treatment for six weeks or so whilst the chemotherapy is administered. If the tumour is not chemosensitive it could grow larger during this time (DeSouza et al. 2004).

Nevertheless, there are a number of reasons why neoadjuvant chemotherapy might be helpful, and why research in this area continues:

(1) Chemotherapy may be more effective if given before tumour blood flow has been disrupted by surgery or radiotherapy (Rein and Kurbacher 2001).
(2) Chemotherapy may be less toxic when given before the bone marrow has been affected by radiotherapy.
(3) Patients with large tumours are at risk of harbouring micrometastases, so early chemotherapy may treat these.
(4) Cervical cancer patients with tumours greater than 4 cm in diameter have the worse outcome (see Chapter 1). Such tumours are difficult to excise surgically and are also difficult to treat with radiotherapy because central hypoxia decreases its effect (Modaress et al. 2005). Early chemotherapy may reduce tumour bulk, rendering radiotherapy more effective or surgery feasible (Moore 2006).

A number of trials have indeed demonstrated good response rates to neoadjuvant chemotherapy ranging between 35% and 100% (Rein and Kurbacher 2001). However, these response rates have not always been associated with increased survival, especially with advanced stage tumours (Rein and Kurbacher 2001). Furthermore, the studies are often small and not randomized (DeSouza et al. 2004, Moore 2006).

The neoadjuvant chemotherapy research is divided into neoadjuvant chemotherapy plus radiotherapy versus neoadjuvant chemotherapy plus surgery. The data on neoadjuvant chemotherapy and radiotherapy is disappointing. A Cochrane review of the literature was recently performed collating information from 18 studies involving 2074 patients. It was concluded that there was no evidence of an effect of neoadjuvant chemotherapy plus radiotherapy on survival, or any other endpoint (NACCCMA 2004).

Despite this overall conclusion, some interesting observations were made in the review. For example, centres administering more intensive chemotherapy (i.e. a shorter cycle length and/or a higher dose intensity) tended to show an advantage for neoadjuvant chemotherapy, whereas those delivering chemotherapy in a less intensive and more prolonged manner (i.e. a longer cycle length or a lower dose intensity) tended to show a detrimental effect of chemotherapy (NACCCMA 2004). The implications of this are uncertain but it confirms that the scheduling of chemotherapy is very important, particularly where it is being used in conjunction with another therapy.

The data supporting neoadjuvant chemotherapy plus surgery is slightly more promising. One important trial is by Sardi et al. (1986) who randomised patients between neoadjuvant chemotherapy plus surgery versus surgery alone. A significantly improved outcome was found in the chemotherapy arm. It has been suggested that the success of this trial is in part because a dose-dense chemotherapy schedule was employed in which cytotoxics were administered every ten days. Such a regimen may have allowed more efficient suppression of tumour cell regrowth (Rein and Kurbacher 2001).

Information about the toxicities associated with neoadjuvant chemotherapy is limited. Tierney found that data about side effects was only recorded in half of the trials he analysed. Overall, a relatively small number of late effects were documented – not really sufficient to warrant formal analysis. However, from the limited amount of information available, neoadjuvant chemotherapy does not seem to be associated with increased toxicity.

Intra-arterial chemotherapy

Some of the chemotherapy studies have administered the cytotoxics intra-arterially. This is thought to selectively increase drug concentrations at tumour level and reduce systemic exposure and toxicity. The chemotherapy is usually administered via percutaneous catheters inserted bilaterally in the hypogastric arteries. To date intra-arterial chemotherapy has not been found to be superior to traditional drug delivery (Moore 2006).

Chemotherapy toxicities

The data available on toxicities associated with chemosensitising chemotherapy is still in its infancy and is discussed in Chapter 4. Similarly, there is limited data on the toxicities associated with neoadjuvant chemotherapy. Thus, the following section focuses on the toxicities of chemotherapy where it is used as a primary treatment, principally in the setting of advanced disease (see Table 5.3).

The section begins with a discussion of two important toxicities which are common to many of the chemotherapy agents which could be employed in the treatment of cervical cancer: bone marrow suppression and nausea/vomiting. This is followed by discussion of some specific toxicities associated with cisplatin, the most commonly used chemotherapy agent in cervical cancer.

Bone marrow suppression

Just as radiotherapy interferes with the process of cell division (see Chapter 4), so does chemotherapy. Different chemotherapy agents affect the cell in different ways and at different stages of mitosis. However, the net result is the same. The tumour cells are unable to repair themselves from the chemotherapy-associated damage and the tumour thus reduces in size and ideally disappears altogether.

As with radiotherapy, chemotherapy associated side effects relate to chemotherapy's lack of specificity. Certain normal cells – particularly those which need to divide rapidly in order to maintain their population – are affected by chemotherapy drugs in the same way that the cancer cells are. Fortunately, most of the normal cells have the capacity to repair

Table 5.3 Ematogenic potential and other toxicities of drugs used to treat cervix cancer (MASCC: www.mascc.org accessed 27/12/06, Baker et al. 2005)

Drug + indication	Ematogenicity	Bone marrow suppression	Alopecia	Other
Cisplatin – chemosensitising (40 mg/m²)	Moderate to low	Y	Possible	Renal failure, ototoxicity, neurotoxicity
Cisplatin – recurrent disease/ relapse (>50 mg/m²)	High	Y	Possible	
Carboplatin	Moderate	Y	uncommon	
Ifosphamide	Moderate	Y	Y	Bladder irritation
Irinotecan	moderate	Y	Y	Cholinergic syndrome, diarrhoea
Paclitaxel	low	Y	Y	Aches, neuropathies
Gemcitabine	low	Y	rarely	Flu-like illness
5 FU	low	mild	rarely	Sore mouth, diarrhoea
Methotrexate	low	Y	rarely	Sore mouth, diarrhoea, gritty eyes
Vinorelbine	low	Y	rarely	Parasthesia, pain in vein during injection

themselves, whereas the cancer cells do not. An optimal chemotherapy dose provides the maximum amount of drug to destroy the cancer cells whilst at the same time maintaining a tolerable rate of toxicity.

Bone marrow suppression is probably the most important potential toxicity associated with many chemotherapy regimens. The three types of blood cell which are affected by chemotherapy are the red and white blood cells and the platelets. Whilst to some degree platelets and red blood cells can be managed by transfusion, white blood cells cannot. Neutrophils are particularly susceptible to the effects of chemotherapy because of their rapid turnover – their lifespan in blood is only about ten hours (Hoffbrand et al. 2001). If the chemotherapy dose causes profound and/or protracted neutropenia it renders chemotherapy patients at risk of contracting infections.

Whilst avoiding pathological micro-organisms is obviously sensible for patients undergoing chemotherapy, in practice this may be difficult and may not necessarily protect them from infections. This is because the majority of infections amongst the neutropenic population are caused by their own, endogenous flora (Schimpff et al. 1972). Thus, rather than avoidance of infections, the mainstay of management for the neutropenic patient is the prompt initiation of antibiotic therapy. More than 70% of neutropenic patients will respond to antibiotics if they are given within the first 24 hours, compared with only 22% if they are delayed to the third day following the development of symptoms (Bodey et al. 1985).

The neutrophil nadir can occur at any time from a few days to weeks after chemotherapy administration, depending on the agents used. Patients receiving chemotherapy are at greatest risk of becoming neutropenic following their first or second cycle (Lyman and Kuderer 2004).

Nausea and vomiting

Different chemotherapy agents are associated with different ematogenic potentials, as illustrated in Table 5.3. A number of chemotherapy drugs used to treat cervix cancer are associated with high levels of nausea and vomiting – cisplatin being one of them. The severity of the symptoms is dose-related and therefore nausea and vomiting are more likely to be a problem with higher doses as used in the salvage setting rather than lower radio-sensitising doses.

Nausea and vomiting are particular problems in today's health care setting in which most chemotherapy is delivered on an out-patient basis. Moreover, a number of studies disappointingly suggest that health professionals underestimate the severity and significance of post-chemotherapy nausea and vomiting amongst their patients (Grunberg et al. 2004).

Fortunately, the introduction of serotonin antagonists in the 1980s significantly improved our management of chemotherapy associated vomiting. Chemotherapy related nausea has also been reduced by this category of drugs, although not completely eradicated. Whereas vomiting was found to be the most severe symptom amongst patients undergoing chemotherapy in 1983 (Coates et al. 1983), by 1993 it had fallen to fifth place and had been replaced by nausea (Griffin et al. 1996).

The mechanism of chemotherapy associated nausea and vomiting

The vomiting centre (VC) is the portion of the brain responsible for coordinating the nausea and vomiting response. It consists of a collection of neurons distributed throughout the medulla oblongata. It is stimulated by a number of different neuroreceptors including dopamine, histamine, acetylcholine, serotonin and substance-P (Baker et al. 2005).

The chemoreceptor trigger zone (CTZ) is a specific location in the brain directly sensitive to agents with ematogenic potential, and is located in the fourth ventricle at the area postrema. The CTZ is responsible for the transmission of most of the ematogenic stimuli to the vomiting centre (Baker et al. 2005).

It is considered unlikely that toxins provide a significant direct stimulus to the CTZ via the systemic circulation. Instead, this function is likely to be mediated by the enterochromaffin cells. These cells are located within the gut and are damaged by the metabolites of chemotherapy agents causing them to release serotonin which stimulates the vagus nerve. The vagus in turn supplies the VC and CTZ (Baker et al. 2005).

There are three phases of chemotherapy associated nausea and vomiting (Baker et al. 2005):

- acute: occurs within 16 to 24 hours after chemotherapy
- delayed: after the acute period and may last as long as six or seven days (can be a problem with cisplatin)
- anticipatory: a learned response related to associations with previous negative chemotherapy experiences. It occurs in approximately 30% of chemotherapy patients (Morrow 2003). It usually begins around the fourth or fifth session (Hockenberry-Eaton and Benner 1990), but can occur after just one round of chemotherapy (Rudd and Andrews 2005).

Management of nausea and vomiting

Adequate management of nausea and vomiting at the beginning of chemotherapy treatment is important not only in improving the patient's quality of life, but also in minimising the risk of the patient developing anticipatory nausea and vomiting – a condition which is notoriously difficult to manage. In most cases nausea and vomiting requires a multiple pathway approach using several different classes of antiemetic agents (Viale 2006) (see Table 5.4).

Box 5.2 Risk factors for chemotherapy associated nausea and vomiting (Viale 2006)

- age less than 50
- history of motion sickness
- high level of anxiety (a variety of 'higher' brain centres can stimulate the vomiting centre, including the limbic system which is involved in emotional responses to events or sensory stimuli)
- significant emesis during prior pregnancy or chemotherapy
- low alcohol consumption
- chemotherapy type/dose

Box 5.3 Other causes of nausea and vomiting in oncology patients

It should not always be assumed that chemotherapy is the sole reason for a patient's nausea and vomiting. There are other potential causes which should considered in the assessment, particularly with intractable nausea and vomiting. These include:

- raised intra-cranial pressure, e.g. from brain metastases
- more generalised disordered gut function, e.g. delayed gastric emptying and anorexia, usually related to chemotherapy as well
- hepatomegaly
- splenomegaly
- adhesions
- bowel obstructions
- hypercalcaemia
- uraemia
- medications

Selection of appropriate medication

During the acute phase many patients have a good response to 5-HT$_3$ antagonists, either as single agents or in combination with other agents such as corticosteroids, although it should be remembered that serotonin antagonists are ineffective in as many as 10–30% of patients (Roila et al. 1991, Manusirvithaya et al. 2004).

As the acute nausea period ends, the role of the serotonin becomes less significant and other anti-emetic agents apart from 5HT$_3$ antagonists have a greater part to play. At this time dexamethasone alone has been found to be just as efficacious as dexamethasone plus a 5HT$_3$ antagonist (Geling and Eichler 2005).

Also, 'anti-dyspepsia' drugs such as maxalon may be useful because the nausea at this time is, at least in part, related to reduced gut motility and altered secretion (Rudd and Andrews 2005).

The recent introduction of NK-1 receptor antagonists which bind to the receptor sites of substance-P (Aprepitant) has been found to give a 20% improvement in emesis control and add a new and highly active drug to the anti-emetic armoury (Massaro and Lenz 2005). Aprepitant is particularly effective in the management of acute and delayed nausea.

A number of organisations have put forward anti-emetic guidelines (see the resources section at the end of this chapter). Whilst some variations exist – for example in drug dosages – most of the recommendations are broadly similar. For highly ematogenic regimens the suggestion is for a 5HT$_3$ antagonist, corticosteroid and NK-1 receptor antagonist. Delayed emesis is a little more problematic, with guidelines cautioning practitioners to be regimen specific.

Table 5.4 Anti-emetics and their mode of action

Class of agent	Examples/dosage	Mode of action	Side effects/precautions	When to use
Phenothiazines	Prochlorperazine, promethazine	Block dopamine receptors located in chemoreceptor trigger zone (CTZ) and other parts of the brain	Sedation, extrapyramidal symptoms	Delayed N&V
Benzamides	Metoclopramide	Block dopamine receptors located in chemoreceptor trigger zone (CTZ) and other parts of the brain	Sedation, extrapyramidal symptoms	Delayed N&V
Benzodiazepines	Lorazepam	Reduce anxiety levels which may be closely linked with experience of nausea and vomiting; have a role in management of anticipatory nausea and vomiting	Sedation, short-term memory loss	Acute/delayed N&V
Corticosteroids	Dexamethasone – guidelines re dosage range from 8 mg to 12 mg for acute nausea (MASCC 2008)	Mechanism of action unknown	Hyperglycaemia, insomnia, gastrointestinal effects, itching, hiccoughs	Acute and delayed N&V
5-HT$_3$ antagonists	Ondansetron, granesitron, tropesitron, palonosetron	Neurotransmitter serotonin antagonists	Headache and constipation	Acute phase N&V
Neurokinin-1 inhibitors	Aprepitant (only available orally); given in three-day regimen, 125 mg for first day and 80 mg for the following two	Mainly centrally –acting at substance P pathway	Caution using with agents metabolised by the CYP3A4/CYP2C9 pathways (e.g. warfarin, cisapride, steroids, oral contraceptives, some benzodiazepines).	Acute and delayed N&V
Antipsychotic (butyrophenone)	Haloperidol	Centrally acting, blocks dopamine	CNS toxicity, dry mouth	Delayed N&V
Antihistamine	Cyclizine	Unknown, possibly acts on CTZ	Dizziness, drowsiness, blurred vision, dry mouth	Delayed N&V

Non-pharmacological control of nausea and vomiting

Disappointingly, there is not a great deal of literature about non-pharmacological methods of controlling nausea and vomiting.

Tipton et al. (2007) reviewed the literature on strategies to reduce chemotherapy induced nausea and vomiting and ranked the interventions according to the level of evidence supporting it (see Box 5.4). It can be seen that further evidence is required in many areas.

Acupuncture has been claimed to have a role in the control of nausea, with P6 being the acupuncture point for nausea. A recent Cochrane review of eleven trials involving 1200 patients examined some of the data on the subject (Ezzo et al. 2006). Interestingly, the type of acupuncture used appeared to be significant. Electro-acupressure (acupuncture point is stimulated with electricity) was found to be superior to manual acupressure for the management of acute vomiting, but did not affect acute nausea. Disappointingly, electrostimulation using wristwatch-like devices showed no benefit over placebo for any nausea and vomiting score.

Guided imagery involves focusing on pleasing images which the individual associates with relaxation (King 1997, Miller and Kearney 2004). It has been found to reduce the severity of nausea but not vomiting (Luebbert et al. 2001).

Progressive muscle relaxation requires the individual learning to recognise tension in various muscle groups and subsequently relax them in order to attain a deep degree of relaxation (Miller and Kearney 2004). It has been suggested that this may delay or prevent the symptoms of radiotherapy associated nausea. A meta-analysis by Luebbert et al. (2001) found it to have a significant impact on nausea but not on vomiting.

Manusirvithaya et al. (2004) looked at the efficacy of ginger for use in chemotherapy induced nausea. The study was small – 48 women receiving cisplatin for gynaecologic cancer were randomised into receiving ginger or placebo. All women also received standard anti-emetics. No benefit was demonstrated either in acute phase or delayed vomiting by the addition of ginger.

Box 5.4 Interventions for nausea and vomiting supported by empirical studies (Tipton et al. (2007) with permission)

Recommended for practice

Pharmacologic interventions including benzodiazepines, $5HT_3$ receptor antagonists, corticosteroids and NK1 receptor antagonists

Likely to be effective

Acupuncture
Acupressure
Guided imagery
Music therapy
Progressive muscle relaxation
Psychoeducational support and information

Benefits balanced with harms

Virtual reality

Effectiveness not yet established

Exercise
Hypnosis
Massage and aromatherapy
Acustimulation with wristband device
Ginger

Box 5.5 Cisplatin – potential toxicities

(MIMS:- http://www.mims.com.au accessed 10/7/07)

Toxicities: these include nephrotoxicity, ototoxicity, neurotoxicity, hyperuricaemia, leucopenia, thrombocytopenia, anaemia, severe nausea, vomiting, hypomagnesaemia, hypocalcaemia, SIADH, peripheral neuropathy, blurred vision, optic neuritis, papilloedema, cortical blindness, cardiac disorders, alopecia, myalgia, decreased fertility (male), pyrexia, injection site reactions such as phlebitis, anaphylactic-like reactions.

Renal toxicity: cumulative and dose related renal insufficiency is the major dose limiting toxicity of cisplatin. At one time acute renal toxicity was its major dose limiting toxicity, but in recent years it has been better controlled by pre- and post-hydration regimens and forced diuresis. However, cumulative toxicity does remain a problem and may be severe. Renal impairment, which is associated with tubular damage, may be noticed during the second week after a dose and is manifested by an increase in serum creatinine and urea. Renal failure has also been reported following intraperitoneal instillation of the drug.

Hypomagnesaemia and hypocalcaemia may also occur during the course of cisplatin therapy and is probably due to renal tubular damage leading to wasting of magnesium ions. Monitoring of electrolytes is necessary and some centres routinely supplement these Mg and Ca in their pre-hydration.

Prior to initial therapy, then before subsequent doses, the following biochemical parameters should be monitored in order to prevent or detect renal toxicity:

* glomerular filtration rate (GFR)
* blood urea nitrogen (BUN)
* serum creatinine
* creatinine clearance
* electrolytes to detect hypomagnesaemia or hypocalcaemia

Pre-treatment and post-treatment hydration and forced diuresis using mannitol reduces nephrotoxicity.

Bone marrow suppression: haematological toxicity is dose related and cumulative. The lowest levels of circulating platelets and leucocytes generally occur two to three weeks after treatment, depending on the dosage. Anaemia also occurs in a significant number of patients, usually after several courses of treatment.

Nausea and vomiting: cisplatin in doses of greater than 50 mg/m is a highly emetogenic drug. It has a unique biphasic pattern of emesis that manifests itself by an acute phase, peaking on the first day of drug administration and a delayed phase peaking 48 to 72 hours after chemotherapy (Viale 2006). Nausea and vomiting may persist for up to a week and may necessitate dosage reduction or discontinuance of treatment.

Neurotoxicity and ototoxicity: ototoxicity is cumulative and occurs mainly with high dose regimens. It is manifest as tinnitus or occasional decreased ability to hear normal conversation. Tinnitus is usually transient, lasting from a few hours to a week after cessation of therapy. Peripheral neuropathy and other neurotoxicities are less common, but have been observed, especially after prolonged cisplatin treatment.

Extravasation: whilst not generally categorised as a vesicant, local effects such as phlebitis, cellulitis and skin necrosis (following extravasation of the drug) have been reported.

Conclusion

It can thus be seen that the role of chemotherapy in the management of cervical cancer is limited by the low chemosensitivity of the disease. However, it is the principal treatment for metastatic cervical cancer and has also been shown to significantly potentiate the efficacy of radiotherapy. The principal chemotherapy agent is cisplatin. Although a number of newer agents have been shown to have some activity in the management of cervical cancer, none has replaced it.

Frequently asked questions

(1) I am going to receive radiosensitizing chemotherapy with cisplatin. Will I lose my hair?

No, cisplatin is not associated with significant hair loss at these doses.

(2) How long will cisplatin chemotherapy take to administer?

You will require intravenous hydration both before and after your chemotherapy because of the potential renal toxicities, so you should allow a whole day for treatment.

(3) Will I need a needle every time?

Yes, the drugs are given intravenously and so you will need a cannula for each treatment. If your veins are difficult to find or you find cannulation particularly stressful, indwelling venous catheters are available for long-term use which reduce the number of cannulations.

(4) Will the chemotherapy make me sick?

This depends on the type and dose of chemotherapy. Cisplatin can cause nausea and vomiting, but only when given at high doses. The nausea and vomiting associated with this drug may also be delayed, occurring a couple of days after the drug has been administered. However, the anti-emetics used today are generally very effective. You will be given anti-nausea drugs both before treatment and to take at home.

Resources

National Comprehensive Cancer Network: www.nccn.org
Multinational Association of Supportive Care in Cancer: www.mascc.org
Oncology Nursing Society: www.ons.org/outcomes/resources/nausea.shtml
American Society of Clinical Oncology: www.asco.org
European Society of Medical Oncology: www.esmo.org

References

Baker P, Morzorati SL and Ellett ML (2005) Pathophysiology of chemotherapy-induced nausea and vomiting. *Gastroenterology Nursing*, 28 (6), 469–480

Bodey G, Jadeja L and Elting L (1985). Pseudomonas bacteremia: retrospective analysis of 140 episodes. *Annals of Internal Medicine*, 145, 1621–1629

Byfield JE, Calabro-Jones P, Klisak I, et al. (1982) Pharmacologic requirements for obtaining sensitization of human tumor cells in vitro to combined 5-fluorouracil or ftorafur and X-rays. *Int J Radiat Oncol Biol Phys*, 8, 1923–1933

Cannistra SA and Niloff JM (1996) Cancer of the uterine cervix. *N Engl J Med*, 334, 1030–1038

Chambers SK, Lamb L, Kohorn EI, Schwarz PE and Chambers JT (1994) Chemotherapy of recurrent-advanced cervical cancer: results of the Yale University PMB-PFU protocol. *Gynaecol Oncol*, 53, 161–169

Coates A, Abraham S, Kaye SB, et al. (1983) On the receiving end: patient perception of the side-effects of cancer chemotherapy. *Eur J Cancer Clin Oncol*, 19, 203–208

DeSouza NM, Soutter WP, Rustin G, et al. (2004) Use of neoadjuvant chemotherapy prior to radical hysterectomy in cervical cancer: monitoring tumour shrinkage and molecular profile on magnetic resonance and assessment of three-year outcome. *British Journal of Cancer*, 90, 2326–2331

Eisenhauer FA and Vermorken JB (1996) New drugs in gynecologic oncology. *Curr Opin Oncol*, 8, 408–414

Eralp Y, Saip P, Sakar B, et al. (2003) Prognostic factors and survival in patients with metastatic or recurrent carcinoma of the uterine cervix. *International Journal of Gynecological Cancer*, 13 (4), 497–504

Ezzo J, Streitberger K and Schneider A (2006) Cochrane systematic reviews examine P6 acupuncture-point stimulation for nausea and vomiting. *Journal of Alternative and Complementary Medicine*, 12 (5), 489–495

Geling O and Eichler HG (2005) Should 5-hydroxytryptamine-3 receptor antagonists be administered beyond 24 hours after chemotherapy to prevent delayed emesis? Systematic re-evaluation of clinical evidence and drug cost implications. *J Clin Oncol*, 23 (6), 1289–1294

Griffin AM, Butow PN, Coates AS, et al. (1996) On the receiving end V: patient perceptions of the side effects of cancer chemotherapy in 1993. *Ann Oncol*, 7, 189–195

Grunberg SM, Deuson RR, Mavros P, et al. (2004) Incidence of chemotherapy-induced nausea and emesis after modern antiemetics: perception versus reality. *Cancer*, 100, 2261–2268

Hockenberry-Eaton M and Benner A (1990) Patterns of nausea and vomiting in children: nursing assessment and intervention. *Oncology Nursing Forum*, 17 (4), 575–584

Hoffbrand AV, Pettit JE and Moss PAH (2001) *Essential Haematology*. Blackwell Science, Oxford, UK. pp. 113

Kallman RF, Bedarida G and Rapacchietta D (1992) Experimental studies on schedule dependence in the treatment of cancer with combinations of chemotherapy and radiotherapy. *Front Radiat Ther Oncol*, 25, 31–44

Keys HM, Bundy BN, Stehman FB, et al. (1999) Cisplatin, radiation, and adjuvant hysterectomy compared with radiation and adjuvant hysterectomy for bulky stage IB cervical carcinoma. *N Engl J Med*, 340, 1154–1161

King CR (1997) Nonpharmacologic management of chemotherapy-induced nausea and vomiting. *Oncology Nursing Forum*, 24 (7, Suppl), 41–48

Lehman M and Thomas G (2001) Is concurrent chemotherapy and radiotherapy the new standard of care for locally advanced cervical cancer. *International Journal of Gynecological Cancer*, 11 (2), 87–99

Loizzi V, Cormio G, Loverro G, Selvaggi L, Disaia PJ and Cappuccinic F (2003) Chemoradiation: a new approach for the treatment of cervical cancer. *International Journal of Gynaecologic Cancer*, 13 (5), 580–586

Luebbert K, Dahme B and Hasenbring M (2001) The effectiveness of relaxation training in reducing treatment-related symptoms and improving emotional adjustment in acute, non-surgical cancer treatment: a meta-analytical review. *Psycho-oncology*, 10, 490–502

Lyman GH and Kuderer NM (2004) The economics of the colony-stimulating factors in the prevention and treatment of febrile neutropenia. *Critical Reviews in Oncology/Haematology*, 50, 129–146

Manusirvithaya S, Sripramote M, Tangjitgamol S, et al. (2004) Antiemetic effect of ginger in gynaecology oncology patients receiving cisplatin. *International Journal of Gynaecological Cancer*, 14 (6), Nov/Dec, 1063–1069

MASCC (2008) http://www.mascc.org/content/127.html (accessed 1/7/08)

Massaro AM and Lenz KL (2005) Aprepitant: a novel antiemetic for chemotherapy-induced nausea and vomiting. *Ann Pharmacother*, 39, 77–85

Medley L and Cullen M (2002) Best supportive care versus palliative chemotherapy in non-small cell lung cancer. *Current Opinion in Oncology*, 14 (4), 384–388

Miller M and Kearney N (2004) Chemotherapy-related nausea and vomiting – past reflections, present practice and future management. *European Journal of Cancer Care*, 13 (1), 71–81

Modarress M, Maghami FQ, Golnavaz M, Behtash N, Mousavi A and Khalili GR (2005) Comparative study of chemoradiation and neoadjuvant chemotherapy effects before radical hysterectomy in stage IB–IIB bulky cervical cancer and with tumour diameter greater than 4 cm. *International Journal of Gynaecological Cancer*, 15 (3), 483–488

Moore DH (2006) Chemotherapy for recurrent cervical cancer. *Current Opinion in Oncology*, 18 (5), 516–519

Morris M, Eifel PJ, Lu J, et al. (1999) Pelvic radiation with concurrent chemotherapy compared with pelvic and para-aortic radiation for high-risk cervical cancer. *N Engl J Med*, 340, 1137–1143

Morrow GR (2003) cited in Baker P, Mozorati SL and Ellet M (eds) (2005) The pathophysiology of chemotherapy-induced nausea and vomiting. *Gastoenterology Nursing*, 28 (6), 469–480

Morrow GR, Roscoe JA, Hickok JT, Andrews PLR and Matteson S (2002) Nausea and emesis: evidence for a biobehavioral perspective. *Supportive Care in Cancer*, 10 (2), 96–105

Neoadjuvant Chemotherapy for Cervical Cancer Meta-analysis Collaboration (NACCCMA) (2004) Neoadjuvant chemotherapy for locally advanced cervix cancer. *Cochrane Database of Systematic Reviews*. Issue 2. Art. No.: CD001774. DOI: 10.1002/14651858.CD001774.pub2

Park TK, Kim SN, Kwon JY and Mo HK (2001) Postoperative adjuvant therapy in early invasive cervical cancer patients with histopathologic risk factors. *International Journal of Gynaecological Cancer*, 11 (6), Nov/Dec, 475–482

Perez C, Kurman R, Stehman F, et al. (1992) Uterine cervix, in Hoskins W, Perez C and Young R (eds) *Principles and Practice of Gynecologic Oncology Group*. Lippincott, Philadelphia, PA. p. 637

Peters WA, Liu PY, Barrett RJ, et al. (2000) Concurrent chemotherapy and pelvic radiation therapy compared with pelvic radiation therapy alone as adjuvant therapy after radical surgery in high-risk early-stage cancer of the cervix. *J Clin Oncol*, 18, 1606–1613

Rein DT and Kurbacher CM (2001) The role of chemotherapy in invasive cancer of the cervix uteri: current standards and future prospects. *Anticancer Drugs*, 12 (10), 787–795

Roila F, Tonato M, Cognetti F, et al. (1991) Prevention of cisplatin-induced emesis: a double-blind multicenter randomized crossover study comparing ondansetron and ondansetron plus dexamethasone. *J Clin Oncol*, 9, 675–678

Roscoe JA, Morrow GR, Hickok JT and Stern RM (2000) Nausea and vomiting remain a significant clinical problem: trends over time in controlling chemotherapy-induced nausea and vomiting in 1413 patients treated in community clinical practices. *J Pain Symptom Manage*, 20, 113–121

Rose PG, Bundy BN, Watkins EB, et al. (1999) Concurrent cisplatin-based radiotherapy and chemotherapy for locally advanced cervical cancer. *N Engl J Med*, 340, 1144–1153

Rose PG and Eifel PJ (2001) Combined radiation therapy and chemotherapy for carcinoma of the cervix. *The Cancer Journal*, 7 (2), 86–92

Rudd JA and Andrews PLR (2005) Chapter 2: Mechanisms of acute, delayed, and anticipatory emesis induced by anticancer therapies, in Hesketh PJ (ed.), *Management of Nausea and Vomiting in Cancer and Cancer Treatment*. Jones and Bartlett Publishers, Sudbury, MA

Saibishkumar EP, Patel FD and Sharma SC (2005) Results of radiotherapy alone in the treatment of carcinoma of uterine cervix: a retrospective analysis of 1069 patients. *Int Jnl Gyne Cancer*, 15 (5), Sept/Oct, 890–897

Sardi J, di Paola G, Sananes C, et al. (1986) A possible new trend in the management of carcinoma of the cervix uteri. *Gynecol Oncol*, 25, 139–146

Schimpff SC, Young VM, Greene WH, Vermeulen GD, Moody MR and Wiernik PH (1972) Origin of infection in acute nonlymphocytic leukaemia. Significance of hospital acquisition of potential pathogens. *Annals of Internal Medicine*, 77, 707–714

Sood, BM, Timmins PF, Gorla GR, et al. (2002) Concomitant cisplatin and extended field radiation therapy in patients with cervical and endometrial cancer. *International Journal of Gynaecological Cancer*, 12 (5), 459–464

Symonds P, Kirwan J, Williams C, et al. (2003) Concomitant hydroxyurea plus radiotherapy versus radiotherapy for carcinoma of the uterine cervix. *The Cochrane Database of Systematic Reviews*, 2, Art. No. CD003918.pub2. DOI: 10.1002/14651858.CD003918.pub2

Symonds RP, Collingwood M, Kirwan J, et al. (2004) Concomitant hydroxyurea plus radiotherapy versus radiotherapy for carcinoma of the uterine cervix a systematic review. *Cancer Treatment Reviews*, 30, 405–414

Tambaro R, Scambia G, Di Maio M, et al. (2004) The role of chemotherapy in locally advaced, metastatic and recurrent cervical cancer. *Critical Reviews in Oncology and Haematology*, 52, 33–44

Tipton J, McDaniel RW, Barbour L, et al. (2007) Putting evidence into practice: nausea and vomiting. *Clinical Journal of Oncology Nursing*, 11 (1), 69–78

Viale PH (2006) Update on the management of chemotherapy-induced nausea and vomiting. *Journal of Infusion Nursing*, 29 (5), 283–291

Whitney CW, Sause W, Bundy BN, et al. (1999) Randomized comparison of fluorouracil plus cisplatin versus hydroxyurea as an adjunct to radiation therapy in stage IIB–IVA carcinoma of the cervix with negative para-aortic lymph nodes: a Gynecologic Oncology Group and Southwest Oncology Group study. *J Clin Oncol*, 17, 1339–1348

Chapter 6

Psychological and social aspects of cervical cancer

Alison Nightingale and Ruth Dunleavey

'Only emotion endures'

Ezra Pound

Introduction

The psychological and social impact of cervical cancer begins at the time of diagnosis and continues for many years afterwards (Ashing-Gawa et al. 2004). Its effects are far-reaching, involving not only the cervical cancer patient, but also her partner, children and family.

Cervical cancer is a disease arising predominantly between the ages of 30 and 50 (see Chapter 1). During this period of their lives women often play a central role in the day-to-day management of the family, the nurturing of children and the care of extended family members (Lowdermilk and Germino 2000). When a woman learns she has a gynaecological cancer, her ability to perform these important roles may be affected, resulting in a negative impact on the whole family system (Yates, 1999).

Depending on their individual circumstances, different women will have different concerns, and over time their needs will change and evolve. For some, fertility will be a major issue, for others body image and sexuality. Others, still, will have more practical worries regarding their role in the home, workplace and/or as a carer. Because cervical cancer is most common amongst those of lower socioeconomic status (Franco et al. 2001), financial considerations may present an additional stress. Moreover, the stigma which is attached to the disease and its connotations with sexual activity can be devastating for some women and their families. The potential impact of this on adjustment, especially sexual adjustment, should not be underestimated.

A number of studies have been carried out to investigate the psychosocial impact of cervical cancer, particularly with regard to sexual dysfunction. In this chapter, we will discuss some of the issues raised by this research with reference not only to the available literature but also drawing on the personal experiences of a number of women. This information has been obtained from Jo's Trust, a patient support charity in the UK for women with cancer and cervical dysplasia (www.jotrust.co.uk.). The comments have been sourced from the online bulletin board and it is hoped that they help illustrate the challenges faced by women as they pass through the treatment trajectory and attempt to resume their everyday lives.

Studies of the psychosocial impact of cervical cancer have examined a number of different factors. For the purposes of this review these have been divided into the following categories:

- cervical cancer, psychological morbidity and quality of life
- relationships

- sexuality and body image
- sexual functioning
- talking to children about cervical cancer
- support groups

Psychological impact of cervical cancer and quality of life

'I felt embarrassed about telling people – like cervical cancer you bring on yourself – someone actually said to me – 'wow you must have really slept around.'

(Jo's Trust)

'Then all of a sudden, like six months later (following treatment) when it finally hit me, I don't think people were prepared for it because I've been so strong. People looked at me and physically I'm fine and I can do everything again, I mean it took me seven months before it hit me.'

(Juraskova et al. 2003, p. 272)

'One of the things I find hard is planning ahead. My bridesmaids have been nagging me to set a date for my hen night but I worry about setting dates as I wonder if IT will come back and I am tempting fate by trying to be normal.'

(Jo's Trust).

The very word 'cancer' is associated with a number of fears, including fear of pain, anaesthesia, surgery and death, fear of dependency or abandonment, fear of possible sexual or reproductive changes, fear of changes in body image as well as fears regarding ability to work, financial matters and family functioning (Turns 2001). Consequently, any cancer diagnosis is associated with high levels of distress and psychological morbidity. Thompson and Shear (1998) found that on being told they had cancer 20% of patients were so distressed that they could have been classified as 'psychiatrically ill'. This provides an indication of the magnitude of the impact the disease can have on psychological wellbeing.

Steginga and Dunn (1997) asked a number of women with gynaecological cancer to describe the main worries or problems they experienced at diagnosis and during treatment. Eighty-one percent reported psychosocial difficulties, the most common of which were depression (49%), anxiety (37%) and fear of dying (35%). This is consistent with other literature in which depression and anxiety are the most frequently mentioned psychological morbidities (Petersen et al. 2005). The prevalence of depression amongst gynaecology oncology patients is cited as ranging from 4% to 90% – levels both lower and higher than population norms. Levels of anxiety are generally reported as higher than in non-cancer populations (Thompson and Shear 1998).

The type and intensity of psychological morbidity changes over time (see Box 6.1). Initially, women commonly experience feelings of shock and disbelief, coupled with concerns about treatment options. Many feel numb and disconnected from their diagnosis. For some, the news that they have cancer may even cause a stress reaction similar to that of a major trauma, with an associated risk of developing post-traumatic stress disorder (Sukegawa et al. 2006).

Feelings of guilt and blame are also common after diagnosis. For several years epidemiological studies have indicated that cervical cancer and sexual intercourse are linked (Slattery et al. 1989). Our more recent understanding of the role of HPV in cervical cancer provides the rationale for this association (see Chapter 1). In the public's perception it seems to be impossible to disentangle cervical cancer from sexual activity. Unfortunately, cervical cancer has therefore been labelled as a disease of the 'promiscuous'. Some women describe feeling 'dirty' following their diagnosis and many experience emotions such as anxiety, anger, shock, guilt and shame at this time (McIntosh 1996). The involvement of a sexually transmitted virus may also raise questions regarding fidelity in long-term partnerships (Wilmoth and Spinelli 2000). Some women – particularly those from certain ethnic minorities – feel too embarrassed to tell others about their illness:

Box 6.1 Timing of psychological and social impact of cervical cancer

Early impact

- shock, disbelief, anger, confusion, anxiety
- concerns over treatment options
- concerns about future fertility
- concerns about survival
- communication with treatment team
- financial worries – ability to work during and after treatment

Three to nine months following treatment

- prognosis
- fertility
- depression and anxiety
- impact on relationships
- resuming sexual activity
- finding support
- expectations of 'getting back to normal'
- reduction in social and professional support
- ability to work
- fatigue
- making plans for the future

Nine to eighteen months following treatment

- depression
- prognosis
- symptoms of recurrence
- attendance at follow-up appointments
- continuing need to de-brief yet reduction in ability to discuss these concerns
- fertility
- sexual activity may decrease even after increasing during the last period
- feeling 'normal' – finding people in the same boat
- ability to work
- fatigue
- lymphoedema
- making plans for the future

More than 18 months following treatment

- prognosis
- fertility
- long-term sexual dysfunction
- long-term physical morbidity
- lymphoedema

Klee et al (2000), Hawighorst-Knapstein et al. (2004),
De Groot et al. (2005), Vistad et al. (2006), Matsushita (2007)

'I have always been very ashamed of having cervical cancer and hardly anyone knows. Feel like it's my fault with the media last year about the HPV and also 'cos I didn't have my smears.'

(Jo's Trust)

A number of quality of life (QOL) studies have attempted to assess not only the psychological, but also the physical, social and functional impact of cervical cancer, using tools such as the EORTC QLQ-CX24 questionnaire. There is no doubt from the literature that at diagnosis and during therapy, quality of life is substantially impaired in women undergoing treatment for cervical cancer and that this impairment may continue for a considerable time (Vistad et al. 2006).

However, some studies indicate that by six to twelve months following treatment QOL scores amongst cervical cancer survivors are significantly improved and do not differ from those of 'healthy controls' (Andersen et al. 1989, Lutgendorf et al. 2002). Conversely, other studies have been published indicating long-term psychological, physical, sexual and social impairment up to five years following treatment (Klee et al. 2000, Greimel et al. 2002).

Paradoxically, some studies have found that a proportion of cancer survivors actually have a *better* quality of life than those who have not had cancer, despite the substantial physical and mental challenges they meet (Wenzel et al. 2005). This apparent improvement in QOL may be the result of 'response shift' (Schwartz and Sprangers 1999). Response shift refers to a process of personal reflection which leads to a change in an individual's expectations over time. This may result in a redefinition of internal standards regarding what constitutes health, a change in values and priorities, and consequently an alteration in perception of quality of life (Schwartz et al. 2004).

Coping

The psychological impact of cervical cancer and the individual's ability to cope with the disease is influenced by a number of 'internal' and 'external' factors. Internal factors refer to the patient's personal coping strategies. External factors include social support, for example from partners, the family, health professionals and support groups.

Looking first at external factors, women who consider their social support to be poor have been found to have a high risk of developing anxiety and depressive symptoms (Petersen et al. 2005). Relationship status in particular has been found to be a significant factor influencing the psychosocial functioning of women with cervical cancer (Schrover et al. 1989, Weijmar Schultz et al. 1992, Chan et al. 2001).

Social support has been described as having three dimensions – emotional, informational and instrumental (Thoits 1986). The principal types of support offered by health professionals are generally 'informational' and 'instrumental' (i.e. the provision of information and of 'practical' support).

Whilst these types of support are undeniably important, the literature suggests that it is emotional support which is most consistently associated with better psychological outcomes for women affected by cancer. Information and help with decision making is important, but it may not be *as* helpful if emotional support is perceived as inadequate (Arora et al. 2006).

Turning to 'internal' factors, patients who adopt maladaptive strategies to cope with their cancer have been shown to have higher levels of emotional distress – even if their prognosis is relatively good (Lutgendorf et al. 1999). Maladaptive coping strategies include use of alcohol, smoking and withdrawal. Healthier coping strategies involve seeking emotional social support in order to reduce their level of distress.

Box 6.2 lists some of the risk factors for poor psychological adjustment to a diagnosis of cervical cancer.

The impact of cervical cancer on relationships

He felt really lost and helpless, I think that he felt really guilty too as if he, you know, in some way contributed to it.

(Juraskova et al. 2003, p. 273)

> **Box 6.2 Factors associated with poor psychological adjustment in women with cancer of the cervix**
>
> Patients, on the whole, welcome being asked about their psychological wellbeing and emotional status by health professionals. In one study 73% of subjects stated that physicians should ask whether or not their cancer patients wanted help in dealing with their emotions and 69% whether they want help dealing with fears (Detmar et al. 2000).
> Factors which have been associated with poor psychological adjustment to the disease include:
>
> - single women and those in unstable relationships
> - women with a history of psychological morbidity (e.g. depression)
> - those with a lack of social support
> - young women
> - those with sub-optimal coping styles (e.g. avoidance, denial, disengagement)
> - those with maladaptive coping strategies such as denial and use of drugs or alcohol
> - those who experienced a significant impact with regards to infertility
> - those experiencing problems with treatment-related menopause
> - those whose ability to work changed following treatment due to physical symptoms
>
> (Chan et al. 2001, Wenzel et al. 2005, Bradley et al. 2006, Constanzo et al. 2006)

'I remember the night I came home from the hospital, crying, and my husband laid up against me, and I felt his erection, and I thought, "This is the best gift he could ever give me."'

(Bruner and Boyd 1999)

'My husband was useless with my cancer, realising that life is too short, I left him six months after I was diagnosed.'

(Jo's Trust)

Cervical cancer impacts a woman's functioning in a variety of roles. Professionally, the disease and treatment may affect her ability to work. As a mother – especially of young children – many women find it significantly compromises their ability to perform their usual tasks. Bruner and Boyd (1999) found that fatigue in particular, interfered with normal role functioning. However, possibly the most significant effects of the disease are on relationships with a partner or spouse.

In a couple with poor communication skills, the disease may cause increased distance and turbulence between partners. Communication difficulties and ambivalent messages can generate stress within a relationship and may lead to emotional withdrawal (Maughan et al. 2002). Approximately 25% of couples separate within the first two years following a cancer diagnosis (Butler-Manuel et al. 1999).

Conversely, couples with stable and supportive relationships have been shown to have better long-term quality of life and emotional adjustment (Fowler et al. 2004). Indeed, for a couple with good communication skills, the diagnosis may result in a stronger, closer relationship.

Women who are not in a relationship at the time of their diagnosis tend to have the poorest outcomes in terms of adjustment to their disease (Weijmar Schultz et al. 1992, Chan et al. 2001). They often have less social and practical support than women who are within partnerships (whether homosexual or heterosexual). If they live alone they may not have adequate assistance and may face logistical problems, for example in attending appointments – especially for long treatment courses such as chemoradiation.

Single women also face the concern that at some point in the future they may want to form new sexual relationships. This may induce a high level of anxiety associated with issues of body image, femininity, the ability to conceive and also worries about re-infection with HPV.

The impact of gynaecological cancer varies for the patient and her spouse and adaptive recovery is only possible if the couple can learn to function effectively with their new circumstances (Maughan et al. 2002). This adaptation is not easy and it has been reported that many husbands find it difficult to cope with their partner's diagnosis of cervical cancer and tend not to discuss their feelings (Juraskova et al. 2003). Partners may also experience feelings of powerlessness and sexual dysfunction in response to their wife's illness (Maughan et al. 2002).

For many women with cervical cancer, sexual intimacy serves as a painful reminder of both the changes in their relationships and the changes in their body which have been brought about by the disease process. Some report feelings of sadness and grief which emerge during sexual experiences, exacerbating sexual dysfunction and feelings of inadequacy (Carter et al. 2005). The effects of the disease and its treatment on sexuality and sexual function are discussed in the following section.

Sexuality

'Just a sense of loss . . . a grieving that I lost my femininity . . . (reproductive organs) they are symbols of womanhood I suppose. (age 30)'

(Juraskova et al. 2003, p. 271)

'I was so angry, I just couldn't control it and I didn't want anybody near me because I felt dirty. I scrubbed my body, I scratched myself that bad that I bled and everything . . . I've got scars. (age 41)'

(Juraskova et al. 2003, p. 271)

'I have had quite a few issues with femininity – couldn't wear flat shoes, obsessed with pink for months after my surgery. I felt asexual.'

(Jo's Trust)

'I feel absolutely de-feminised and very, very ashamed.'

(Jo's Trust)

In caring for women who have cervical cancer, sexuality and sexual function are important issues that will arise at many phases of treatment, from diagnosis to the end of therapy and beyond. The effects of cervical cancer treatment on sexuality and sexual functioning have been shown to be significant, incorporating both physical and psychological components. In order to achieve informed consent for cervical cancer treatment, it is essential that the potential sexual implications of any proposed intervention are discussed (Wilmoth and Spinelli 2000).

The terms 'sexuality' and 'sexual function' are not interchangeable. Sexual function refers to the sexual act – although this need not be restricted to intercourse alone. Sexual behaviour may also include masturbation, kissing, mutual body caressing and oral sex (Skye Caldwell 2003). 'Sexuality' is a broader term incorporating a range of concepts such as self-esteem, body image, gender and identity (Carr 1991). Even women who are no longer sexually active are sexual beings and may have issues with their sexuality following treatment. To quote Wilmoth and Spinelli (2000) p. 413:

Sexuality is more than the ability to have sexual intercourse. To many women, sexuality includes feelings about their body appearance, their femininity, their ability to bear children, and their ability to function sexually. Sexuality is an integral aspect of a woman's personality, with emotional, intellectual, and sociocultural components.

One important aspect of sexuality is body image. This can be defined as 'general and enduring positive and negative attitudes about the body' (Andersen and LeGrand 1991). Treatment for gynaecological cancer can result in the 'loss and mutilation of body parts' – an experience which leaves some feeling 'incomplete', 'freakish' or 'damaged'

(Skye Caldwell 2003). Scars, oedema or incontinence may all diminish an individual's feelings of attractiveness (Bos-Branolte 1991). Those who require a stoma are likely to be particularly vulnerable to problems with femininity (Weijmar Schultz et al. 1991).

Whilst it should not be assumed that treatments offered for cervical cancer will *inevitably* result in a negative body image, this is certainly an issue for a proportion of women (Price 1998). For these individuals a diagnosis of gynaecological cancer may touch the very core of their identity. For some it is an intact uterus which identifies them as female and therefore loss of the uterus affects their very sense of self.

The first section of this chapter has outlined some of the psychological, relationship and sexuality changes brought about by the diagnosis and treatment of cervical cancer. The combination of these factors may also impact another important aspect of a woman's wellbeing – that is her sexual function.

Sexual function

'Physically I had no problems. I think most of it was dealing with emotional pain. There were times when I actually just detached myself . . . like at the beginning there were a lot of time I don't even remember . . . like I just blanked myself out from it, when we were actually having sex.'

(Juraskova et al. 2003, p. 272)

'I don't feel anything . . . I don't feel anything except fear.'

(Juraskova et al. 2003, p. 271)

'Before we did it all the time . . . now . . . sometimes I feel like I'm not doing my duty.'

(Juraskova et al. 2003, p. 272)

'I have no sexual desire. I force myself. He's just on top of me and I wait until he's finished.'

(Ashing-Gawa et al. 2004, p. 717)

Adequate sexual functioning involves the combination of a number of factors which come together to form the 'sexual response cycle'. This consists of three phases: desire, arousal and orgasm (Kaplan 1979).

Desire is thought to be the most complex part of the sexual response. It is mediated by testosterone and luteinising hormone, but is also significantly affected by higher centres and can be inhibited by emotions such as anger, anxiety and concerns over body image and self-esteem. Conversely, it is enhanced by touch, visual imagery and fantasy (Wilmoth and Spinelli 2000). Lack of desire is one of the commonest sexual problems after treatment for women with cervical cancer (Corney et al. 1993).

The next steps in the sexual response cycle are arousal to orgasm and orgasm itself. Both require an intact parasympathetic nervous system plus a combination of psychic and somatic stimulation (Wilmoth and Spinelli 2000).

Both the physical and psychological changes associated with cervical cancer and its treatment can contribute to sexual dysfunction. The physical changes have already been discussed in Chapters 3 and 4 and include vaginal stenosis, post-coital bleeding and dyspareunia (Klee et al. 2000, Juraskova et al. 2003). Bladder and bowel dysfunction may also negatively impact sexual function. Inextricably linked with such changes are the psychological and social factors mentioned above (Thranov and Klee 1994). These include anxiety, depression, changes in self-image and relationship changes.

The combination of physical, social and psychological factors can impact sexual function in a variety of ways resulting in:

- dyspareunia
- ovarian failure leading to an early menopause
- a reduced frequency of intercourse
- a compromised ability to become sexually aroused

- impaired orgasm
- reduced ease and spontaneity of sexual pleasuring activities
- altered sexual self-esteem
- altered body-image

(Andersen et al. 1989, Bruner and Boyd 1999, Gamel et al. 2000).

The complexity of the sexual response cycle makes assessment of sexual functioning after treatment for cervical cancer difficult and it is an area of research which has been associated with significant methodological problems. One common shortcoming is the use of sub-optimal assessment tools. A number of scales have been developed to assess sexual function, including the Sexual Adjustment Questionnaire (SAQ), the Sexual Behaviors Questionnaire (SBQ), the Sexual Function After Gynecologic Illness Scale (SFAGIS), Watt's Sexual Functional Questionnaire (WSFQ) and the Sexual function – Vaginal changes questionnaire (SVC) (Bruner and Boyd 1999, Jensen et al. 2004). However, not all studies have utilised such scales, preferring instead to adopt unvalidated tools. For example, some have simply used the frequency of sexual contact or orgasm. Unfortunately frequent sexual intercourse does not necessarily indicate a healthy or fulfilling sexual life.

Another important factor in considering the impact of cervical cancer on sexual function is consideration of pre-morbid sexual wellbeing. A number of women have pre-treatment sexual problems which need to be accounted for when determining the effects of cervical cancer and its therapy (Meston and Bradford 2004). Corney et al. (1993) found that 19% of women receiving treatment for gynaecological cancer reported pre-operative sexual problems. This figure rose to 76% post-operatively.

Despite these methodological issues, there is general consensus that women treated for cervical cancer have significantly higher levels of sexual problems than 'healthy' controls (van de Wiel et al. 1988). When Corney et al. (1993) interviewed a number of women with gynaecological cancer about sexual function they found that amongst those with no pre-existing sexual morbidity, 66% had sexual problems at six months post-treatment and 15% of these never resumed sexual intercourse.

Resuming sexual activity following treatment for cervical cancer is a source of significant concern for many women. Some fear that they will hurt themselves, bleed, or that their vagina will be too small. Others are worried that it will feel different for themselves and/or their partner or that they will no longer be able to have an orgasm (Wilmoth and Spinelli 2000, Zegwaard et al. 2000). Frequently, these concerns are not discussed with the partner, who in turn may have their own anxieties about sex (Zegwaard et al. 2000). It has been reported that partners worry about hurting their spouse and wait for the women to initiate intimate activities (Jursakova et al. 2003).

Indeed, generally the first intercourse post-treatment is instigated by the woman. Many women recall this experience vividly, comparing it with their 'first time', and describing feelings of stress and fear of the unknown (Zegwaard et al. 2000). It is not uncommon for women to feel 'detached' when resuming sexual contact again. Others lose all interest in sex following treatment and participate simply because they feel that they 'should do'.

Although a significant proportion of sexual relationships have been shown to be compromised as a result of cervical cancer, this does not automatically mean that all are threatened. Corney et al. (1993) found half of the women they interviewed felt their sexual relationship had deteriorated, but only 16% felt that their marriage had worsened. Thus, the association between sexual contact and the quality of relationships is a complex one.

Talking about sex

Although many comments can be found in the nursing literature about the importance of the nurse in caring for the psychosexual needs of patients, guidance on precisely what this role should be is less clear. In a study by Wilson and Williams (1988), 91% of nurses agreed that discussion of sexuality should be a routine part of nursing care. However, only 58% felt happy initiating such a discussion.

Many nurses report being happier talking about sex if the discussion has been opened by the patient (Cartwright-Alcaresse 1995). However, it is more than likely that patients are just as uncomfortable as their nurse when it comes to discussing sexual issues. Some will not even have an adequate sexual vocabulary to express their concerns (Corney et al. 1993).

Broaching sexual matters with a newly diagnosed patient may well feel uncomfortable and inappropriate, and at diagnosis many women will not consider sexual function to be of prime importance. However, it is thought that early discussion of sexual morbidity can be helpful in the long term. This is because it paves the way for women to raise the issue of sexuality later, at a time that is comfortable to them. It also makes it easier for the treatment team to bring up the subject during follow-up appointments.

Who, then, should be talking about sexual issues with patients? Is it the role of all nurses or just 'specialists'? Certainly the role of the specialist nurse in caring for the psychosocial and psychosexual needs of the cervical cancer patient would seem to be an important one. For example, Maughan and Clarke (2001) demonstrated that the intervention of a nurse specialist substantially improved the quality of life of women in their recovery from gynaecological cancer.

Skills and experience will largely determine the ability of the nurse to discuss topics of sexuality with patients. It is probably unreasonable to expect newly qualified or inexperienced nurses to broach highly sensitive aspects of sexual dysfunction with patients – particularly when they are unlikely to have the knowledge to offer helpful advice. However, nurses with higher levels of experience and training are better equipped to open discussion in this area.

PLISSIT (Annon 1976) provides a useful tool for nurses wishing to address matters of sexuality with patients. This model identifies different levels of communication regarding sexual function. The depth of communication reached is determined by the assessor's level of experience, knowledge and comfort. Examples of how this model may be employed for communication with women with cervical cancer are given in Box 6.3.

Box 6.3 The PLISSIT model

The PLISSIT (Permission, Limited Information, Specific Suggestion, Intensive Therapy) model (Annon 1976, Wilmoth and Spinelli 2000)

P = Permission: this gives the client permission to talk about sexual issues and should be a comfortable level of discussion for most nurses.
Example: 'Women undergoing this treatment often have questions or concerns about sexuality. Is there anything you would like to discuss?'
LI = Limited information: this refers to factual information given in response to a question or observation. Once again, most nurses would probably feel able to function at this level.
Example: 'While you should not have penetrative intercourse until you have had your six week post-medical check-up, it's fine to kiss and cuddle with your partner. Don't worry if you become aroused . . . it is not harmful and may speed up healing.'
SS = Specific suggestions: this requires a slightly greater level of expertise.
Example: 'If you find penetrative intercourse painful, particularly deep thrusting, you may want to suggest to your partner that you use a side-on position.'
IT = Intensive therapy: this suggests the requirement for more specific intervention and would probably require referral to an appropriate specialist.
Example: 'It sounds to me that the sexual abuse you describe has had long-lasting effects on you. I would like to refer you to a specialist in this area.'
Adapted from Katz (2002)

Management of psychosexual morbidity

The provision of information has been shown to be important in reducing stress and preparing women for the possible psychological sequelae of cervical cancer (Andersen 1992). Unfortunately, there is evidence to suggest that health care professionals are failing to meet all the informational psychosexual needs of gynaecological cancer patients (Bourgeois-Law and Lotocki 1999).

In order to address this deficiency a number of institutions have set up formal sexual health programmes which provide both psychological support and information to patients undergoing treatment for gynaecological malignancies (Robinson et al. 1999). The establishment of a well-structured sexual health programme in a cancer setting has been shown to result in a 70% subjective improvement in sexual health complaints (Amsterdam and Krychman 2006).

As well as providing information in the context of a formal educational programme, nurses are also in a position to offer informal support and advice about intimate sexual topics because of the unique relationships they are able to develop with patients. These relationships can be particularly close and open not only because of the large amount of time nurses spend in close contact with patients but also because of the sensitive nature of some of the activities they have to perform.

There is little research that has specifically aimed to determine *when* different types of psychosexual support should be offered to women with cervical cancer, and it is likely that different information and interventions are required at different times. Gamel et al. (2000) identified three distinct phases in cervical cancer treatment and follow-up, each requiring different types of support:

(1) Diagnosis and treatment period
   In the diagnosis and treatment period, women have questions about the effects of treatment on sexuality, although they may have difficulty retaining information because they are often in a state of shock (Weijmar Schultz et al. 1992).
(2) Recovery and first intercourse
   The second phase encompasses early recovery and the first intercourse. At this time many women seek practical guidance and advice regarding resuming sexual relationships. For example, they want to know whether pain and bleeding will occur during or after intercourse, or whether physical complications such as incontinence and radiation changes in the vagina will influence sexual activities (Gamel et al. 2000, Zegwaard et al. 2000).

   This is also a time when practical information about sexual activity might be useful. For example, in the early stages of treatment it is sometimes suggested that women resume limited intimate activities before engaging in full sexual intercourse (Juraskova et al. 2003). Couples may also wish to explore different methods of sexual expression such as massage, mutual masturbation and the use of sex aids. Advising the use of extended foreplay may help with arousal (Robertson 2005).

   Patients experiencing difficulties with symptoms may be helped by practical advice. For example, dyspareunia is a common problem but may be alleviated by pelvic floor exercises and the use of water-based lubricants. A change of sexual position may also be helpful. Some women who have received radiotherapy report a burning sensation when semen touches some of the vaginal tissues, which may be alleviated by using condoms (Robertson 2005).
(3) The period of rebuilding sexual life
   Rebuilding a sex life is a process that may continue for several years and is often still ongoing at two years after the diagnosis of cervical cancer (Gamel et al. 2000). The process is significantly influenced by the experience of their first intercourse after treatment (Zegwaard et al. 2000). During this period ongoing information is required about potential long-term problems that may be encountered.

> **Box 6.4 Nursing management of psychosexual needs of patients with cervical cancer**
>
> - identifying women with high risk coping styles and offering more nursing follow-up to these women
> - giving information about support groups and sources of information at diagnosis, six and twelve months after diagnosis
> - ensuring that leaflets and posters about support are readily available at clinic locations
> - focusing on symptom control
> - ensuring that sexual functioning is discussed and that there are mechanisms by which women with significant dysfunction can be treated

Support for partners and families

'At the end of the day, I will never know what she has been through, but perhaps in a way she will never know what I have been thinking . . . We talk about things . . . But, you know, sometimes you can never talk about your darkest fears.'

(Maughan et al. 2002, pp. 33)

The impact of the disease on partners, children and families is almost as great as the impact on the patient themselves and for this reason they require considerable support (Maughan et al. 2002). It is therefore unfortunate that partners and families sometimes seem to be overlooked during cervical cancer treatment. Lalos et al. (1995) found that most partners had not been given even basic information about the cancer and its treatment. Some wrongly believed that they had given the cancer to their partner through sexual intercourse (Carlsson and Strang 1998).

The research available on useful support interventions for men is limited. However, it would appear that men and women are interested in different types of support. Specifically, looking at self-help groups, male partners seem more likely to participate in those with more educational aspects (Taylor et al. 1998 cited in Carlsson and Strang 1998).

Partners will benefit from information about what to expect from treatment and should also be prepared for the fact that even if a full physical recovery has been made the emotional impact of the disease on the couple may be only just beginning. It is important to offer joint counselling to the couple, especially with regards to sexual functioning following treatment. It might also be useful to discuss sexual functioning with partners separately to discuss any concerns that they may not wish to share with their spouse.

Talking to children

The very word 'cancer' provokes anxiety amongst most people, and children who are old enough to understand are no different. Many women choose not to disclose their diagnosis to their children. This is not necessarily 'wrong' except that children may well overhear discussions with other family members and it might be better to tell them directly rather than them hearing the news second-hand.

News of their mother's diagnosis will affect children differently depending on their age and developmental stage. For example, young children may be concerned about the family staying together whereas older school-aged children may be worried about the disruptions caused by the illness (Lowdermilk and Germino 2000). Adolescents may want to be supportive and help care for the woman, or they may not want to be involved at all and may resent having to help. They may also be concerned about heredity and whether or not they will also be at risk of developing cancer (Lowdermilk and Germino 2000). Hence, children of different ages need to have their mother's illness discussed with them according to their individual and developmental needs (See Box 6.5).

No matter how old the children are, their mother's illness and treatment will disrupt life for a substantial period of time. She will have a reduced ability to carry out her normal roles, and is likely to require considerable support in order to care for her children. Where the woman experiences psychological morbidity this support may be required for months or even years following treatment.

Long-term support and the role of support groups

'Well, the way I got through it was by talking to people . . . I've got other friends who had breast cancer . . . I think what helps you to cope with it sometimes is when you know somebody who got through it, I think that helps.'

(Juraskova et al. 2003, p. 274)

'I was treated two years ago, I have never talked to anyone about it. I haven't met anyone else with cervical cancer. I felt like I was put in the middle of a field and left to find my own way home.'

(Jo's Trust)

At diagnosis, a woman with cervical cancer will receive support from the multidisciplinary team and from friends and family. During treatment, this level of social and professional support remains – the patient is in 'fighting' mode. On news that margins are clear, lymph nodes are unaffected or chemoradiation seems to be shrinking the tumour, the treatment team act in a positive way, and friends and family may celebrate, but for the patient this news may or may not be so well received. Whilst for some, celebration of the end of treatment may herald the beginning of their recovery, for others it may signify the abrupt removal of major social and professional support and the beginning of coming to terms with the fact that they have been diagnosed with cancer (Arora et al. 2006).

Although clinical follow-up regimens for women with cervical cancer are well established, psychological follow-up is less formalised and is entirely dependent on the skills of the clinical staff in both recognising psychological difficulties and providing appropriate counselling. Those who seek support are unlikely to be at the highest risk – it is women who do not seek support due to the employment of denial and avoidance as coping mechanisms who are most likely to need proactive management (Chan et al. 2001). For a small proportion of these women, referral to a clinical psychologist may be necessary.

Some – but not all – women may benefit from support groups to help them to come to terms with their cancer. For some it may be a time when contact with others 'in the same boat' may be useful. In this way they can find out more about treatments from those who have experienced them. It also provides a forum for the discussion of other practical concerns which may not seem important to health professionals but are important to patients, such as what to wear in hospital post-surgery.

For others a support group at the time of diagnosis may be the last thing that they want. Attending meetings or seeing other women in a similar situation may be perceived as too difficult. Many women do not join internet support groups such as Jo's Trust or Hystersisters until two years or more following their initial diagnosis. At this time they think they should be 'over' their cancer and 'getting back to normal' and yet they do not seem to be. Indeed, it has been found that although the need to discuss their cancer continues for at least two years following the end of initial treatment, the ability to discuss this with others decreases rapidly after the first six months (Klee et al. 2000).

Information about the availability of support groups locally, nationally and internationally should be given to the woman and her family at diagnosis.

Box 6.5 Talking to children – some tips for mothers

The information in this section is general – each child will have different needs at each stage. Helping children understand your experience of cancer needs sensitivity and a good sense of timing. Your children may go through some of the feelings that you may have, such as disbelief, anger, uncertainty, hope, fear and acceptance. They may have special needs because of their ages, and these may change at different stages of your illness.

(1) Five years and under

The youngest children fear separation, strangers and being left alone. If you are in hospital, arrange for a familiar person to stay with them. Talk to them and assure them you are coming home from hospital soon and that you think of them when you are apart. If they come to visit you, suggest they bring a well-loved toy with them. You can give them something special (such as a toy or a blanket) that they can keep with them when they are at home, to remind them that you are thinking of them and that you care about them.

Young children often feel they have magical powers and that what they wish will come true. They may feel guilty that a parent is ill, or that they have had bad thoughts about a parent. Assure them that nothing they have done, said or thought could have caused your illness. They may also worry that they too will get cancer, and it is helpful to let them know that cancer is not 'catching'.

(2) Ages 6–11

Children between six and eleven may be very concerned about a parent's health. It is important not to put pressure on them or worry them with details.

Many children of this age have a basic knowledge of body parts and their functions, and can understand simple explanations about the cancer and its effects on the body.

Children may show their worry or concern through disturbances in eating, sleeping, schoolwork or friendships. Children at any age may start behaving like younger children. Sometimes it is just their way of saying 'I'm here too'.

Let the children's teachers and school nurse know about your illness, as their suggestions and understanding may help if there are any problems. You could also ask your child if there is anyone they would like you to tell about the cancer, such as their brownie or cub scout leader or their friends' parents.

(3) Teenagers

Teenagers can have an especially hard time – adolescence is not an easy phase of growing up in any case. Their emotions are sometimes complicated and troublesome. They may find it hard to talk to you or to show you how they feel, and at times their behaviour may be difficult for everyone to deal with.

At a time when they are probably struggling to be grown-up they may feel that it will be seen as childish to show their emotions or to ask for help. They may stop talking to you because they are trying to appear strong for you, or are worried that they will be misunderstood.

It may help to reassure them that talking about their feelings and worries is a positive way of coping and is how adults often deal with stressful situations. If they are finding it hard to talk to you, encourage them to talk to someone close who can support them, such as a relative or family friend.

Your illness may mean that they are asked to take on more responsibility than they had before. This can be a positive experience for them if they feel that their efforts are helpful and recognised. However, difficulties can arise if they feel over-burdened with responsibility to the point of not having their own needs met. Teenagers need to be included and consulted as adults, but will continue to need guidance, support and reassurance.

Boys may have difficulty dealing with women's cancers due to self-consciousness around the time of puberty, and girls may worry that they will develop the same type of cancer.

Types of 'support group'

One-to-one support

For some women, discussing their worries one to one with someone who has also been through cervical cancer treatment may be very helpful. In order to facilitate this it may be useful to have a list of patients who are willing to talk to women who have just been diagnosed with cervical cancer. However, it should be remembered that this is an intensive and potentially difficult activity for those who have been treated in the past and it is necessary to keep checking that these women are still happy to carry out this type of support.

General cancer support groups (local)

The benefit of a group is that it can offer social support and friendship which may not be accessible elsewhere. However, it is important to bear in mind that the issues surrounding genital cancer are difficult to discuss openly and therefore general cancer support groups, whilst offering help with dealing with cancer as a disease may be of limited use in terms of the longer term sexual sequelae of cervical cancer. Many women with cervical cancer feel that breast cancer, for example, is a more socially acceptable cancer. Both diseases are associated with changes in body image and sexuality, but the specific issues are very different in cervical cancer and cannot necessarily be discussed with breast cancer patients. Additionally, the success of support groups – even those dedicated to the gynaecological cancers – may be dependent on the similarity of women attending them in terms of life experience and age. Many young women with cervical cancer express a difficulty with being able to relate to older women with the disease.

Internet support groups

These have the benefit of being internationally available. There are several Internet sites that deal specifically either with gynaecological cancer (Hystersisters, DipEx) or one that is cervical cancer-specific (Jo's Trust). Internet support groups allow women to gain support and information whilst remaining completely anonymous (unless the woman wishes to make herself known, either using her name or a pseudonym). Participation in discussions can be as involved or remote as required and women can visit the sites as often or seldom as they want.

The disadvantages of Internet support groups are that participants cannot always meet face to face (although this facility is offered by some). Additionally, some women find themselves accessing the site excessively, potentially at the expense of seeking help from friends and family. Furthermore, whilst useful in providing long-term support these sites may also trigger an unhelpful emotional dependency because of the ease of access. Nevertheless, many women find the support gained from Internet sites hugely beneficial.

Conclusion

The impact of cervical cancer on psychological wellbeing, social functioning, sex and sexuality is significant. Some women will experience long-term psychological morbidity and sexual dysfunction as a result of the disease and its treatment. Support from both within and outside the family is essential to overcome these effects. The role of the nurse is important in the psychosocial assessment of patients, in the provision of support and in facilitating onward referral to specialist services for those women who would benefit from more protracted or intensive counselling or psychosexual therapy.

Frequently asked questions

(1) When will I start to feel 'back to normal'?

This is a highly individual thing and for some women the definition of 'normal' will alter irrevocably. However, whilst it is to be hoped that you make a full recovery within weeks and months of finishing your treatment this is not the case for a number of women and you should not feel abnormal or inadequate if you do not return to normal for some years. That said, if you feel your progress is too slow you may benefit from some counselling or from joining a support group. Discuss these possibilities with your doctor.

(1) What happens at follow-up appointments?

At follow-up appointments you will be seen by your consultant or registrar who will ask you questions about your wellbeing and any symptoms. They will conduct a physical examination and will usually conduct a vaginal examination. If your treatment left you free of disease it is unlikely that scans will be necessary unless you are experiencing symptoms which require further investigation.

(3) How do I talk to my partner about how I am feeling?

Broaching the subject of feelings with a partner, especially when it comes to sensitive issues such as sex and sexuality, can be difficult. It is probable that your partner will be experiencing a wide range of fears and emotions too. If you are finding it hard to discuss these matters it may be helpful to employ a third party. Your doctor should be able to help you find a counsellor to assist with this.

(4) I am worrying about every ache and pain. How do I deal with it?

First of all be assured that as difficult as this problem is it is extremely normal. And it is something that will remain with you for a long time. Maybe even for ever. However, most women do find that as time passes these fears become more manageable. Once again, if you feel you are preoccupied with fears about your body it may be helpful to seek help from a counsellor.

(5) How will I know if my menopause starts if I don't have periods any more?

It is possible that you will experience some of the symptoms associated with menopause such as flushes and mood swings. It is unlikely that you will pass through the menopause without feeling anything at all.

(6) Will sex ever feel the same again?

The treatment you have undergone for your cancer has a significant physical and psychological impact. Not only does it change your body but it also changes the way you think and can lead to significant relationship changes. In the light of this it is unlikely that sex will feel the same as it felt before. This does not, however, have to mean that sex will feel worse, just different.

(7) What do I tell people about my cancer?

This is a very subjective and private matter. Some people chose to disclose details of their disease openly whereas others conceal it even from their closest friends. The stigma that has traditionally been associated with cancer of the cervix may make disclosure of the disease more difficult for many women. This is a matter for you, and perhaps for your partner, to discuss and decide.

Resources

Jo's Trust: www.jotrust.co.uk
CancerBacup: www.cancerbacup.org.uk
TellHer: www.tellher.com
Eyes on the Prize: www.eyesontheprize.org

References

Amsterdam A and Krychman ML (2006) Sexual dysfunction in patients with gynaecologic neoplasms: a retrospective pilot study. *Journal of Sexual Medicine*, 3 (4), 646–649

Andersen BL and LeGrand J (1991) Body image for women: conceptualization, assessment and a test of its importance to sexual dysfunction and medical illness. *The Journal of Sex Research*, 28 (3), 457–477

Andersen BL (1992) Psychological interventions for cancer patients to enhance the quality of life. *Journal of Consulting and Clinical Psychology*, 60 (4), 552–568

Andersen BL, Anderson B and de Prosse C (1989) Controlled prospective longitudinal study of women with cancer. I. Sexual functioning outcomes. *J Consult Clin Psychol*, 57 (6), 683–697

Annon JS (1976) *The Behavioural Treatment of Sexual Problems*. Vol 1, *Brief Therapy*. Harper and Row, New York

Arora NK, Finney Rutten LJ, Gustafson DH, et al. (2006) Perceived helpfulness and impact of social support provided by family, friends and health care providers to women newly diagnosed with breast cancer. *Psycho-oncology*, 16, 474–486

Ashing-Gawa KT, Kagawa-Singer M, Padilla GV, et al. (2004) The impact of cervical cancer and dysplasia: a qualitative multiethnic study. *Psycho-oncology*, 13, 709–728

Bergmark K, Avall-Lundqvist E, Dickman PW, Henningsohn L and Steineck G (2002) Patient-rating of distressful symptoms after treatment for early cervical cancer. *Acta Obstet Gynecol Scand*, 81, 443–450

Bishop T (2004) Female sexual dysfunction. *Practice Nurse*, 28 (9), 62–67

Booth K, Beaver K, Kitchener H, O'Neill J and Farrell C (2005) Women's experiences of information, psychological distress and worry after treatment for gynaecological cancer. *Patient Education and Counselling*, 56, 225–232

Bos-Branolte G (1991) Gynaecological cancer: a psychotherapy group, in Watson, Maggie (ed.) *Cancer Patient Care: Psychosocial Treatment Methods*. Cambridge University Press, Cambridge. pp. 260–280, 320

Bourgeois-Law G and Lotocki R (1999) Sexuality and gynaecological cancer: a needs assessment. *The Canadian Journal of Human Sexuality*, 8 (4), 231–240

Bradley S, Rose S, Lutgendorf S, Constanzo E and Anderson B (2006) Quality of life and mental health in cervical and endometrial cancer survivors. *Gynaecol Oncol*, 100, 479–486

Bruner DW and Boyd CP (1999) Assessing women's sexuality after cancer therapy: checking assumptions with the focus group technique. *Cancer Nursing*, 22 (6), 483–447

Butler-Manuel SA, Summerville K, Ford A, et al. (1999) Self-assessment of morbidity following radical hysterectomy for cervical cancer. *J Obstetrics Gynaecology*, 19 (2), 180–183

Carlsson ME and Strang PM (1998) Educational support programmes for gynaecological cancer patients and their families. *Acta Oncologica*, 37 (3), 269–275

Carr G (1991) Sexuality – a topical issue for nursing. *Nursing Standard*, 6 (1), 52–55

Carter J, Rowland K, Chi D, et al. (2005) Gynecologic cancer treatment and the impact of cancer-related infertility. *Gynecologic Oncol*, 97, 90–95

Cartwright-Alcaresse F (1995) Addressing sexual dysfunction following radiation therapy for a gynaecologic malignancy. *Oncology Nursing Forum*, 22, 1227–1232

Chan YM, Ngan HYS, Li BYG, et al. (2001) A longitudinal study on quality of life after gynaecologic cancer treatment. *Gynecologic Oncol*, 83, 10–19

Constanzo ES, Lutgendorf SK, Rothrock NE and Anderson B (2006) Coping and quality of life among women extensively treated for gynaecologic cancer. *Psycho-oncology*, 15, 132–142

Corney RH, Crowther ME and Howells A (1993) Psychosexual dysfunction in women with gynaecological cancer following radical pelvic surgery. *British Journal of Obstetrics and Gynaecology*, 100, 73–78

De Groot JM, Mah K, Fyles A, et al. (2005) The psychosocial impact of cervical cancer among affected women and their partners. *Int J Gynecol Cancer*, 15, 918–925

Detmar SB, Aaronson NK, Wever LVD, Muller M and Schornagel JH (2000) How are you feeling? Who wants to know? Patients' and oncologists' preferences for discussing health-related quality-of-life issues. *J Clin Oncol*, 18, 3295–3301

Edgren G (2007) Risk of anogenital cancer after diagnosis of cervical intraepithelial neoplasia: a prospective, population based study. *Lancet Oncology*, 8 (4), 311–316

Fowler J, Carpenter K, Gupta P, Golden-Kreutz D and Andersen B (2004) The gynecologic oncology consult: symptom presentation and concurrent symptoms of depression and anxiety. *Obstetrics and Gynecology*, 103 (6), 1211–1217

Franco EL, Duarte-Franco E and Ferenczy A (2001) Cervical cancer: epidemiology, prevention and the role of human papilloma virus infection. *CMAJ*, 164 (7), 1017

Gamel C, Hengeveld M and Davis B (2000) Informational needs about the effects of gynaecological cancer on sexuality: a review of the literature. *J Clin Nurs*, 9, 678–688

Greimel E, Thiel I, Peintinger F, Cegnar I and Pongratz E (2002) Prospective assessment of quality of life in female cancer patients. *Gynecologic Oncol*, 85, 140–147

Hawighorst-Knapstein S, Fusshoeller C, Franz C, et al. (2004) The impact of treatment for genital cancer on quality of life and body image – results of a prospective, longitudinal one-year study. *Gynaecologic Oncology*, 94, 398–403

Jensen PT, Klee MC, Thranov I and Groenvold M (2004) Validation of a questionnaire for self-assessment of sexual function and vaginal changes after gynaecological cancer. *Psycho-oncology*, 13, 577–592

Juraskova I, Butow P, Robertson R, Sharpe L, McLeod C and Hacker N (2003) Post-treatment sexual adjustment following cervical and endometrial cancer: a qualitative insight. *Psycho-oncology*, 12, 267–297

Kaplan HS (1979) *Disorders of Sexual Desire*. Simon & Schuster, New York

Katz A (2002) Sexuality after hysterectomy. *JOGNN*, 31 (3), May/June, 256–262

Klee M, Thranov I and Machin D (2000) Life after radiotherapy: the psychological and social effects experienced by women treated for advanced stages of cervical cancer. *Gynaecol Oncol*, 76, 5–13

Lalos A, Jacobsson L, Lalos O and Stendahl U (1995) Experiences of the male partner in cervical and endometrial cancer – a prospective interview study. *J Psychosom Obstet Gynaecol*, 16, 153–165

Lowdermilk D and Germino B (2000) Helping women and their families cope with the impact of gynaecologic cancer. *Journal of Obstetric, Gynaecologic and Neonatal Nursing*, 29 (6), pp. 653–660

Lutgendorf SK, Anderson B, Larsen K, Buller RE and Sorosky J (1999) Cognitive processing, social support coping, and distress in gynaecologic cancer patients. *Cancer Res Ther Control*, 8, 123–137

Lutgendorf SK, Anderson B, Ulrich P, et al. (2002) Quality of life and mood in women with gynaecologic cancer. *Cancer*, 94 (1), 131–140

McIntosh H (1996) Patients wrestle with anxiety and fear in treatment choices affecting sexuality. *JNCI*, 88 (22), 1618–1620

Matsushita T, Murata H, Matsushima E, Sakata Y, Miyasaka N and Aso T (2007) Quality of life in gynecological inpatients undergoing surgery. *Health Care for Women International*, 28 (9), Sep, 828–842

Maughan K and Clarke C (2001) The effect of a clinical nurse specialist in gynaecology oncology on quality of life and sexuality. *Journal of Clinical Nursing*, 10 (2), 221–229

Maughan K, Heyman B and Matthews M (2002) In the shadow of risk: how men cope with a partner's gynaecological cancer. *International Journal of Nursing Studies*, 39, 27–34

Meston CM and Bradford A (2004) A brief review of the factors influencing sexuality after hysterectomy. *Sexual and Relationship Therapy*, 19 (1), 5–12

Miller BE, Pittman B and Strong C (2003) Gynaecologic cancer patients' psychosocial needs and their views on the physician's role in meeting those needs. *International Journal of Gynaecological Cancer*, 13 (2), 111–119

Petersen RW, Graham G and Quinlivan JA (2005) Psychologic changes after gynaecologic cancer. *The Journal of Obstetrics and Gynaecological Research*, 31 (2), 152–157

Price B (1998) Cancer: altered body image. *Nursing Standard*, 12 (21), 49–55

Robertson R (2005) Sexuality and body image, in Lancaster T and Nattress K (eds) *Gynaecological Cancer Care*. Ausmed Publications, Melbourne. pp. 289–302

Robinson J, Faris P and Scott C (1999) Psychoeducational group increases vaginal dilatation for younger women and reduces sexual fears for women of all ages with gynaecological cancer treated with radiotherapy. *International Journal of Radiation Oncology Biology and Physics*, 44, 497–506

Schrover LR, Fife M and Gershenson DM (1989) Sexual dysfunction and treatment for early stage cervical cancer. *Cancer*, 63, 204–212

Schwartz CE and Sprangers MAD (1999) Methodological approaches for assessing response shift in longitudinal quality of life research. *Social Science and Medicine*, 48, 1531–1548

Schwartz CE, Merriman MP, Reed GW and Hammes BJ (2004) Measuring patient treatment preferences in end-of-life care research: applications for advance care planning interventions and response shift research. *Journal of Palliative Medicine*, 7 (2), 233–245

Slattery ML, Overall JC, Abbott TM, French TK, Robinson LM and Gardner J (1989) Sexual activity, contraception, genital infections and cervical cancer: support for a sexually transmitted disease hypothesis. *Am J Epidemiol*, 130 (2), 248–258

Skye Caldwell R (2003) An exploration of the unique experience of survivors of gynaecologic cancer: sexuality and body image. PhD dissertation, Institute of Transpersonal Psychology, Palo Alto, California

Steginga SK and Dunn J (1997) Women's experiences following treatment for gynecologic cancer. *Oncol Nurs Forum*, 24, 1403–1406.

Sukegawa A, Miyagi E, Suzuki R, et al. (2006) Post-traumatic stress disorder in patients with gynaecologic cancers. *J Obstet Gynecol Res*, 32 (3), 349–353

Thoits PA (1986) Social support as coping assistance. *J Consult Clin Psychol*, 54, 416–423

Thompson DS and Shear MK (1998) Psychiatric disorders and gynecological oncology: a review of the literature. *Gen Hosp Psychiatry*, 20, 241–247

Thranov I and Klee M (1994) Sexuality among gynaecologic cancer patients: a cross-sectional study. *Gynaecologic Oncology*, 52, 14–19

Turns D (2001) Psychosocial issues: pelvic exenterative surgery. *Journal of Surgical Oncology*, 76, 224–236

Vistad I, Fossa SD and Dahl AA (2006) A critical review of patient-related quality of life studies of long-term survivors of cervical cancer. *Gynecologic Oncol*, 102, 563–572

Weijmar Schultz WCM, van de Wiel HBM and van Son-Schoones N (1991) Sexuality and chronic somatic illness. *Tijdschrift voor Seksuologie*, 15, 114–122

Weijmar Schultz WCM, van de Wiel HBM, Hahn DEE and Bouma J (1992) Psychosexual functioning after treatment for gynaecological cancer: an integrative model, review of determinant factors and clinical guidelines. *Int J Gynaecol Cancer*, 2, 281–290

Wenzel L, DeAlba I, Habbal R, et al. (2005) Quality of life in long-term cancer survivors. *Gynecologic Oncol*, 97, 310–317

van de Wiel HBM, Weijmar Schultz WCM, Hallensleben A, Thurkow FG and Bouma J (1988) Sexual functioning following treatment of cervical carcinoma. *European Journal of Gynaecologic Oncology*, 4, 275–281

Wilmoth MC and Spinelli A (2000) Sexual implications of gynaecologic cancer treatments. *Journal of Obstetric, Gynaecologic and Neonatal Nursing*, 29 (4), 413–423

Wilson ME and Williams HA (1988) Oncology nurses' attitudes and behaviours related to sexuality of patients with cancer. *Oncology Nursing Forum*, 15, 49–53

Yates P (1999) Family coping: issues and challenges for cancer nursing. *Cancer Nursing*, 22 (1), 63–71

Zegwaard MI, Gamel CJ, Dugris DJ and Logmans A (2000) De beleving van seksualiteit en informatie vourziening van vrouw en partner na behandeling van cervixcancer (The experience of sexuality and information received in women with cervical cancer and their partners). *Verpleegkunde*, 15 (1), 18–27

Chapter 7

Fertility and menopause

Mary Ryan and Ellen Barlow

'Even though I am dealing with a life threatening disease it is dealing with infertility that is the hardest thing!! I think it is because that we have been robbed of our future dreams of our own family.'

(Jo's Trust)

Introduction

Many women diagnosed with cervical cancer will not only have to deal with the burden of having a life-threatening illness but will also be confronted with the prospect of treatment-related infertility and premature menopause. This chapter provides an overview of the options available to women of childbearing potential who wish to maintain their fertility, and pre-menopausal women who want to ameliorate the unpleasant symptoms associated with a premature menopause.

Fertility

Recent decades have seen marked advances in cancer management. No more evident are these advances than when we consider the preservation of fertility amongst women of childbearing age with cancer in their reproductive organs.

The diagnosis of cancer causes a tremendous upheaval for a woman, and when the possibility of infertility is added the result can be devastating. We have learnt from Chapter 1 that the average age for developing cancer of the cervix is 30 to 50 years, with around 30% percent of women developing the disease before the age of 45 years. An increasing number of women – particularly in Western countries – are delaying having children until they are well into their thirties or early forties (Marhhom and Cohen 2006). For such women a diagnosis of cervical cancer may arrive just at the time when fertility issues become relevant to them.

When a person is diagnosed with cancer the paramount goal is to treat the disease. Within the field of gynaecological oncology there are now a number of surgical options which preserve a woman's fertility while treating her cervical cancer. In some cases it might be necessary to combine these surgical options with Assisted Reproductive Technology (ART) in order to give the woman the best chance of becoming a mother.

To ensure the woman is able to make an informed choice about her childbearing options, referral to a fertility clinic early in the diagnostic period is necessary (Pearce 2005). The American Society of Clinical Oncology in 2006 published the following recommendations regarding management of fertility options in cancer treatment:

'As part of the education and informed consent before cancer therapy, oncologists should address the possibility of infertility with patients treated in their reproductive years and be prepared to discuss possible fertility preservation options or refer appropriate and interested patients to reproductive specialists.'

(ASCO 2006)

Psychological effects of infertility

Apart from radical trachelectomy virtually all treatments for cervical cancer cause infertility. Sudden unanticipated loss of reproductive potential is known to have long-term negative consequences for women who have been treated for cervical cancer (Wenzel et al. 2005). For some, the impact of this is even greater than that of the diagnosis of cancer. The prospect of treatment related infertility may further compound the stigmatisation already felt from a cancer diagnosis.

Loss of fertility has a particularly powerful effect on women who equate their ability to conceive with their sense of femininity and it may take many years to come to terms with – if at all. In one study, 80% of women were frequently distressed by their infertility 12 months following treatment for cervical cancer and 50% were unable to accept their infertility at all (Carter et al. 2005).

Issues concerning the potential loss of reproductive function are not restricted to women who are childless. The inability to complete a family can impact women who already have children but who may have desired more (Wenzel et al. 2005). Those whose families are completed might also mourn a loss of reproductive function. However, probably the most powerful challenges face those women who wish for a family and have not yet begun to have one. For these individuals the desire to conceive a child can be almost all-consuming. Some may even choose a less toxic treatment regime to preserve fertility despite the fact that it could confer less protection from recurrence.

Conversely, not all women of childbearing potential will want to have children. For some, the diagnosis of a life-threatening illness may result in considering different ways of including children in their life.

Employing methods to conserve fertility in the presence of a cancer diagnosis is also likely to have a considerable emotional impact, although unfortunately this is an area which is not well described in the literature (Carter et al. 2007a). Some of the fertility-preserving options available to women with cervical cancer are discussed below. It is important to remember that not all countries will have access to such technologies. An extreme lack of services exists, for example, in certain African countries (Cooke 2007). Furthermore, while most developed countries will have access to the technologies, availability will vary from centre to centre. With some of the more controversial interventions such as surrogacy, governing statutes will also vary within the country, depending on local and state laws (Gossfeld and Cullen 2000, Pearce 2005).

Surgical options

The fertility-preserving surgical options available will depend on the stage of the cervix cancer at diagnosis (Gershenson 2005) and are discussed below.

Cone biopsy

A woman diagnosed with an early stage invasive cancer (IA1), where there is no extensive lymph vascular space invasion, may be treated with cone biopsy alone therefore preserving her uterus and ovaries (Hacker 2005). It is vital that the surgical margins of a cone biopsy are clear to ensure minimal risk of recurrence of the cancer. A cone biopsy alone is not adequate treatment where the cancer extends beyond stage IA1. However, for women with stage IA2 cervical cancer with no lymph vascular space invasion and clear margins, a large cone biopsy with lymph node dissection could be recommended. For more advanced cancers a radical trachelectomy would be considered.

Radical trachelectomy

Prior to radical trachelectomy the only options available to women with early stage invasive cervical carcinoma were surgery which involved the removal of the uterus, or radiotherapy, both of which significantly reduced childbearing options. Radical trachelectomy (either vaginal or abdominal) is an important advance in fertility-preserving surgery and is appropriate for women with stage IA1 cervical cancer with extensive lymph vascular space invasion or with stage IA2 or IB1 when the lesions are less than or equal to 2 cm (Stehman et al. 2003) (see Chapter 3).

The option of radical trachelectomy may not be available to all women, because it is a relatively new procedure and surgeons are still developing skills and experience. Furthermore, radical trachelectomy as fertility preserving surgery does not guarantee the future reproductive ability of a woman. Referral for counselling at a fertility clinic would still be advisable to determine any existing fertility issues between the woman and her partner. Women commonly describe fears about their reproductive ability following this surgery (Carter et al. 2007b). These fears are not unfounded, as a pregnancy following radical trachelectomy is considered high risk following reports of second trimester loss and prematurity at rates higher than that of the general population (Leitao and Chi 2005).

Neoadjuvant chemotherapy (followed by radical surgery, see Chapter 5)

When the cervical cancer lesion exceeds 2 cm, or when the local disease is more advanced, the option of radical trachelectomy is not recommended. Another option for these women is neoadjuvant chemotherapy followed by radical surgery. This form of treatment is particularly relevant for women who are diagnosed with advanced cervical cancer during pregnancy. The benefit of this treatment is that the woman does not have to have radiotherapy, therefore reducing the risk of premature loss of ovarian function without increased toxicity or loss of survival benefit (Benedetti-Panici et al. 2002). Neoadjuvant chemotherapy which is given prior to definitive treatment has the potential of reducing or eliminating the cancer while preserving ovarian function and therefore fertility (Plante and Roy 2006). Usually, the woman is treated with a combination of platinum based chemotherapeutic agents, or cisplatin may be given as a single agent, (see Box 7.1). The long-term effects of using neoadjuvant chemotherapy followed by radical surgery instead of using conventional radiotherapy have not been the subject of definitive clinical trials. However, available data suggests that this method of treatment for women who wish to preserve their fertility or avoid premature menopause is promising (Plante and Roy 2006).

Ovarian transposition

For women who do not have the option of conservative surgery, transposition of the ovaries will protect their ovarian tissue, giving them the opportunity to undergo embryo creation and freezing, egg freezing or ovarian tissue freezing. Despite ethical and legal obstacles, pregnancies can result from fertilised eggs retrieved from transposed ovaries following hysterectomy, radiotherapy and chemotherapy (Steigrad et al. 2005). Ovarian transposition is discussed more fully later in this chapter.

Box 7.1 Cancer in pregnancy, a case study

Brenda (not her real name) is 31 years old and has been in a stable relationship with her partner, James, for some years. Soon after stopping the oral contraceptive pill Brenda fell pregnant but unfortunately suffered a miscarriage. Another positive pregnancy test was soon returned. It was during this pregnancy that a routine Pap smear revealed a high grade abnormality. Referral for a colposcopically directed biopsy showed an invasive squamous cell carcinoma. Stage IB1 squamous cell carcinoma with extensive lymph vascular space invasion and positive ectocervical and endocervical margins was diagnosed following cone biopsy.

When Brenda was referred to a gynaecological oncologist she was 24 weeks pregnant. Brenda and James were very keen to continue with this pregnancy despite the inherent risks. Recommendation was made for:

(1) Radical hysterectomy and pelvic lymphadenectomy to offer Brenda the best prognosis.
(2) Neoadjuvant chemotherapy to allow the pregnancy to continue to near term, followed by a caesarean section and radical hysterectomy plus lymph node dissection.

Brenda and James, after careful informed consideration, chose the option of neoadjuvant single agent cisplatin under the supervision of a medical oncologist.

Brenda received three cycles of intravenous cisplatin at three-weekly intervals. The treatment was tolerated reasonably well in terms of toxicity and no foetal distress was noted. Brenda was prepared for surgery and a healthy baby boy was delivered at 33 weeks via a classical caesarean section. Following the birth of her baby the operation proceeded to a radical hysterectomy, lymphadenectomy, transposition of the ovaries and insertion of a supra-pubic catheter. The surgical findings were of a grade II squamous cell carcinoma of the cervix with extensive lymph vascular space invasion. All of the lymph nodes were negative for cancer. Brenda went on to receive some external beam radiotherapy and now several years later she is doing well with no signs suggestive of a recurrence of her cancer and her son is thriving.

Assisted Reproductive Technology (ART) options

'Assisted Reproductive Technology is the application of laboratory or clinical technology to gametes and/or embryos for the purposes of reproduction.'

(NHMRC 2007)

There are an increasing number of ART options available to women undergoing cancer treatments. These include cryopreservation of embryos, oocytes and ovarian tissue. An important consideration in employing ART is that it might involve a delay in definitive cancer treatment. The desire to maintain fertility must therefore be balanced against the chance of compromising cure. This results in ethical, medical and social dilemmas. The use of ART might be necessary for women even when the uterus has been conserved, such as following trachelectomy.

Some of the different assisted reproduction technologies are discussed below.

Embryo cryopreservation

Embryo cryopreservation is the most widely used method of preserving fertility (Lee et al. 2006). The procedure is more commonly used for those who are in an established relationship, unless the woman is willing to use donor sperm (Roberts and Oktay 2005). Usual IVF stimulation regimes may be used except where time is limited.

Stimulation usually commences at the start of the menstrual cycle, meaning that a delay in cancer treatment of two to six weeks may be required. The process involves stimulation of the ovaries to produce adequate oocytes. Stimulation of the ovaries requires commitment from the woman to administer hormones to suppress ovulation and to stimulate follicle production. The follicles are then aspirated from the ovary via the vagina, under the guidance of ultrasound (Pearce 2005). The whole cycle will take around three weeks (Pearce 2005). Following retrieval the oocytes are fertilised in vitro and the resulting embryos are frozen indefinitely (Pearce 2005).

Embryo cryopreservation will not be appropriate for all women because of the necessity to delay cancer treatment (Marhhom and Cohen 2006). The procedure also carries significant ethical implications regarding how to manage the unused frozen embryos (Bankowski et al. 2005). For example, what happens to frozen embryos if the 'parents' separate or the cancer treatment has been unsuccessful? These issues not only apply to embryo cryopreservation but also the fate of frozen oocytes and ovarian tissue. Bankowski and colleagues (2005) have recognised the need for further exploration of these implications.

Oocyte cryopreservation

The option of freezing eggs in the presence of a cervical cancer diagnosis is available to women who are not in an established relationship, or choose not to use donor sperm to create and store frozen embryos. The success of this technique remains low (Seli and Tangir 2005) with the chance of having a child using frozen oocytes reported to be around 2% per oocyte (Lieberman and Wood 2007). Debate continues around the most appropriate method to cryopreserve mature oocytes. A factor contributing to the low pregnancy rate from this procedure is the sensitivity of the oocytes to freezing (Maltaris et al. 2006). However, the procedure offers hope to a select group of women and further studies are required to develop ways of protecting oocytes with an aim of producing successful fertilisation and subsequent pregnancy. Once again, this procedure involves ovarian stimulation and therefore a delay in cancer treatment will be required.

Ovarian tissue cryopreservation

Ovarian tissue cryopreservation involves the removal and freezing of ovarian tissue (Seli and Tangir 2005) and is also considered to be experimental (Salle and Lornage 2007). The benefit of ovarian tissue cryopreservation is that the procedure does not require ovarian stimulation prior to collection of the tissue (Practice Committee of the American Society for Reproductive Medicine and Practice Committee of the Society for Assisted Reproductive Technology 2006); therefore it is not necessary to delay definitive cancer treatment.

The problem with storing ovarian tissue for fertility preservation in patients with cancer is that it carries the possible risk of malignant cells remaining in the tissue which could lead to recurrence of cancer after reimplantation. The procedure can therefore only be recommended when the risk of reseeding cancer cells following transplantation can be eliminated (Oktay et al. 2001) (e.g. women diagnosed with a squamous cell carcinoma of the cervix which carries a low risk of metastasis to the ovary (Landoni et al. 2007)).

The tissue is removed at the time of radical surgery or via a laparoscope as a day only procedure. The tissue is then frozen and when required can be transplanted either orthotopically or heterotopically (Lee et al. 2006). When the tissue is grafted orthotopically it is returned to its normal site in the pelvis; heterotopically, it is grafted elsewhere such as the forearm (Roberts and Oktay 2005). Orthotopically grafted ovarian tissue has the potential to restore normal reproductive function (Salle and Lornage 2007). However, the woman with cervical cancer who has undergone hysterectomy or radiotherapy will be more suited to heterotopically grafted tissue. This procedure does not require surgery and the grafted tissue can restore ovarian secretion, which can be used for *in vitro* fertilisation (Salle and Lornage 2007).

Live birth following orthotopic transplantation of cryopreserved ovarian tissue has been reported (Donnez et al. 2004) and it is to be anticipated that in the near future an increasing number of cured patients will request re-implantation of stored ovarian tissue. Methods and molecular techniques to detect tumour and minimal residual disease to exclude possible presence of cancer are essential to increase the safety of cryopreservation-reimplantation procedure.

Surrogacy

Where there is no uterus (i.e. post-hysterectomy), embryos which have resulted from ART may be transferred into a surrogate carrier's uterus. The use of a surrogate carrier, or in other words a third party, has emotional, legal and ethical implications and surrogate carriers undergo intense medical and psychological screening procedures prior to being accepted onto a programme (Gossfeld and Cullen 2000). Surrogacy is not universally available and its financial costs are prohibitive to many women and couples. The use of a surrogate carrier is therefore restricted to women who have sufficient financial resources to meet the associated costs.

Because international, national and state laws vary, the surrogacy procedure can be complicated. For example, in Australia on the birth of the baby the woman and her partner must apply to adopt legally as the birth mother is considered the legal mother (Pearce 2005). However, this is not the case in every country.

The global differences in legal surrogacy practices have given rise to a phenomenon referred to as 'reproductive tourism' (Ferraretti et al. 2007). As an example of this Steigrad et al. (2005) describe a case of a woman who, despite suffering premature ovarian failure following radical hysterectomy with transposition of the ovaries and radiotherapy for an invasive cervical cancer, was able to achieve her desire of becoming a mother. The woman recovered ovarian function and underwent ovarian stimulation; subsequent oocyte retrieval resulted in successful IVF with her husband's sperm. The frozen embryos were transported from Australia to America and transferred to a surrogate carrier. The result was the birth of live twin boys (Steigrad et al. 2005). By using a surrogate carrier in America the biological mother was considered the legal mother as opposed to Australia where, as mentioned before, the biological mother would have been legally required to adopt the babies.

Other reasons for 'reproductive tourism' include a lack of experience and expertise between state and country borders, requiring women and couples to cross borders to have access to the best available technologies (Ferraretti et al. 2007).

As a result of the advances in surgical techniques and artificial reproductive technologies described above, the potential for women to realise their hopes for starting or completing a family have become a viable option. Other benefits of advanced surgical techniques include the potential to prevent premature menopause and the associated effects. The next section of this chapter will explore ways to manage the premature menopause associated with cancer treatment.

Cervical cancer and menopause

Menopause has been described as the progression from the reproductive to the non-reproductive stage of a woman's life (Bertero 2003), and is an inevitable consequence of ageing. However, ageing is not always the pathway to menopause. Of all the women treated each year for cervical cancer, over one half are diagnosed in women less than fifty years of age (Feeney et al. 1995, Australian Institute of Health and Welfare Statistics 2007). As the average age for menopause is 50 to 51 years, these younger women may experience prematurely induced menopause due to surgery, radiotherapy to the pelvic region, or possibly chemotherapy (Biglia et al. 2004).

As already discussed, there are two standard treatments for cervical cancer: primary surgery, which includes a radical hysterectomy with or without bilateral salpingo oophorectomy (removal of both fallopian tubes and ovaries), combined with pelvic lymph-adenectomy, or primary chemoradiation. Pre-menopausal women treated for cervical cancer with radical hysterectomy who have had their ovaries retained will cease menses but maintain ovarian function. Those women who have their ovaries removed, or later ablated by radiotherapy will not only be amenorrhoeic, but will also experience symptoms of ovarian failure.

Due to increased life expectancy, and improved survival following treatment for cervical cancer, women will live for many years with the physiological and psychological conse-quences of early menopause (Duska et al. 1999). Appropriate management of these women is critical in helping to reduce those factors that may adversely affect their future health and quality of life (Peck et al. 2007).

Menopause is literally the cessation of menses as a result of ovarian failure. Ovarian failure may occur naturally, or be induced by:

- surgical removal of the ovaries
- ovarian ablation from radiotherapy
- ovarian ablation from chemotherapy

The climacteric is the combination of symptoms, including cessation of menses associated with ovarian failure. Loss of ovarian function results in a decline in the ovarian production of estradiol and progesterone and the increased production of follicle stimulating hormone from the pituitary gland (Zacur 1999, DeMasters 2000, Gold and Greendale 2007).

Primary surgery

For women with cervical cancer who have not yet reached natural menopause the removal of both ovaries (bilateral oophorectomy) at the time of hysterectomy causes a significant reduction in the production of oestrogen and progesterone, resulting in surgically induced menopause (Allina and Suthers 2006). For younger women wishing to preserve subsequent hormonal function, many authors recommend the option of ovarian preservation, with or without transposition, to protect the ovaries in the event that post-operative radiation is required. Ovarian transposition can be performed at the time of radical hysterectomy in patients with early stage disease and macroscopically normal ovaries and is described in the following section (Feeney et al. 1995, Morice 2000, Hacker 2005, Landoni et al. 2007).

The major concern with ovarian preservation is that occult ovarian metastases from the cervical cancer may remain. In order to identify risk factors associated with ovarian metas-tases in women with cervical cancer, Landoni et al. (2007) retrospectively studied 1695 patients who had their ovaries conserved at the time of treatment. They found that early stage squamous cell carcinoma of the cervix rarely metastasised to the ovary (0.9%), and concluded that ovarian conservation could be safely performed in women under 45 years with early stage disease and macroscopically normal ovaries.

Further contraindications to ovarian preservation would be a proven BRCA 1 or 2 mutation, or HNPCC (hereditary non-polyposis colon cancer), and anyone who has a strong family history of breast or ovarian cancer. Relative contraindications would be a past history of endometriosis or pelvic inflammatory disease.

The literature reports that radical hysterectomy with bilateral ovarian preservation without transposition does not significantly reduce the age of menopause for this group of women, as long as adjuvant radiation is not given (Feeney et al. 1995, Van Eijkeren et al. 1999, Morice et al. 2000).

Primary radiotherapy for cervical cancer

When radiotherapy is used to treat cervical cancer the ovaries are exposed to doses in excess of 50 Gy. This has a well recognised adverse effect on ovarian function, causing complete ovarian failure. Most young pre-menopausal women experience ovarian failure after a radiation dose of 20 Gy. In older pre-menopausal women as little as 5 to 10 Gy can induce menopause (Eifel 2005).

Preservation of ovarian function may be achieved for pre-menopausal women by the transposition of either one or both ovaries to the right or left paracolic gutter, prior to radiotherapy, at the time of laparotomy or laparoscopy. This technique places the ovaries out of the pelvic radiation field, avoiding radiation induced ovarian failure (Van Eijkeren et al. 1999). The literature identifies a failure rate for preserving ovarian function in this group of women of 28% to 50% (Feeney et al. 1995, Van Eijkeren et al. 1999, Morice et al. 2000). For women who have had unilateral oophorectomy, and the other ovary transposed, the incidence of retained ovarian function is further reduced. This has been attributed to the combined loss of ovarian volume and possible vascular compromise associated with the transposition (Buekers et al. 2001).

Chemotherapy

Chemotherapeutic agents, particularly alkylating agents, may produce either temporary or permanent ovarian failure (Rebar 2007). Because the effects of chemotherapy on the ovaries usually occur over several months, this disruption to ovarian function may only be temporary, and is dependent on the dose and duration of the treatment. It is proposed that women closer to menopause having chemotherapy are most likely to experience induced menopause (Elson and Noone 2006).

Symptoms of menopause

Menopausal symptoms vary among individuals and ethnic groups, with about 75% of women experiencing some form of menopausal symptom (Bertero 2003). The symptoms of surgical or treatment induced menopause are often sudden, and can be more pronounced than in a natural menopause (DeMasters, 2000).

Box 7.2 Ovarian preservation, a case study

Jenny (not her real name), a 30-year-old mother of one presented with post-coital bleeding. Biopsy confirmed adenocarcinoma of the cervix, staged as IB1. Jenny and her husband were counselled regarding the need for a radical hysterectomy. The issue of whether to preserve the ovaries was discussed. Jenny had no history of ovarian, bowel or breast cancer, and had no prior history of endometriosis or pelvic inflammatory disease.

It was therefore recommended that the ovaries be conserved at the time of radical hysterectomy, unless they appeared abnormal.

One week later, Jenny underwent a radical hysterectomy, and a bilateral pelvic lymphadenectomy. Both ovaries were conserved, and the left transposed above the pelvic brim, in case of the need for adjuvant pelvic radiotherapy.

Jenny made an uneventful recovery from surgery, returning to work six weeks later. The lymph nodes were negative and the surgical margins clear and she did not require adjuvant pelvic radiation.

Jenny remains well nine years after her surgery and her conserved ovaries still function as normal. Her only regret is that she was able to have only one child.

Hot flushes

The most commonly reported early symptoms of the menopausal transition are associated with the reduction in circulating oestrogen and progesterone, and increases in follicle stimulating hormone (FSH) affecting the central nervous system. This results in vasomotor instability, causing hot flushes and night sweats (Bertero 2003, Freeman et al. 2007). During a hot flush an intensely warm sensation, with sweating and erythema radiates upward from the chest to the face. These episodes vary in length and frequency and are more intense for women who have experienced surgical menopause (Zacur 1999, Dormire 2003, Rogers 2006). For some women hot flushes are accompanied by palpitations and feelings of panic.

Physiologically night sweats are the same as hot flushes, although many women deny hot flushes but admit to night sweats when asked. Hot flushes occurring at night may over time cause sleep deprivation, precipitating fatigue, irritability and depressed mood (Zacur 1999, Rogers 2006, Freeman et al. 2007). Hot spicy foods, alcohol, smoking, exertion and stress have been reported to precipitate an episode. Although the medical community considers hot flushes to be benign, most women who seek advice regarding this menopausal symptom do so because of the associated discomfort, inconvenience, and disruption to their lives (Dormire 2003).

Urogenital symptoms

Tissues that contain receptor sites for oestrogen are affected by the reduction in circulating oestrogen. The vagina, vulva, urethra and trigone of the bladder have large numbers of oestrogen receptors, and depletion of oestrogen at menopause causes atrophy of the urogenital epithelium. These symptoms usually develop over time with vaginal atrophy (thinning of the skin of the vulva and vagina) causing decreased vaginal elasticity, and shortening. Thinning of the vaginal epithelium and decreased lubrication can lead to sensations of itching, irritation, and painful intercourse (dyspareunia). Vaginal dryness causing dyspareunia is a significant risk factor for decreased libido (Freeman 2007). For women who experience either surgical or natural menopause, decreased levels of endogenous testosterone could also precipitate a decrease in libido (Warren and Valente 2004). Oestrogen depletion also affects urinary sphincter tone due to atrophy of the periurethral tissues, with resultant increased stress incontinence, frequency, urgency and an increased incidence of urinary tract infections.

Longer-term symptoms of menopause

Osteoporosis

Due to the loss of ovarian hormone production at menopause, women are at an increased risk for osteoporosis. Bone density is regulated by sex hormones which control the flow of calcium into and out of the bones. When these hormone levels decline during menopause, calcium metabolism is affected, resulting in bone resorption exceeding bone formation (Smith 1998). This subsequent decrease in bone density increases the risk of fracture, particularly of the vertebrae, hips and wrist (Paterson 2005). By 50 years of age a Caucasian woman's lifetime risk for hip fracture is 15%, and by 85 years, 33% of women will have sustained a hip fracture (Warren and Valente 2004). Factors contributing to a higher incidence of osteoporosis are earlier age at menopause, family history, thin body build, fair complexion, decreased exercise, cigarette smoking, heavy alcohol use and a lack of dietary intake of vitamin D and calcium. Medications such as glucocorticoids and anticonvulsants can also increase the lifetime risk of fracture (Paterson 2005).

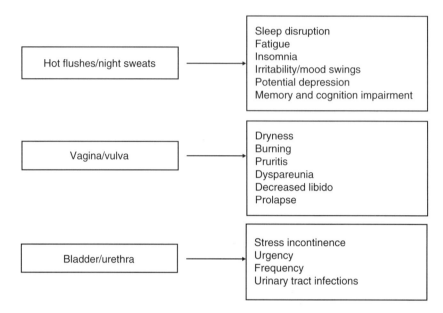

Figure 7.1 Symptoms of the menopause.

Cardiovascular disease

Cardiovascular disease is one of the leading causes of female mortality in most developed countries. The likelihood of developing cardiovascular disease increases with age. Oestrogen deficiency at menopause has been strongly implicated in the development of the disease in women. Menopause initiates changes in cholesterol, causing total cholesterol to rise by about 6%, low density lipoprotein by 10%, and triglycerides by about 11% (Hsia et al. 2006). This unfavourable change in lipoprotein profile results in an increased risk of atherosclerosis (Paterson 2005).

Memory, cognition and dementia

Many women complain of memory and cognitive difficulties associated with changes in their ovarian hormone levels, while other post-menopausal women taking hormone therapy comment on the positive effect it has on their memory and cognition. However, the mechanisms through which these hormones affect cognition remain confusing (Craig and Murphy 2006, Silva and Naftolin 2007). It is thought the decline of oestrogen at menopause may contribute to the neurodegenerative process associated with dementia. Alzheimer's disease occurs more often in women than in men, and those women who do develop the disease have a lower body mass index than other women. This supports the theory that obese women might well be afforded some protection by increased oestrogen produced from endogenous androgen occurring in adipose tissue (Silva and Naftolin 2007).

Management of menopausal symptoms

Women treated for cervical cancer are particularly vulnerable to the physiological consequences of early menopause. For this reason they need to be well informed of their emerging health risks following menopause, made aware of their options for managing menopausal symptoms, and also the potential hazards and benefits of hormone therapy. Additionally, information on other treatment options such as phytoestrogens, lifestyle modifications including diet, exercise, cessation of smoking, and modification of alcohol intake should be provided (Dormire 2003). Well-informed nurses involved in the care of these women are ideally placed to discuss the implications of treatment and provide information on current management strategies.

Hormone therapy

Hormone therapy (HT) has been used to treat menopausal symptoms since the 1950s (Kelsey and Marcus cited in Dormire 2003), and is considered the most effective tool in alleviating many of the symptoms of menopause that negatively impact quality of life. Often post-menopausal women taking HT will abruptly discontinue it when diagnosed with cervical cancer, assuming it contributed to the development of their disease. There is no known association between the use of HT and the incidence of squamous cell carcinomas of the cervix. However, according to some, the use of oestrogen has been positively associated with cervical adenocarcinomas (Lacey et al. 2000, Biglia et al. 2004). Likewise, some women treated for cervical cancer are reluctant to take HT, fearing a recurrence of their disease. The use of HT in women following treatment for cervical cancer has not been shown to negatively affect either survival, or five-year disease free survival (Ploch 1985, Biglia et al. 2004).

In 2002, the first randomised prevention trial of menopausal hormones, the Women's Health Initiative Trial (WHI) was stopped early due to adverse outcomes. The purpose of this study was to determine the long-term risks and benefits of hormone therapy on chronic disease prevention in post-menopausal women (Warren and Valente 2004). Early results indicated that combined oestrogen and progesterone actually increased women's risk for breast cancer, heart attack, stroke and blood clots (Allina and Suthers 2006). The subsequent media attention, with exaggerated interpretation of the results, caused many women to abruptly discontinue hormone therapy. Since this time the use of HT has become increasingly controversial and commonly avoided by both menopausal women and their clinicians (Barlow 2007).

Benefits of hormone therapy

Vasomotor and urogenital symptoms

The general consensus in the literature regarding the benefits associated with the use of HT is that it is effective in reducing or eliminating hot flushes in about 80% to 90% of women. HT has also been shown to significantly reduce vaginal and urogenital atrophic symptoms, sleep disturbances and other complaints associated with insomnia (van der Mooren and Kenemans 2004, Warren and Valente 2004).

Osteoporosis

There is good clinical evidence that HT will reduce the risk of fractures that are a consequence of osteoporosis. The WHI trial reported five fewer hip fractures per 10,000 women who were taking HT (Warren and Valente 2004). In studies conducted to determine bone mineral density, oestrogen therapy has been shown to prevent bone loss (Barlow 2007). However, there is debate in the literature as to the benefit of taking HT for the reduction of fracture risk. Most of the protective benefit of HT is lost once it is stopped and accelerated bone loss will occur (De Masters 2000). Therefore, for a woman in her eighties, when falls and osteoporotic fractures are most likely, it seems improbable that HT stopped 15 to 20 years earlier would have any protective effect (Brockie 2001). However, randomised controlled trials have shown that taking HT for two to five years, more than ten years earlier, significantly reduced the fracture rate (Barlow 2007).

Colorectal cancer

The incidence and mortality of colon cancer is lower in females than males, and has been attributed to the protective effect of oestrogen. According to a majority of studies, HT reduces the risk of colon cancer. The WHI trial showed that combined oestrogen plus progestogen therapy was associated with six fewer cases of colon cancer per 10,000 women. However, there is considered to be insufficient evidence to support the recommendation of long-term HT in the prevention of colon cancer (Biglia et al. 2004, Warren and Valente 2004).

Alzheimer's disease

Several studies have reported the effects of HT on the incidence of dementia and Alzheimer's disease. The Cache County Study was a longitudinal study conducted to determine the incidence of Alzheimer's disease and dementia relative to environmental factors. Results showed that this disorder varied with the duration of HT use, the longer use of HT (greater than ten years), was associated with a greater reduction in the incidence of Alzheimer's disease (Zandi et al. 2002). The WHI Memory Study showed no apparent benefit in preventing mild cognitive impairment in women taking combined HT. Surprisingly, these results indicated a probable increased risk of dementia in women older than 65 years taking HT (Schumaker et al. 2003). Clearly, the long-term benefit of HT in providing protection for dementia is controversial. There is considered to be no benefit in initiating HT as a secondary prevention for dementia in older post-menopausal women. For younger women, however, the primary prevention benefit should be considered when determining the risk benefit ratio for the use of HT (AACE Menopause Guidelines Revision Taskforce 2006).

Cardiovascular disease

The long-term protective benefit of oestrogen against the development of cardiovascular disease is no longer considered an indication for initiating, or continuing HT (AACE Menopause Guidelines Revision Taskforce 2006). The WHI trial showed combined HT had no beneficial effect on coronary heart disease risk in post-menopausal women. These results are controversial when compared to earlier observational data, which indicated a cardiovascular protective benefit of HT (van der Mooren and Kenermans 2004). It has been suggested that the older population of the WHI study, who had more cardiac risk factors, and were ten years or more away from menopause, could explain the differences in these results (Lobo 2007). In younger post-menopausal women the protective benefit of HT against cardiovascular disease may still be considered relevant (AACE Menopause Guidelines Revision Taskforce 2006, Lobo 2007).

The risks of hormone therapy

Endometrial cancer

Endometrial cancer has been shown to be increased in women with an intact uterus taking unopposed oestrogen, and should be avoided. However, with the addition of progestogen, the incidence of endometrial cancer in women is no different to placebo rates (Anderson et al. 2003).

Breast cancer

Breast cancer risk is influenced by length of exposure to oestrogen and progestogens. However, some authors argue this risk may be isolated to older women with longer exposure to oestrogen. Several observational case control studies have reported oestrogen alone to have no significant increased risk of breast cancer, but an increased risk with combined HT. The WHI study suggested that oestrogen plus progesterone does increase the risk of breast cancer. This risk has been determined to be small, but does cause considerable anxiety among patients and clinicians (Creasman 2005, AACE Menopause Guidelines Revision Taskforce 2006).

Venous thrombosis

There is evidence from several studies that HT significantly increases the relative risk of thromboembolism. This increased risk is concentrated in the first two to three years of initiating HT. However, the actual risk of developing venous thromboembolism is quite low, due to the already low frequency of this event. This risk can be further reduced with the use of statins and aspirin (Speroff 2005).

Stroke

In the WHI study cerebrovascular accidents (stroke) were more common in the treated group than the placebo group. However, the survey of an older population in this study has prompted questions about the significance of these results to younger women taking lower doses of HT (AACE Menopause Guidelines Revision Task Force 2006).

The main types of hormone therapy

- Oestrogen only therapy: this is often referred to as unopposed oestrogen, and is only recommended for women who have had a hysterectomy, as unopposed oestrogen is associated with an increased risk of endometrial cancer.
- Combination therapy: this is a combination of oestrogen plus progestogen.
- Tibolone (Organon, Livial): a synthetic steroid, with a mixed profile of oestrogenic, progestogenic and androgenic effects. It is effective in reducing vasomotor symptoms, and has also been shown to reduce depressive symptoms, and improve libido (Cancer-BACUP 2005).
- Progestogens (Medroxyprogesterone Acetate (MPA)): this is considered the most effective drug therapy after HT in reducing vasomotor symptoms. The use of this medication is limited by the side effects of weight gain and withdrawal bleeding (CancerBACUP 2005, AACE Menopause Guidelines Revision Taskforce 2006).
- Testosterone: there is some evidence that testosterone has a positive effect on improving libido in post-menopausal women. However, there has been limited research on the safety of its use (North American Menopause Society cited in Allina and Suthers 2006).

Administration

Hormone therapy can be administered in a number of different ways. Most women using HT take it orally. However, it can also be administered through the skin in the form of skin patches and gels, or transdermally. Both oestrogen only and combination oestrogen, and progestogen patches are available. Oestradiol implants can be inserted subcutaneously under local anaesthetic with the oestrogen being released over many months, depending on the dose. These implants can be effective in controlling menopausal symptoms for three to four years. Vaginal oestrogen creams and pessaries can also be used to alleviate vaginal dryness and thinning of the vaginal epithelium; however, these have not proven to be effective against hot flushes or night sweats. As these preparations are not absorbed systemically to any significant degree they can be used in women with a contraindication to HT (Brockie 2001, Allina and Suthers 2006).

Alternatives to hormone therapy

Some women have contraindications to taking HT, and many women are reluctant to use it. Therefore, it is important to make these women aware of other therapeutic options:

- Antidepressants (Venlafaxine, Fluoxetine): evidence exists that serotonin reuptake inhibitors are effective in reducing vasomotor symptoms (van der Moorens and Kenemans 2004). Side effects of these medications include nausea, dry mouth, insomnia, and gastrointestinal disturbances, often leading to therapy withdrawal (AACE Menopause Guidelines Revision Taskforce 2006).
- Gabapentin: this medication is currently in use for seizures and neuropathic pain, but has shown efficacy in the reduction of hot flushes. It is not currently available outside specialist centres (Royal College of Obstetricians and Gynaecologists 2006).
- Selective oestrogen receptor modulators (SORMs): these preparations are considered effective in the prevention of osteoporotic fractures. Raloxifene, a second generation SORM has also been found to have some beneficial effect in reducing the risk of breast cancer. It has not been found to decrease vasomotor symptoms (Brockie 2001, van der Mooren and Kenemans 2004).
- Bisphosphonates: like the SORMs these preparations are effective in preventing bone loss and reduce the risk of new and recurrent fractures, particularly of the hip and lumbar vertebrae. The side effects are mainly limited to the gastrointestinal tract (Brockie 2001, van der Mooren and Kenemans 2004).
- Phytoestrogens: these plant oestrogens have a weak oestrogenic effect in women. The most common of these, black cohosh, is widely used for reducing menopausal symptoms. The commercial preparation of black cohosh is Remifemin. Other sources of phytoestrogens include soybeans, flaxseed, and red clover (Dennehy 2006).
- Supplements: those that have been recommended for the relief of menopausal symptoms include evening primrose oil, dong quai, wild yam, and vitamin E (Dennehy 2006).

So that it can be seen that the consequences of oestrogen deprivation can cause significant problems for women following treatment for cervical cancer, and hormone therapy remains an important therapeutic option. For women who use HT following surgical menopause, relief of menopausal symptoms has been reported as comparable to the relief experienced by women after natural menopause (Allina and Suthers 2006). The decision as to whether or not to use hormone therapy should be individualised and flexible, involving the clinician and the patient (Lobo 2007). The consideration of benefits and risks in respect to dosage, duration of HT, and a risk benefit analysis of the patient's medical history in relation to the side effects of hormone therapy are essential (Warren and Valente 2004). The provision of information to these women regarding the management of menopausal symptoms, and long-term disease prevention is also important to ensure future quality of life, and should be an integral part of holistic nursing cancer care.

Conclusion

The diagnosis of cervical cancer in women who are pre-menopausal and who have not realised their childbearing potential presents a double burden in terms of loss of fertility and premature menopause. It is reassuring to know that there are options available to preserve fertility, and in some cases prevent the sudden onset of menopause. With ongoing research into ART and the treatment of menopause, health professionals are able to guide women to make informed choices. It is the responsibility of health professionals to recognise a multidisciplinary approach to care to ensure that women have access to the available information.

Frequently asked questions

(1) How will you make sure there are no cancer cells in my stored ovarian tissue?
   The most common type of cervix cancer does not normally spread to the ovaries. Portions of the ovarian tissue will be examined closely by a pathologist to make sure there are no cancer cells before the tissue is stored (Sonmezer et al. 2005).
(2) How long can you store frozen embryos?
   This will depend on local, state and national laws. In Australia, guidelines from the National Health and Medical Research Council (NHMRC) recommend that the maximum time embryos are kept in storage is five years, with the possibility of extending this consent a further five years (NHMRC 2007).
(3) Will ovarian stimulation cause my cancer to recur?
   This is considered unlikely because cervix cancer is not hormone related.
(4) Does taking hormone therapy increase my chance of developing breast cancer?
   The WHI study suggested that oestrogen plus progesterone does increase the risk of breast cancer. This risk has been determined to be small, but does cause considerable anxiety among patients and clinicians (Creasman 2005, AACE Menopause Guidelines Revision Taskforce 2006).
(5) How long should I take hormone therapy?
   Hormone therapy can be taken for as long as debilitating menopausal symptoms persist, but is not now advocated for chronic disease prevention. The consideration of benefits and risks in respect to dosage, duration of HT, and a risk benefit analysis of the patient's medical history in relation to the side effects of hormone therapy are essential and should be individualised for each woman (Warren and Valente 2004).

Resources

Gynecologic Oncology Group: www.gog.org
Australian New Zealand Gynaecological Oncology Group: www.anzgog.org.au
National Cervical Cancer Coalition: www.nccc-online.org
Women's Cancer Network: www.wcn.org
Jo's Trust: www.jotrust.co.uk
Gynaecological Cancer Support: www.gynaecancersupport.org.au
IVF Australia: www.ivf.com.au
Access Australia: www.access.org.au
Cancerbacup: www.cancerbacup.org.uk

References

Allina A and Suthers K (2006) Hormone Treatment, in Stephenson H (ed.) *The Boston Women's Health Book Collective, 'Our Bodies, Ourselves: Menopause'*. Simon & Schuster, New York. pp. 99–122

American Association of Clinical Endocrinologists (AACE) Menopause Guidelines Revision Task-force (2006) American Association of Clinical Endocrinologists medical guidelines for clinical practice for the diagnosis and treatment of menopause. *Endocrine Practice*, 12 (3), 315–337

American Society of Clinical Onclogy (ASCO) (2006) Recommendations on fertility preservation in cancer patients. *Journal of Clinical Oncology*, 24 (18), 2917–2931

Anderson G, Judd H, Kaunitz A, et al. (2003) Effects of estrogen plus progestin on gynecologic cancers and associated diagnostic procedures: the Women's Health Initiative randomized trial. *JAMA*, 290 (13), 1739–1748

Australian Institute of Health and Welfare (2006) Cancer age specific data cube. *Cancer Data Online*: http://www.aihw.gov.dataonline.cfm (accessed 20/7/07)

Bankowski B, Lyerly A, Faden R and Wallach E (2005) The social implications of embryo cryopreservation. *Fertility and Sterility*, 84 (4), 823–832

Barlow D (2007) Individualisation of HRT treatment, in Kruger T, van der Spuy Z and Kempers R (eds) *Advances in Fertility Studies and Reproductive Medicine – IFFS 2007*. Juta and Co Ltd, Cape Town

Benedetti-Panici P, Greggi S, Colombo A, et al. (2002) Neoadjuvant chemotherapy and radical surgery versus exclusive radiotherapy in locally advanced squamous cell cervical cancer: results from the Italian multicentre randomized study. *Journal of Clinical Oncology*, 20 (1) 179–188

Bertero C (2003) What do women think about menopause? A qualitative study of women's expectations, apprehensions and knowledge about the climacteric period, International Council of Nurses. *International Nursing Review*, 50, 109–118

Biglia N, Gadducci A, Ponzone R, Roagna R and Sismondi P (2004) Hormone replacement therapy in cancer survivors. *Maturitas*, 48, 333–346

Brockie J (2001) The climacteric, in Gangar E (eds) *Gynaecological Nursing: a Practical Guide*. Churchill Livingstone, London. pp. 317–337

Buekers T, Anderson B, Sorosky M and Buller R (2001) Ovarian function after surgical treatment for cervical cancer. *Gynecologic Oncology*, 80, 85–88

CancerBACUP website: www.cancerbacup.org.uk (accessed 7/12/2005)

Carter J, Lewin S, Abu-Rustum N and Sonada Y (2007a) Reproductive issues in the gynecologic cancer patient, *Oncology*, 21 (5, 30 April) 598, Expanded Academic ASAP (22 August 2007). Thomson Gale. University of Sydney

Carter J, Sonada Y and Abu-Rustum NR (2007b) Reproductive concerns of women treated with radical trachelectomy for cervical cancer, *Gynecologic Oncology*, 105, 13–16

Carter J, Rowland K, Chi D, et al. (2005) Gynecologic cancer treatment and the impact of cancer-related infertility. *Gynecologic Oncology*, 97, 90–95

Cooke I (2007) The globalisation of reproductive technology, in Kruger TF, Van Der Spuy Z and Kempers RD (eds) *Advances in Fertility Studies and Reproductive Medicine – IFFS 2007*, Juta & Co Ltd, Cape Town. pp. 234–240

Craig MC and Murphy DG (2006) Oestrogen, cognition and the maturing female brain. *Journal of Neuroendocrinology*, 19, 1–6

Creasman W (2005) Hormone replacement therapy after cancers. *Current Opinion in Oncology*, 17 (5), 493–499

Dennehy C (2006) The use of herbs and dietary supplements in gynecology: an evidence-based review. *Journal of Midwifery Women's Health*, 51 (6), 402–409

DeMasters J (2000) HRT 7 menopause: a clinician's guide to understanding the dilemma. *Association of Women's Health, Obstetric and Neonatal Nurses*, 4 (2), 26–35

Donnez J, Dolmans MM, Demylle D, et al. (2004) Livebirth after orthotopic transplantation of cryopreserved ovarian tissue. *Lancet*, 364, 1405–1410

Dormire S (2003) What we know about managing menopausal hot flashes: navigating without a compass. *JOGNN*, 32, 455–464

Durna EM (2001) Studies on the use of hormone replacement therapy in women with breast cancer, PhD thesis, University of New South Wales, Australia

Duska L, Trimble C and Trimble E (1999) Ovulation, menstruation, and contraception in the cancer patient, in Trimble E and Trimble C (eds) *Cancer Obstetrics and Gynecology*. Lippincott, Williams & Wilkins, Philadelphia. pp. 1–19

Eifel P (2005) Radiation therapy, in Berek J and Hacker N (eds) *Practical Gynecologic Oncology*. Lippincott, Williams & Wilkins, Philadelphia. pp. 119–161

Elson J and Noone P (2006) Sudden and early menopause, in Stephenson H (ed.) *The Boston Women's Health Book Collective, 'Our Bodies, Ourselves: Menopause'*. Simon & Schuster, New York. pp. 57–73

Feeney D, Moore D, Look K, Stehman F and Sutton G (1995) The fate of the ovaries after radical hysterectomy and ovarian transposition. *Gynecologic Oncology*, 56, 3–7

Ferraretti AP, Gianaroli L, Magli MC, et al. (eds) (2007) *Advances in Fertility Studies and Reproductive Medicine – IFFS 2007*, Juta & Co Ltd, Cape Town. pp. 241–249

Freeman E, Sammel M, Lin H, et al. (2007) Symptoms associated with menopausal transition and reproductive hormones in midlife women. *Obstetrics & Gynecology*, 110 (2), 230–240

Gershenson DM (2005) Fertility-sparing surgery for malignancies in women. *Journal of the National Cancer Institute Monographs*, 34, 43–47

Gold E and Greendale G (2007) Epidemiology of menopause: demographics, environmental influences and ethnic and international differences in the menopausal experience, in Lobo R (ed.) *Treatment of the Post Menopausal Woman, Basic and Clinical Aspects*, third edition. Academic Press, San Diego, CA. pp. 77–96

Gossfeld LM and Cullen ML (2000) Sexuality and fertility issues, in Moore-Higgs G, Almadrones L, Eriksson J, Gossfeld L and Huff B (eds) *Women and Cancer: a Gynecoloic Oncology Nursing Perspective*. Jones and Bartlett publishers, Sudbury. pp. 186–232

Hacker NF (2005) Cervical cancer, in Berek JS and Hacker NF (eds) *Practical Gynecologic Oncology*, fourth edition. Lippincott Williams & Wilkins, Philadelphia. pp. 337–395

Hsia J, Levin G, Abramson J and Casey A (2006) Heart health, in Stephenson H (eds) *The Boston Women's Health Book Collective, 'Our Bodies, Ourselves: Menopause'*. Simon & Schuster, New York. pp. 246–263

Kruger T, van der Spuy Z and Kempers R (2007) *Advances in Fertility Studies and Reproductive Medicine – IFFS 2007*, Juts and Co Ltd, Cape Town

Lacey J, Brinton L, Barnes W, et al. (2000) Use of hormone replacement therapy and adenocarcinomas and squamous cell carcinomas of the uterine cervix. *Gynecological Oncology*, 77, 149–154

Landoni F, Zanagnolo V, Lovato-Diaz L, et al. (2007) Ovarian metastases in early-stage cervical cancer (IA2–IIA): a multicenter retrospective study of 1965 patients (a Cooperative Task Force study). *Int J Gynecol Cancer*, 17, 623–628

Lee SJ, Schover LR, Partridge AH, et al. (2006) American Society of Clinical Oncology recommendations on fertility preservation in cancer patients, *Journal of Clinical Oncology*, 24 (18), 2917–2931

Leitao MM and Chi DS (2005) Fertility-sparing options for patients with gynaecologic malignancies. *Oncologist*, (10), 613–622

Lieberman BA and Wood MJ (2007) Strategies for preservation of ovarian function: an overview, in Kruger TF, Van Der Spuy Z and Kempers RD (eds) *Advances in Fertility Studies and Reproductive Medicine – IFFS 2007*, Juta & Co Ltd, Cape Town. pp. 398–402

Lobo RA (2007) The future of therapy and the role of hormone therapy, in Lobo R (ed.) *Treatment of the Post Menopausal Woman, Basic and Clinical Aspects*, third edition. Academic Press, San Diego, CA. pp. 875–880

Maltaris T, Boehm D, Dittrich R, Seufert R and Koelbl H (2006) Reproduction beyond cancer: a message of hope for young women, *Gynecologic Oncology*, 103, 1109–1121

Marhhom E and Cohen I (2006) Fertility preservation options for women with malignancies. *Obstetrical and Gynecological Survey*, 62 (1), 58–72

van der Mooren M and Kenemans P (2004) Postmenopausal hormone therapy: impact on menopause-related symptoms, chronic disease and quality of life. *Drugs*, 64 (8), 821–836

Morice P, Juncker L, Rey A, El-Hassan J, Haie-Meder C and Castaigne D (2000) Ovarian transposition for patients with cervical carcinoma treated by radiosurgical combination. *Fertility and Sterility*, 74 (4), 743–748

NHMRC (2007) *Ethical Guidelines on the Use of Assisted Reproductive Technology in Clinical Practice and Research*. National Health and Medical Research Council, www.nhmrc.gov.au (accessed 29/04/08)

Oktay K, Kan M and Rosenwaks Z (2001) Recent progress in oocyte and ovarian tissue cryopreservation and transplantation. *Current Opinion in Obstetrics and Gynecology*, 13, 263–268

Paterson G (2005) Menopause, in Lancaster T and Natress K (eds) *Gynaecological Cancer Care A Guide to Practice*. Ausmed Publications, Melbourne. pp. 201–211

Pearce E (2005) Fertility, in Lancaster L and Nattress K (eds) *Gynaecological Cancer Care A Guide to Practice*. Ausmed Publications, Melbourne. pp. 187–199

Peck A, Chervenak J and Santoro N (2007) Decisions regarding treatment during the menopause transition, in Lobo R (ed.) *Treatment of the Post Menopausal Woman, Basic and Clinical Aspects*, third edition. Academic Press, Massachusetts. pp. 157–167

Plante M and Roy M (2006) Fertility-preserving options for cervical cancer. *Oncology* (30 April), 479. Expanded Academic ASAP (18 June). Thomson Gale, University of Sydney

Ploch E (1985) Hormonal replacement therapy in patients after cervical cancer treatment. *Gynecologic Oncology*, 26, 169–177

Practice Committee of the American Society for Reproductive Medicine and Practice Committee of the Society for Assisted Reproductive Technology (2006) Ovarian tissue and oocyte cryopreservation. *Fertility and Sterility*, 86 (suppl 4), S142–S147

Rebar R (2007) Premature ovarian failure, in Lobo R (ed.) *Treatment of the Post Menopausal Woman, Basic and Clinical Aspects*, third edition. Academic Press, San Diego. pp. 99–109

Roberts JE and Oktay K (2005) Fertility preservation: a comprehensive approach to the young woman with cancer. *Journal of the National Cancer Institute Monographs*, 34, 57–59

Rogers J (2006) Hot flashes, night sweats, and sleep disturbances, in Stephenson H (ed.) *The Boston Women's Health Book Collective, 'Our Bodies, Ourselves: Menopause'*. Simon & Schuster, New York. pp. 74–98

Royal College of Obstetricians and Gynaecologists (2006) Alternatives to HRT for management of symptoms of the menopause. *Scientific Advisory Committee Opinion, Paper 6*

Salle B and Lornage J (2007) Ovarian tissue transplantation, in Kruger TF, Van Der Spuy Z and Kempers RD (eds) *Advances in Fertility Studies and Reproductive Medicine – IFFS 2007*. Juta & Co Ltd, Cape Town. pp. 403–407

Seli E and Tangir J (2005) Fertility preservation options for female patients with malignancies. *Current Opinion in Obstetrics and Gynecology*, 17, 299–308

Shumaker S, Legault C, Rapp S, et al. (2003) Estrogen plus progestin and the incidence of dementia and mild cognitive impairment in post-menopausal women. The women's health initiative memory study: a randomized controlled trial. *JAMA*, 289 (20), 2651–2661

Silva I and Naftolin F (2007) Clinical effects of sex steroids on the brain, in *Treatment of the Post Menopausal Woman, Basic and Clinical Aspects*, third edition. R. Lobo R (ed.), Academic Press, Massachusetts. pp. 199–215

Smith A (1998) Women's health issues of middle age, in Rodgers-Clark C and Smith A (eds) *Women's Health A Primary Care Approach*. Maclennan & Petty, Sydney. pp. 189–204

Sonmezer M, Shamonki MI and Oktay K (2005) Ovarian tissue cryopreservation: benefits and risks. *Cell and Tissue Research*, 322, 125–132

Speroff L (2005) Clinical appraisal of the Women's Health Initiative. *J Obstet Gynaecol Res*, 31 (2), 80–93

Stehman FB, Rose PG, Greer BE, et al. (2003) Innovations in the treatment of invasive cervical cancer. *Cancer*, 98 (9, suppl), 2052–2063

Steigrad S, Hacker NF and Kolb B (2005) *In vitro* fertilization surrogate pregnancy in a patient who underwent radical hysterectomy followed by ovarian transposition, lower abdominal wall radiotherapy, and chemotherapy. *Fertility and Sterility*, 83 (5), 1547e7–1547e9

Van Eijkeren M and Van Der Wijk I (1999) Benefits and side effects of lateral ovarian transposition (LOT) performed during radical hysterectomy and pelvic lymphadenectomy for early stage cervical cancer. *International Journal of Gynecological Cancer*, 9 (5), 396–400

Warren M and Valente J (2004) Menopause and patient management. *Clinical Obstetrics and Gynecology*, 47 (2), pp. 450–470

Wenzel L, Dogan-Ates A, Habbal R, et al. (2005) Defining and measuring reproductive concerns of female cancer survivors. *Journal of the National Cancer Institute Monographs*, 34, 94–98

Zacur H. (1999) Hormone therapy, menopause and malignancy, in Trimble E and Trimble C (eds) *Cancer Obstetrics and Gynecology*. Lippincott Williams & Wilkins, Philadelphia. pp. 33–51

Zandi P, Carlson M, Plassman B, et al. (2002) Hormone replacement therapy and incidence of Alzheimer's disease in older women: The Cache County study. *JAMA*, 288 (17), 2123–2129

Chapter 8

Cervical screening

'The object of screening is to discover those among the apparently well who are in fact suffering from disease.'

(Wilson and Jugner 1968, p. 7)

Introduction

Most developed nations have some kind of cervical screening programme and each one has the same goal, which is the early detection and treatment of cervical cancer precursors (and sometimes cervical cancer itself). In order to implement an effective screening programme it has been suggested that a number of criteria should be fulfilled (see Box 8.1). These principles were put forward by Wilson and Jugner back in the 1960s when cervical cancer screening was very much in its infancy. Whilst most of them are clearly applicable to cervical cancer, arguably some are not.

Ever since the concept of screening was first mooted there has been debate over the optimal format of screening programmes. Thus, although many schemes have now been in place for well over a decade, there is still a surprisingly large disparity between different practices in different countries. For example, there are different screening intervals, different policies regarding management of low grade abnormalities and different views on the adoption of liquid based cytology and HPV testing (see Box 8.2).

In part, these differences can be explained by the often idiosyncratic evolution of screening. In many countries programmes have developed in an ad hoc way, without a clear sense of direction or order. A good analogy is provided by Muir Grey (2001) who compared the UK cervical screening programme with 'Brownian motion'.

Brown was a botanist who noticed that pollen grains when examined under a microscope were in a state of perpetual motion; motion that was full of energy but without purpose or direction. Muir Grey comments that cervical cancer screening had drifted into practice in the 1960s without either a sound evidence base or a programme of implementation. In the late 1980s and 1990s it resembled Brownian motion, with a growing number of smears each year but no systematic approach to programme management or quality assurance. Inevitably, there followed a number of problems (see Box 8.3) resulting in a review of the system and a look at some quality control issues.

The UK is not alone in this pattern of evolution. In many other developed nations, cervical screening programmes have arisen in a less than orderly manner. The USA provides another example of a country in which cervical screening guidelines have been confusing and are still the subject of considerable individual interpretation (Waxman 2005).

Box 8.1 Principles of early disease detection (Wilson and Jugner 1968, pp. 26–27, reproduced with permission)

(1) The condition sought should be an important health problem.
(2) There should be an accepted treatment for patients with recognised disease.
(3) Facilities for diagnosis and treatment should be available.
(4) There should be a recognisable latent or early symptomatic stage.
(5) There should be a suitable test or examination.
(6) The test should be acceptable to the population.
(7) The natural history of the condition, including development from latent to declared disease, should be adequately understood.
(8) There should be an agreed policy on whom to treat as patients.
(9) The cost of case-finding (including diagnosis and treatment of patients diagnosed) should be economically balanced in relation to possible expenditure on medical care as a whole.
(10) Case-finding should be a continuing process and not a 'once and for all' project.

Although it can be seen that in the case of cervical screening most of these conditions are met, there are nevertheless a few which are not. Even today there is confusion as to 'whom to treat as patients' (8), particularly amongst the young. Furthermore, cost factors (9) are a source of constant concern, particularly with the introduction of new technologies such as liquid-based cytology.

Box 8.2 Cervical screening programmes in Europe

The current diversity of screening practices within the developed world can be illustrated by looking at different programmes within Europe. Anttila et al. (2004) recently reviewed the cervical screening programmes in 18 European countries. He concluded that 'in general there are large variations in European cervical cancer screening policies and in the organisation of programmes.'

To begin with, not all European countries have cervical screening programmes. Several Eastern European countries have established cancer registries but have not implemented formal screening. Unfortunately, cervical cancer mortality rates are uniformly increasing in some of these countries (Anttila et al. 2004).

Linos and Riza (2000) compared the screening programmes within the European Union countries in 2002 and also found widely disparate practices. Although the EU has changed significantly since then, the paper still provides a good illustration of the variety of screening measures that can co-exist.

National cervical screening programmes were then operating in six states: Finland, England, Germany, Luxembourg, the Netherlands and Sweden. In Austria, Belgium, France, Greece, Italy, Portugal, Denmark and Spain cervical cancer screening was performed regionally.

Whilst the majority of countries invited women for screening via personal invitation utilising a national database, some places left the responsibility to GPs or gynaecologists. All countries utilised the cervical smear as the main screening tool, although Italy also combined this with colposcopy.

The target age group ranged from 20–25 up to 59–64 years in most countries. Finland and the Netherlands addressed a smaller target age group, 30–60 years, and Luxembourg applied a lower age limit of 15 years. Whilst the recommended screening interval was three years in most countries, in some it was extended to three to five years (England, Finland, Ireland, the Netherlands). In Austria, Germany and Luxembourg the screening interval was only one year.

There was great variability between states regarding the professional background of the smear taker. In Denmark and Portugal smears were taken only by the GP whereas GPs and/or other physicians took smears in Belgium, France, Luxembourg and Spain. Finland, Sweden,

England, Greece, Ireland, Italy and the Netherlands also utilised nurses and other health professionals.

Most countries received at least partial financial support for their campaign from their government, with the EU providing some financial assistance for quality control purposes. The UK appeared to be unusual in its financial incentive scheme for screening. (See Box 8.6)

Box 8.3 Errors, audit and litigation

In February 1999, three women were declared the victims of medical negligence in the Kent and Canterbury region, England, because they had apparently had negative smears and then preceded to contract cervical cancer. The judge made his finding despite evidence from two cytologists called by the former East Kent Health Authority stating that they would not have expected such abnormalities to be picked up in a routine screening programme at that time.

Thus the 'Bolam test' was effectively overruled. The 'Bolam test' is the standard in British law which is applied to cases of apparent medical negligence. Alleged negligence can be defended if a responsible body of medical opinion agrees with the manner and standard in which the disputed task was conducted (Slater 1998).

In 1996, the trust had decided to audit its cervical screening and re-examined 91000 smears. Eight women had died, 30 others developed cancer and had hysterectomies, and hundreds of women needed treatment for abnormalities that had been undetected. Out-of-court settlements paid equalled 1.6 million (Dyer 1999a). An independent inquiry in 1997 found a catalogue of mismanagement and failings in the service, which was subsequently transferred to another hospital (Dyer 1999b). Many other hospitals followed suit by instigating internal audit and today much more formal systems of quality control have been implemented throughout the UK.

Another such audit was conducted in Leicester in the late 1990s and attracted considerable attention at the time. This case highlights some of the ethical and legal aspects of medical audit (Symonds et al. 2003).

The cervical smear histories of 403 women who developed invasive cervical cancer in Leicester between January 1993 and September 2000 were reviewed in a retrospective audit, the aim of which was 'to ascertain whether diagnosis could potentially have been made sooner and to identify improvements that could have been made within the laboratory aspect of the screening service'.

Before diagnosis, 324 (80%) of the women had had a cervical smear. Of these, 122 were given a wrong diagnosis. A false negative report had been issued for 84 women and in 38 the cytological abnormality had been undergraded. The consequences of these misclassifications were serious: 20 of the 122 women died, diagnostic delay being a factor in 14 of these deaths. Similarly, a diagnostic delay led to 64 women requiring more radical treatment than would have been necessary if they had received the correct diagnosis and therapy earlier. During this time Leicester conducted 80,000 cervical smears a year.

The interesting issue about this case was how it was dealt with by the health authority. The managers were informed of the results before they were submitted to a scientific journal, leading to an internal debate about what to do with the information. Eventually, advice was sought from the Department of Health and a decision was made at ministerial level to release these data at a press conference and to tell the women or their bereaved relatives the results of individual reviews of previous cytological examinations (Symonds et al. 2003).

A number of issues arose from this unfortunate episode. Principally, did it breach the principle of confidentiality which is imperative to an audit? And what was the impact of this disclosure on the relatives of the affected women? 'A false negative smear is not necessarily evidence of negligence' (Symonds et al. 2003). How helpful, therefore, was this information to the individuals concerned and to their families?

The differences could also reflect a paucity of high level evidence regarding optimal screening practices. Another surprising feature of cervical screening programmes is the dearth of relevant large-scale clinical trials. This is in spite of the fact that they have been running for long periods of time with large patient populations and an apparent infra-structure to facilitate good quality research. This deficit was commented on in Australia when the cervical screening guidelines were revised in 2006. It was apparent that there had been no formal Australian research studies of relevance at all during the previous decade – and this was despite comments in the 1994 guidelines expressing disappointment at the lack of data on which recommendations could be based (Mitchell 2006).

Finally, the differences could be a reflection of other country-specific factors such as political or financial considerations. For example, to quote Mitchell (2006), 'the intense medico-legal pressures in the United States' health system means their policies may not be appropriate elsewhere. The funding arrangements of the National Health Service in the United Kingdom means their guidelines may not be relevant to other countries.'

Below there follows an examination of cervical screening programmes with particular emphasis on the programmes in the UK and Australia.

Cervical screening programmes – do they work?

In today's era of 'evidence based medicine' it is perhaps of interest that cervical screening programmes which are well established and respected in much of the developed world, have never been evaluated in the context of a randomised, controlled trial. Furthermore, they probably never will be. It is now widely accepted that screening is effective and con-stitutes a valuable public health intervention (Sasieni and Adams 1999). The data to support this comes from looking at cervical cancer rates following the introduction of screening programmes. For example, an analysis of trends in mortality from cervical cancer before and after screening was introduced in England suggests that the programme saves up to 4500 lives each year (Peto et al. 2004).

A recent evaluation by the International Agency for Research on Cancer (IARC) con-cluded that there is sufficient evidence that screening women ages 35 to 64 for cervical cancer precursors by conventional cytology every three to five years within high quality programmes reduces the incidence of invasive cervical cancer by at least 80% amongst those screened (IARC 2005). Sasieni et al. (2003) calculate that if 80% of women between 25 and 64 were screened a reduction in death rates of 95% is achievable.

Problems with cervical screening programmes

False positives and negatives

All screening programmes must have false positives and negatives. It is impossible to run a screening programme without false positives and negatives. This information should be made clearly available to women being offered screening.

(Muir Gray 1995, quoted in Slater 1998, p. 151)

The terms 'sensitivity' and 'specificity' as applied to cervical screening were mentioned in Chapter 2: 'Sensitivity is the proportion of truly diseased persons in the screened popu-lation who are identified by the screening test. Specificity is the proportion of truly non-diseased persons who are so identified by the screening test' (Karnon et al. 2003).

Thus, the sensitivity of the test is its ability to avoid false negatives which can arise from inadequate collecting or reporting. Its specificity is its ability to avoid false positives – that is identifying someone as having a cervical abnormality when in fact their smear result is normal. The sensitivity of conventional smears has been estimated to be 55–65% and their specificity 65–70% (Fahey et al. 1995). The impact of false positives and negatives is discussed more fully below.

Clearly a *false negative* result – that is being told that a cervical smear is satisfactory when it in fact indicates that further action is required – is a worrying possibility in any cervical screening campaign and there have been a number of well publicised cases throughout the world illustrating that the test is not failsafe and mistakes can be made (see Box 8.3).

What, therefore, are the safeguards against false negatives? In recent years considerable effort has gone into implementing quality assurance strategies in order to improve both the collection and processing of cervical smears. Stringent quality measures also apply to laboratories. Furthermore, new technologies such as liquid based cytology aim to further improve the reliability of smear results.

It should also be remembered that the sensitivity of one test does not necessarily reflect the sensitivity of the whole programme. For example, one false negative may be of no significance if the abnormality is picked up at the next test. Thus, the sensitivity and specificity also have to be accounted for in the *frequency* of screening.

A *false positive* result is one that comes back positive when in fact the cervix is normal or only slightly abnormal, without requiring any action. False positives can clearly result in significant psychological morbidity. The psychological sequelae of a positive cervical smear are discussed more fully later in this chapter. False positives will also expose the recipient to unnecessary further testing and procedures. The issue of over-testing and over-treating has been a particular problem amongst younger age groups diagnosed with an HPV infection.

The natural history of HPV has already been described in Chapter 1. It has been established that infection with the virus is very common, with 75% of women being exposed to either low risk or high risk HPV at some time in their lives (Koutsky 1997). In most cases a woman will only be transiently positive and will clear the infection using her own, cell-mediated immunity after an average of 8 to 11 months (Ho et al. 1998).

Women in their teens and twenties have an immature transformation zone and are particularly efficient at acquiring high risk HPV (Waxman 2005). This will usually result in a low grade cervical cytology abnormality. Such women have a minimal risk of developing cancer (Moscicki et al. 1999, Ries et al. 2000). It is females in their thirties and older who still test positive for high risk HPV that are at greatest risk of developing neoplastic changes (Waxman 2005).

Thus, the management of younger women and adolescents with low grade abnormalities raises problems. Positive cytology and positive HPV testing is not unusual but is probably no cause for concern. Nevertheless, many women will proceed to have further investigation – either a repeat smear or colposcopy. In women younger than 24 there is a 1 in 13 chance of being referred for a colposcopic examination (Kavanagh et al. 1996). Not only does this have the potential to cause discomfort and anxiety, but it also places a significant strain on the system. To quote Dickinson (1999): 'Taking smears too often not only may cause harm by giving unnecessary referrals, creating emotional stress, and even performing unnecessary operations, but also swamps the follow-up services with work that does not need to be done.'

In the USA, the American College of Obstetricians and Gynaecologists (ACOG) and the American Cancer Society have released revised guidelines on the management of adolescents with abnormal smears in an attempt to address this issue (Saslow et al. 2002, Wright et al. 2003). Their current recommendations are that adolescents should undergo their first screening pap smear three years after first intercourse or at the age of 21. They advise that the decision about beginning cervical screening in an adolescent should take into account:

(1) age of first sexual activity
(2) behaviours that may place the adolescent at greater risk of HPV infection
(3) risk of non-compliance with follow-up visits

They suggest that the optimal management of younger women involves a less structured approach than that of older women and rather their care should be individualised, with an emphasis on taking of an accurate sexual history in order to gauge level of risk and of compliance.

In the UK cervical screening does not begin until after the age of 25 in order to reduce this problem.

Screening intervals

One of the principal areas in which there appears to be considerable disparity between different screening programmes is in the frequency of testing (see Table 8.1). Within the UK the recommendation is for three to five-yearly screening whereas Australia has a two-yearly policy. The USA applied an annual screening policy for many years and although there have been recent efforts to move to less frequent cervical smears, this has been met with resistance by a lot of American women (Smith et al. 2003).

The obvious question is which country is correct? Surely there must be an 'optimal' screening period. However, in practice this issue is extremely complex and involves balancing a number of factors including the sensitivity of the test, the natural history of the disease and, of course, the cost. As screening frequency increases, the cost-effectiveness decreases dramatically due to increased detection of transient cervical abnormalities and associated low-grade CIN lesions, particularly in the young (Kulasingham et al. 2006). Furthermore, screening does not appear to be as effective against the relatively rare aggressive cancers that do occur in younger women (Kulasingham et al. 2006).

In 1986, the IARC attempted to address the problem of screening interval in a large, international study and this data has subsequently been used to guide practice in a number of countries. The study aimed to estimate:

(1) the risk of invasive cervical cancer among women who had had one or more negative cytology results
(2) the degree to which the risk of developing invasive cancer was related to the time elapsed since the last negative result and the number of previous negative results

The IARC (1986) conclusions were:

• little is gained by screening every year rather than every two or even three years
• screening every five years also offers a high degree of protection but appreciably less than screening every three years
• screening every ten years (option for lower resourced countries) is still associated with reducing the risk of cervical cancer by nearly two thirds

When should screening be instigated and terminated?

Once again this is a contentious issue and one that the IARC also attempted to address in the above paper. It has already been established that invasive cancer is exceedingly rare in women younger than 25 (Moscicki et al. 1999, Ries et al. 2000). After that its incidence increases until a plateau is reached either at age 35–40 in populations of moderate incidence or some ten years later in populations of high incidence. The plateau continues until aged 60 or over, after which some decline may occur (IARC 1986). The IARC thus suggested that regular screening of women aged 35 to 60 should form the core of organised screening but optimally screening should probably start some years before the age of 35.

Table 8.1 Cervical cancer screening recommendations (adapted from Tiffen 2006)

Country	When to begin screening	Screening interval	When to finish screening	After hysterectomy	LBC?	HPV testing?
UK	Twenty five Women who are not sexually active are not excluded but are informed that their risk is very low, and they may wish to decline.	25–49 = 3 yearly 50–64 = 5 yearly abnormal tests	Women aged 65 and over who have had three consecutive negative smears are taken out of the call recall system.	Normally would not require one but confirm with surgical team.	Yes – should be nationwide by 2008.	Role being examined in UK for management of low grade lesions.
Australia	All women who have ever been sexually active should start having Pap smears between the ages of 18 and 20 years, or one or two years after first having sexual intercourse, whichever is later. In some cases, it may be appropriate to start screening before 18 years of age.	Two-yearly	Pap smears may cease at the age of 70 years for women who have had two normal Pap smears within the last five years. Women over 70 years who have never had a Pap smear, or who request a Pap smear, should be screened.	Probably not necessary for total hysterectomy but may be for partial – discuss with doctor.	Not currently supported by Australian screening system. Women choosing to have LBC will need to pay an additional charge of approximately $30.	HPV testing is recommended to confirm cure in cases of high grade abnormalities where cytology has returned to normal.

Box 8.4 Reasons for non-attendance of cervical screening

(1) do not know about the services
(2) do not realise they qualify for them
(3) fear the screening itself
(4) believe in erroneous cultural myths
(5) lack free time to pursue self-care activities
(6) psychological factors such as fatalism
(7) lack knowledge about the efficacy of early detection
(8) fear they already have cancer
(9) believe that there is no treatment for cancer
(10) have general (possibly unrealisitic) confidence in their health
(11) fear male physicians and are dissatisfied with physicians' attitudes
(12) are constrained for financial reasons
(13) have a misconception that women visiting gynaecologists have sexually transmitted diseases
(14) are elderly
(15) live in a rural area
(16) are below the poverty index
(17) have less than a high school education
(18) embarrassment
(19) family difficulties/personal circumstances

(Austoker 1994, Jepson et al. 2000, Tseng et a. 2001, Kiger 2003, Park et al. 2005, Forbes et al. 2006)

Problems with access

No matter how well designed a screening programme might be, it is of little value if women do not attend. This has been – and still is – a considerable obstacle to effective cervical screening in both developed and developing countries. Cervical cancer mainly occurs in unscreened or under-screened women who either fail to attend for initial cervical screening or who do not come for follow-up. Current estimates suggest that 50% of women diagnosed with cervical cancer have never had a cervical smear and 10% have not had one in the last ten years (Nuovo et al. 2001).

There are a number of reasons for poor uptake of cervical screening, some of which are listed in Box 8.4. The most highly represented groups of non-attenders are those on low incomes and those from ethnic minorities whose attendance may be further hindered by cultural and language issues (Coughlin et al. 2003, Owusu et al. 2005). Conversely, individual studies have shown a relationship between higher cervical smear attendance and those who are married, employed, or premenopausal (Bowman et al. 1995). Other factors which increase the likelihood of having a cervical smear are:

- being fluent in English
- having a higher education
- being recommended by a physician
- having had prior family planning or obstetric care
- having had a regular health care provider

(Lin-Lee and Menon 2005)

Improving screening uptake amongst minority groups

If you want to build partnerships these have to be equal. People have to be encouraged to share experiences, knowledge and skills. People have to try and understand where you are coming from and they want to know about one's difference ... And it is insult-ing to expect us to 'fix it' if nobody from the community has been involved until then ... plus it makes us people look like we are the troublemakers when it could all be avoided in the first place.

Community Elder, Walgett, NSW (NHMRC 2004, p.13)

In 2004 the National Health Service Cervical Screening Programme (NHSCSP) pub-lished a report called *Woman to Woman* (Chiu 2004). This piece of action research had been commissioned in order to explore the issues involved in promoting cervical screening amongst minority ethnic women. The researchers felt that much of the previous work in the area stereotyped women and failed to reflect the 'diversity and fluidity of minority groups in the contemporary British context'. They considered there was a difference in perceptions between smear takers and ethnic minority women which had not been suffi-ciently explored in previous studies.

Focus groups were employed to discuss these issues further and disturbingly it was found that, 'compounded by language differences, the majority of [minority] women had under-gone smear testing with understanding neither of the screening programme nor the pro-cedure of the test.'

A number of solutions were put forward including:

(1) the training of smear takers in intercultural communication
(2) the delivery of pre-screening health education to minority ethnic women
(3) the employment of bilingual Community Health Educators

Australia has faced similar difficulties regarding cervical screening uptake amongst minority groups. Although the incidence of cervical cancer in Australia is now one of the lowest of the developed countries (Ferley et al. 2004), still cervical screening uptake is low amongst certain parts of the population.

Two groups within Australia which have significantly poorer cervical smear uptake (and outcome) are indigenous women and those living in rural and remote areas. Indigenous residents comprise 29% of the Northern Territory population, two thirds of whom live in remote and rural areas. The incidence of cervical cancer is 2.6 times higher amongst these women and their mortality 8.6 times higher than other Australian women (Binns and Condon 2006). Epidemiological data from Queensland indicates that in some areas the death rate from cancer of the cervix among aboriginal women is 13.3 times higher than the state average (Coory et al. 1999).

In 1988, Kirk et al. produced a report indicating that screening services in Australia were failing to meet the needs of Aboriginal women. For example, screening was often operated out of locations that were not considered to be culturally safe or effective. A number of measures were subsequently implemented, including the appointment of Indigenous Health Workers who work alongside the registered nurses in Well Women's Health Screening. Five key principles of practice (NHMRC 2004) were formulated in order to make the service more acceptable. These were:

(1) Respond promptly to client, community member and staff needs.
(2) Encourage ongoing participation of clients, community members and staff in service design and delivery.
(3) Be courteous and respectful to all clients, community members and staff.
(4) Operate efficiently and effectively.
(5) Work towards best practice standards.

Other programmes have been implemented around the world in order to improve screen-ing uptake amongst minority groups, many of which have involved the use of volunteers. Kiger (2003) describes a number of such initiatives used in California. 'The African Ameri-can Tell a Friend Programme' recruits and trains groups of women to call five of their friends and encourage them to have a mammogram or Pap smear. Volunteers are given incentive gifts to participate. Other schemes such as the Witness Project utilise spiritual communities as a forum for promotion of women's health issues. Volunteers are trained to conduct presentations in churches and community centres. The Witness Project incorporates spiritual concepts, faith components, storytelling and experiential learning techniques to address the needs of African American women (Kiger 2003). 'Survivors' are included amongst the volunteers who are useful at promoting the concept that cancer is not necessarily a death sentence.

Black et al. (2006) describes a Canadian volunteer scheme which was set up to target Chinese and Vietnamese women. Volunteer 'health educators' were trained to provide education to women from these groups. They began by arranging tea parties in which they discussed healthy living, risk factors for cancer, cancer screening and how to access health care services. Meetings were held in churches, libraries and YMCAs. At baseline approximately 40% of women had never undergone a Pap smear, a figure which fell by 20% at four months follow-up.

Another group which is underrepresented in cervical screening populations is women with learning difficulties. As few as 8% of women with learning difficulties attend for cervical screening in the UK compared with 85% of the general female population (Band 1998). Broughton and Thomson (2000) interviewed a group of women with learning difficulties and their carers about cervical screening and one of the key issues identified for this patient population was the need for adequate preparation and education about the screening procedure. Another reason that women with learning difficulties are less likely to be screened is that they are deemed to be unable to give consent (Djuretic et al. 1999). The issue of consent is a pertinent one across the screening programme and is discussed more fully below.

Information and consent

For some time the emphasis of many cervical screening programmes has been on encouraging higher levels of participation. One potential casualty of this is adequate informed consent – particularly where financial incentives are being offered in order to boost screening numbers. In recent years there has been growing concern that women are attending for screening without having a proper understanding of the procedure and that they are therefore not providing fully informed consent. Whilst it has already been recognised that this is the case amongst some minority groups, there is also research to suggest that even where language differences do not exist, poor understanding of the cervical screening procedure can be found. A number of participants appear to adopt a passive acceptance of screening procedures without fully realising what is happening. To quote one woman in a Swedish study (Idestrom et al. 2006): 'I have not quite understood what part of the genitals they have examined. I have been a patient that shall be examined.'

In this study many of the participants were unaware of the purpose of screening, a finding which is in keeping with previous studies in Sweden, indicating that only 32% to 60% of women knew that the cervical smear aimed to detect precursors of/or cervical cancer (Idestrom et al. 2002). Despite their lack of understanding most of the women were regular screening attendants. A number of women seemed to adopt a paternalistic approach to the system and were prepared to simply 'put themselves into the hands of the professionals'.

The same would appear to be true in the UK. Philips et al. (2005) looked at the level of understanding of cervical screening amongst a cohort of British women. They distributed a questionnaire via GPs to 1244 women who were eligible for screening (see Box 8.5). They found that many women had a poor understanding of the cervical screening programme and concluded that fully informed consent was not being achieved. They identified two main issues:

(1) The quality of public knowledge about cervical cancer risk factors is variable. Women are especially unsure about HPV. Many people incorrectly considered there to be a

---

Box 8.5 Participant knowledge of cancer and screening

This shows the result of a survey distributed to women in the UK in order to assess their level of knowledge about cervical cancer screening (Phillips et al. 2005, reproduced with permission).

Question	Percentage of women who thought this answer correct

(1) How common do you think cervical cancer is in the UK?

1 in 100 women get cervical cancer each year	25.1
1 in 1000 women get cervical cancer each year	34.8
1 in 5000 women get cervical cancer each year	24.3
1 in 10,000 women get cervical cancer each year	12.6
1 in 20,000 women get cervical cancer each year	3.3

(2) Approximately what proportion of women in the UK receive an abnormal cervical smear result each year?

1%	3.8
5%	17.9
10%	34.5
20%	27.6
30%	16.2

(3) At what ages are women most likely to receive an abnormal smear result?

18–25 years	7.6
25–35 years	31.8
35–50 years	50.8
50 + years	9.9

(4) How accurate is the cervical smear test?

99% or better?	16.3
75–98%	71.8
50–74%	11.1
Less than 50%	0.8

(5) Approximately how many cases of cervical cancer are prevented each year as a result of the screening programme?

Less than 1000	5.3
Between 1000 and 4000	39.8
Between 4000 and 9000	35.3
More than 10,000	19.6

The correct answers are:

(1) 1 in 10,000 women get cervical cancer each year	12.6
(2) 10% (7.7%)	34.5
(3) 18–25 years	7.6
(4) 50–74% (estimates vary 30–90%)	11.1
(5) Between 1000 and 4000	39.8

---

familial link with cervical cancer. Also, many women considered excess weight to be a risk (this is a risk for breast cancer but has not been linked with an increased risk of cervical cancer).

(2) The population risk of cervical cancer is overestimated by the majority of women. Women are also overly optimistic about the preventative potential of the screening programme.

Information leaflets

The provision of written material has long been regarded as an important and useful method of information giving within the cervical screening programme (Somerset and

Peters 1998). Each campaign has its own collection of information leaflets. Whilst often not subjected to formal evaluation, such literature is generally assumed to be helpful to patients in understanding the cervical screening procedure.

In order to assist in uptake amongst minority groups many countries have attempted to provide translations of such information leaflets. This is not always as simple as it may appear. Kiger (2003) describes attempting to translate an education brochure from English to Spanish. Five different translations were produced, depending on the translator's educational level, where they learned Spanish, and their own interpretation of the material. Similar anecdotes are given in *Woman to Woman*, where a number of information leaflets were reviewed and mistranslation and misinformation was found in most of them. For example, in one Chinese leaflet a 'colposcopy' was described as 'examination by a small camera' (Chiu 2003).

Psychological sequelae of cervical screening

I don't know what she [the physician] said, so I said 'Speak Swedish . . . because I don't understand what you are saying. *What is it that I have? What is this?'* And then she said 'Yes, well there is no sign of cancer at all' . . . '*Yes, but what is it I have?'*

(Ebba, 40 years old, italics added, Forss et al. 2004)

There is clearly a psychological cost associated with any screening procedure, regardless of whether the result is positive or negative. Cervical screening is widely perceived as anxiety provoking, the anxiety beginning with the initial invitation to participate (Rostad 2002). Furthermore, a negative result may not necessarily alleviate fears raised by the screening procedure (Rostad 2002).

The above quotation comes from a qualitative study performed in Sweden which looked at the psychological impact of receiving an abnormal smear result. Most women interviewed in this study indicated that they had no expectation of an abnormality and therefore the result was often received with confusion. An abnormal cervical smear was seen to signify both 'something' and 'nothing'. The authors concluded that receiving notification of an abnormal smear 'can be seen as an unintentional transition from routine confirmation of health to ambivalence . . . as the women expected to have health confirmed but instead neither health nor disease was confirmed or excluded' (Forss et al. 2004).

Doherty et al. (1991) looked at the psychological response of women who had a positive screening test. Women's distress following a positive smear result was classified as: 68% 'a little', 21% 'moderately' and 8% 'severely'. Their main fears were of how the abnormality was caused, whether the treatment would be effective and whether it was cancer. A significant number of women feared that things would get worse in the period whilst they were waiting for appointments, and had concerns about their fertility. There were also anxieties that the disease could be passed on, leading to worries about their sex life.

Gath et al. (1995) found that 51% of women experienced shock, panic or horror on receiving an abnormal cervical smear result. In the first week following the news, 90% of women reported feeling fear and worry, 67% depression, 44% poor concentration and 29% sleep disturbance. Anxiety continued until colposcopy – indeed, one of the most important influences on anxiety was the interval between receiving notification of an abnormal smear and undergoing a colposcopy. Posner and Vesey (1988) found this the most anxious time for more than 50% of women, with the anxiety level unrelated to the severity of the abnormal smear. Furthermore, the colposcopy procedure itself is associated with significant apprehension amongst a large number of women – in fact there is almost as much anxiety about the colposcopy procedure as there is about the outcome (Marteau et al. 1990).

Whilst adverse psychological sequelae are perhaps to be expected in cases of high grade dysplastic changes, similar levels of anxiety have also been reported for women receiving notification of low grade changes and even unevaluable smears (French et al. 2004, Gray et al. 2006).

These high levels of psychological distress are largely a reflection of a poor level of understanding of cervical screening. There appears to be a similar knowledge deficit regarding HPV infection (see Chapter 11). A qualitative study performed in Australia looked at the reaction of women to a positive diagnosis of HPV (McCaffrey and Irwig 2005). A number of themes were revealed, one of the most important being a general level of confusion regarding HPV – even after it had been explained by health professionals. There was a poor understanding of the implications of the infection for partners and its impact on sexual relationships. There were also questions about its effect on fertility. To quote one participant: 'Whether it was an STD or not, I still don't know to this day'. McCaffrey et al. (2003) also looked at attitudes towards HPV testing amongst a number of different ethnic groups in the UK. Similarly, there were a number of concerns regarding relationship issues. HPV positivity carried connotations of infidelity and sexual misconduct. Women were anxious to know who to 'blame' for the infection.

McCaffrey and Irwig (2005) identify a number of informational needs of women regarding HPV including:

- HPV viral types (high risk versus low risk)
- Mode of transmission
- Implications for sexual relationships and partners
- Prevalence, latency and regression of HPV
- Management and treatment options
- Implications for cancer risk and fertility

One important influence on the reaction to a diagnosis of HPV appears to be the way in which the information was given. Disclosure by letter was perceived as most anxiety provoking, with clinician delivery of the information being perceived as optimal (McCaffrey and Irwig 2005).

However, a diagnosis of HPV infection is not perceived as universally negative. Kahn et al. (2005) interviewed a cohort of adolescents in a teen health clinic all of whom were positive for HPV. They found that although many women felt distressed at receiving the result, they also described feelings of empowerment, reflecting a sense of control over their ability to prevent future sexually transmitted diseases and cervical cancer (Kahn et al. 2005).

Box 8.6 Cervical screening UK

Since the inception of the cervical screening programme the incidence of cervical cancer in the UK has fallen more than any other cancer. The death rate is now falling at an accelerated rate of 7% a year, rendering it an increasingly uncommon disease (Lowndes and Gill 2005).

Cervical cytology testing was first introduced into the UK in the early 1960s in a piecemeal fashion, initially directed principally at the over thirty-fives (Bentley et al. 2006). At this time colposcopy was not generally available so women with suspicious smears would be referred to a gynaecologist and the smears would be repeated until normal. Treatment for positive smears was by hysterectomy or latterly cone biopsy. When the oral contraceptive pill became available in the mid-1960s it brought with it a new population of young women seeking cervical cytology testing.

In 1985, district health authorities were made responsible for the introduction of computerised call and recall systems for cervical screening (Department of Health and Social Security 1985). The formal UK screening programme began in 1988 and its national office was set up in Sheffield in 1994. Its remit is to:

- Develop systems and guidelines which will assure a high quality of cervical screening throughout the country.
- Identify important policy issues and help resolve them.
- Improve communications within the programme and to women.

In the decade following its inception there were a number of well publicised errors within the programme (see Box 8.3). Partly as a result of these a range of correctional measures were implemented to ensure comprehensive quality assurance testing. In 1996 the NHSCSP published national quality assurance guidelines. These included improvements in training, proficiency testing and performance standards for reporting (Canfell et al. 2006). Of particular importance a working party was convened to ensure adequate laboratory standards (Johnson and Patnick 2000). Their remit was to:

- Reinforce and where necessary revise existing guidelines for reporting cervical smears and clarify areas of potential misunderstanding.
- Propose new performance indicators for the reporting of negative, inadequate and abnormal categories of cervical smears.
- Identify pitfalls in cytological diagnosis that may lead to false positives and negatives.
- Propose criteria for evaluating performance and effectiveness of cervical cytopathology.
- Reassess the guidance in light of experience and better data quality, and in the context of the 'new NHS' to enable the setting, delivery and monitoring of quality standards in cervical cytopathology.

Today, regional directors of public health are appointed who are responsible for the quality assurance network in their region. This includes monitoring health authority activities, laboratories, colposcopy and primary care. Their function is to:

- Set quality assurance standards.
- Monitor and review performance against these quality assurance standards.
- Identify training needs and advise on how they should be met.
- Identify research needs.
- Advise the programme on professional matters.

                        http://www.cancerscreening.nhs.uk/cervical/quality-assurance.html (28/2/07)

Details of the screening programme are outlined in Table 8.1. Until 2003, the screening interval varied between different health authorities from three to five years, with more than half issuing screening invitations every three years, but this has now been standardised and is age-specific.

Practice incentive schemes were introduced into the UK in the 1990s to encourage promotion of cervical smear testing. Each practice received the maximum payment if more than 80% of registered, eligible women had been screened in the previous five years (Canfell et al. 2006).

NHSCSP statistics

(NHSCSP 2006, p. 5)

- NHSCSP invited 4.7 million women for screening in 2004–2005.
- In 2004–2005 3.3 million women aged 25–64 were tested in England.
- In 2004–2005 3.6 million women of all ages were tested in England.
- In 2004–2005, 80.3% of eligible women aged 25–64 resident in England had been screened at least once in the previous five years.
- Laboratories across the country examined an estimated 4 million samples in England in 2004–2005.
- Cervical screening, including the cost of treating cervical abnormalities, is estimated to be £157 million pa in England.

Box 8.7 Cervical screening Australia

Today, Australia has the second lowest incidence of cervical cancer and the lowest mortality rate among developed countries with comparable registration systems (Ferlay et al. 2004). However, this has not always been the case.

A national cervical screening programme was introduced in Australia in 1991; prior to this screening had been organised in separate states, but there was concern about its efficacy. In 1987 a committee was convened to assess why the cervical cancer rate in Australia did not appear to be diminishing. Problems were delineated at various stages of programme, from the recruitment of appropriate women, to the availability of pathology services and choice of treatment of the abnormalities detected (Dickinson 1999).

A national policy was generated to produce clear guidelines for action. A screening interval was stipulated so that there was no confusion with different regulations. Two years was chosen – a conservative approach to the IARC recommendations (IARC 1986). Over the following decade each state or territory set up its own cervical smear registry.

Standards were established for taking smears, interpreting smears, performing lab processes and reporting test results. Educational standards were developed to improve quality of smear-takers, cytotechnicians and cytopathologists. Quality assurance programmes were developed in smear-taking and the Australian College of Gynaecologists was asked to establish a quality assurance programme in colposcopy. Most importantly, feedback systems were established to ensure women were well informed about their results and reminder programmes were instituted.

In October 1991, the National Advisory Committee to the National Cervical Screening Program was established. This committee was replaced in 2004 by the Australian Screening Advisory Committee (ASAC), which provides advice on national screening policies to the Australian and State and Territory Governments through the Australian Health Ministers' Advisory Council (AHMAC).

Members of the ASAC are drawn from the Australian Government Department of Health and Ageing and State and Territory Health Departments. The ASAC also includes people with expertise in epidemiology, population health, gastroenterology, gynaecological oncology and general practice, and Aboriginal and Torres Strait Islander and consumer representatives (NCSP 2007).

The most recent revision of cervical screening practices in Australia occurred in 2001 when a multidisciplinary committee chaired by Professor Ian Hammond was convened to review the NHMRC 1994 guidelines for the management of asymptomatic women with screen detected abnormalities on a Pap smear (NHMRC 2005). The Guideline Review Group (GRG) identified several key areas for consideration and six major changes resulted for implementation from mid-2006. These were:

(1) The reporting terminology was changed to the Australian Modified Bethesda System (see Chapter 1).
(2) Repeat cervical smears were recommended for most women with LSIL/possible LSIL within 12 months.
(3) Recommendations were made not to treat women who had only biopsy proven CIN1 or HPV lesions.
(4) It was recommended that all women with atypical glandular cells should be referred for colposcopy.
(5) HPV testing was recommended in conjunction with cytology to confirm cure of women treated for CIN 2 and 3.
(6) It was recommended not to report normal endometrial cells in post-menopausal women.

Today, the Australian Cervical Screening Organisation issues an annual report looking at the national achievements of the campaign.

In 2001, practice incentive payments were introduced for screening eligible women who had not been re-screened for four years. In 2005, other incentives were introduced to allow practice nurses to take smears in women who had not been re-screened in four years in regional, rural and remote areas (Canfell et al. 2006).

Australian cervical screening statistics

Australian Screening Website (NHMRC: http://www.cancerscreening.gov.au/internet/screening/publishing.nsf/Content/facts accessed 20/2/07)

- Cervical cancer is the eighteenth most common cause of cancer mortality in Australian women, dropping from eighth place since the introduction of the screening programme.
- From January 2002 to December 2003 3,382,825 Australian women had Pap smears. Of these 3,318,354 (98%) were in the target age group 20–69 years.
- The participation rate for the National Cervical Screening Program was 60.7% of women in the target age group in 2002–2003.
- In 2003, the National Cervical Screening Program detected 14,745 women in the target age group with high grade abnormalities.
- The number of new cases of cervical cancer in Australia has continued to decline. There were 735 new cases in Australia in 2001 compared with 1078 detected in 1990, prior to the start of the organised screening program.
- About half of the new cases of cervical cancer diagnosed each year are in women over 50 years of age as women in this age group are less likely than younger women to have regular Pap smears. More women over 50 years of age die from cervical cancer because their cancer is diagnosed later when treatment is more difficult (HPV booklet).
- The lifetime probability to age 75 years of a woman in Australia developing cervical cancer is 1 in 183. In 2003, 238 women died from the disease (HPV booklet).
- In 2002 the age standardised incidence rate in Australia was 6.8 per 100,000 and in 2004 the mortality rate 1.9 per 100,000. There are approximately 750 cases, 1800 hospitalisations and 250 deaths pa.
- Mortality from cervical cancer declined by nearly 53% between 1982 and 2001 (from six deaths per 100,000 women in 1982 to three deaths per 100,000 women in 2001).

(http://www.aihw.gov.au/mediacentre/2003/mr20031219.cfm)

Conclusion

Cervical cancer is characterised by a long pre-invasive phase which facilitates early disease detection through cervical screening programmes. Within the developed world such programmes have helped reduce cervical cancer levels significantly. However, screening is not without its problems, and schemes vary, sometimes quite widely, between countries. In recent years some countries such as the UK and Australia have instigated formal audit and quality control measures to ensure higher quality results. Cervical screening uptake is an ongoing issue and tends to be poor amongst some minority groups. A number of educational and nursing initiatives have been set up to improve this.

Frequently asked questions

(1) How common are abnormal smears?
This varies between countries. In the UK, nine out of ten smears are normal. About 1 in 20 show mild or borderline changes – most of which will resolve spontaneously. One in 100 show moderate cell changes and 1 in 200 severe changes which will necessitate colposcopy. Less than 1 in 1000 smears will show invasive cancer.
http://www.cancerhelp.org.uk/help/default.asp?page=2756#frequency   (accessed 28/2/07)
(2) At what age is cervical cancer most commonly diagnosed?
In the forties and fifties. It is unusual amongst women in their teens and early twenties, at which time pre-cancerous abnormalities are more common.

(3) How many women die from cervical cancer?

In 2002, 927 deaths from cervical cancer were registered in the UK, with mortality rates increasing with increasing age.

(*Health Statistics Quarterly*, Summer 2003, Office for National Statistics)

(4) I have been through the menopause – do I still need a cervical smear?

Yes, cervical cancer is still a risk in post-menopausal women.

http://www.cancerscreening.gov.au/internet/screening/publishing.nsf/Content/papsmear#1 (accessed 17/6/07)

(5) I am not sexually active – do I still need a cervical smear?

If you have never been sexually active with a man, your risk of cervical cancer is thought to be low and you may choose to decline. If you have been sexually active in the past but are not at the moment you should still continue with cervical screening.

(NHSCSP 2004 *Cervical Cancer: a Pocket Guide*, DOH Publications)

(6) I am a lesbian – do I still need a cervical smear?

Once again, if you or you partner have never been sexually active with a man, your risk of cervical cancer is thought to be low and you may chose to decline. However, if you have had sexual contact with men in the past, or if your partner has, you are still at risk of cervical cancer and should be screened (Rankow and Tessaro 1998).

(7) I've had a hysterectomy – do I still need cervical screening?

Some types of hysterectomy remove the cervix whereas others do not. The surgical team who performed the operation will decide what kind of follow-up is appropriate and you should talk it over with them. Normally, if you do not have a cervix, then you do not need cervical screening.

http://www.cancerscreening.nhs.uk/cervical/faqs.html (accessed 17/6/07)

Resources

Australian Cancer Council: http://www.cancer.org.au/

Australian Institute of Health and Welfare: http://www.aihw.gov.au/

Australian Government Dept of Health and Aging: http://www.cancerscreening.gov.au/internet/screening/publishing.nsf/Content/cervical

National Health Service Cervical Screening Programme (NHSCSP): http://www.cancerscreening.nhs.uk/

References

Anttila A, Ronco G, Clifford G, et al. (2004) Cervical cancer screening programmes and policies in 18 European countries. *British Journal of Cancer*, 91, 935–941

Austoker J (1994) Cancer prevention in primary care: screening for cervical cancer. *BMJ*, 309 (6949), 241–248

Band R (1998) *The NHS – Health for All? People with Learning Disabilities and Health Care.* Mencap, London

Bentley E and TOMBOLA group (2006) Refining the management of low-grade cervical abnormalities in the United Kingdom National Health Service and defining the potential for human papillomavirus testing: a commentary on emerging evidence. *Journal of the Lower Genital Tract Disease*, 10 (1), 26–38

Binns PL and Condon JR (2006) Participation in cervical screening by indigenous women in the Northern Territory: a longitudinal study. *Medical Journal of Australia*, 185, 490–494

Black MEA, Frisina A, Hack T and Carpio B (2006) Improving early detection of breast and cervical cancer in Chinese and Vietnamese immigrant women. *Oncology Nursing Forum*, 33 (5), 873–876

Bowman J, Sanson-Fisher R, Boyle C, Pope S and Redman S (1995) A randomized controlled trial of strategies to prompt attendance for a Pap smear. *J Med Screening*, 2, 211–218

Broughton S and Thomson K (2000) Women with learning disabilities: risk behaviours and experiences of the cervical smear test. *Journal of Advanced Nursing*, 32 (4), 905–912

Canfell K, Sitas F and Beral V (2006) Cervical cancer in Australia and the United Kingdom: comparison of screening policy and uptake, and cancer incidence and mortality. *Medical Journal of Australia*, 185, 482–486

Chiu L (2003) *Woman to Woman*. National Health Service Cervical Screening Programme, University of Leeds

Coory M, Thompson A and Muller J (1999) *Cervical Cancer and the Queensland Cervical Cancer Screening Program*. Information Circular 49, Health Information Centre, Queensland Health, Australia

Coughlin S, Uhler RJ, Richards T and Wilson K (2003) Breast and cervical cancer screening practices among hispanic and non-hispanic women residing near the United States-Mexico border, 1999–2000. *Family and Community Health*, 26 (2), 130–139

Department of Health and Social Security (1985) *Cervical Cancer Screening*. (HC(85)8). DHSS, London

Dickinson JA (1999) Cervical screening: lessons from the Australian experience. *Hong Kong Medical Journal*, 5 (3), Sept, 226–228

Djuretic T, Lang-Morton T, Guy M and Gill M (1999) Concerted effort is needed to ensure these women use preventive services. *British Medical Journal*, 318, 537

Doherty IE, Richardson PH, Wolfe D and Raju KS (1991) The assessment of the psychological effects of an abnormal cervical smear and the subsequent medical procedures. *J Psychosom Obstet Gynaecol*, 12, 319–324

Dyer C (1999a) Health authority appeals on screening negligence. *British Medical Journal*, 318 (7188), 3 April, 895

Dyer C (1999b) Three women win in cancer screening case. *British Medical Journal*, 318 (7182), Feb 20, 484

Fahey MT, Irwig L and Macaskill P (1995) Meta-analysis of Pap test accuracy. *American Journal of Epidemiology*, 141, 680–689

Ferlay J, Pisani P, Bray F and Parkin DM (2004) *Globocan 2002: Cancer Incidence Mortality and Prevalence Worldwide* (CD-ROM). International Agency for Research on Cancer, Lyon. CancerBase No. 5, version 2.0: http://www-dep.iarc.fr/ (accessed 2/3/07)

Forbes C, Jepson R and Martin-Hirsch P (2003) Interventions targeted at women to encourage the uptake of cervical screening. *Cochrane Database Systematic Review*, 4

Forss A, Tishelman C, Widmark C and Sachs L (2004) Women's experiences of cervical cellular changes: an unintentional transition from health to liminality? *Sociology of Health and Illness*, 26 (3), 306–325

French DP, Maissi E and Marteau TM (2004) Psychological costs of inadequate cervical smear test results. *British Journal of Cancer*, 91, 1887–1892

Frazer IH, Cox JT, Mayeaux EJ, Franco EL, et al. (2006) Advances in prevention of cervical cancer and other human papillomavirus-related diseases. *Paediatric Infectious disease Journal*, 25 (2), Supplement, February, S65–S81

Gath DH, Hallam N, Mynors-Wallis L, et al. (1995) Emotional reactions in women attending a UK colposcopy clinic. *Journal Epidemiol Community Health*, 49, 79–83

Gray NM, Cotton SC, Masson LF, et al. on behalf of TOMBOLA group (2006) Psychological effects of a low-grade abnormal cervical smear test result: anxiety and associated factors. *British Journal of Cancer*, 94, 1253–1262

Ho GY, Bierman R, Beardsley L, et al. (1998) The natural history of cervical papillomavirus infection in young women. *N Engl J Med*, 338, 423–428

Idestrom M, Milsom I and Andersson-Ellstrom A (2002) Knowledge and attitudes about the Papsmear screening program: a population-based study of women aged 20–59 years. *Acta Obstet Gynecol Scand*, 81 (10), 962–967

Idestrom M, Milsom I, Andersson-Ellstrom A and Athlin E (2006) Cervical cancer screening – 'for better or worse . . .' women's experience of screening. *Cancer Nursing*, 26 (6), 453–460

International Agency for Research on Cancer (IARC) Working Group on Evaluation of Cervical Cancer Screening Programmes (1986) Screening for squamous cervical cancer: duration of low risk after negative results of cervical cytology and its implication for screening policies. *British Medical Journal*, 293, September, 659–664

International Agency for Research on Cancer (2005) IARC Handbooks of Cancer Prevention Vol. 10. *Cervix Cancer Screening*. IARC Press, Lyon

Jacob M, Bradley J and Barone M (2005) Human papillomavirus vaccines: what does the future hold for preventing cervical cancer in resource-poor settings through immunization programs? *Sexually Transmitted Diseases*, 32 (10), October, 635–640

Jepson R, Clegg A, Forbes C, Lewis R, Sowden A and Kliejnen J (2000) The determinants of screening uptake and interventions for increasing uptake: a systematic review. *Health Technology Assessment*, 4 (14)

Johnson J and Patnick J (2000) *Achievable Standards, Benchmarks for Reporting, and Criteria for Evaluating Cervical Cytopathology*. NHSCSP Publication No 1

Kahn JA, Slap GB, Bernstein DI, et al. (2005) Psychological, behavioural and interpersonal impact of human papillomavirus and Pap test results. *Journal of Women's Health*, 14 (7), 650–659

Kahn JA and Bernstein DI (2005) Human papillomavirus vaccines and adolescents. *Current Opinion on Obstetrics and Gynaecology*, 17, 476–482

Karnon J, Peters J, Chilcott J, McGoogan E and Platt J (2003) Liquid based cytology in cervical screening; an updated and systematic review. NICE: http://www.nice.org.uk/page.aspx?o=65586 (accessed 7/7/07)

Kavanagh A, Santow G and Mitchell H (1996) Consequences of current patterns of Pap smear and colposcopy use. *J Med Screening*, 3, 29–34

Kiger H (2003) Outreach to multiethnic, multicultural, and multilingual women for breast cancer and cervical cancer education and screening. *Community Health*, 26 (4) 307–318

Kirk M, Hoban E, Dunne A and Manderson L (1998) *Barriers to Appropriate Delivery Systems for Cervical Cancer Screening in Indigenous Communities*. Queensland Health, Brisbane

Koutsky L (1997) Epidemiology of genital human papillomavirus infection. *Am J Med*, 102, 3–8

Koutsky LA, Ault KA, Wheeler CM, et al. (2002) A controlled trial of human papillomavirus type 16 vaccine. *New England Journal of Medicine*, 347, 1645–1651

Kulasingham SL, Myers ER, Lawson HW, et al. (2006) Cost-effectiveness of extending cervical cancer screening intervals among women with prior normal Pap results. *Obstetrics and Gynaecology*, 107 (2, part 1), Feb, 321–328

Lin-Lee F and Menon U (2005) Breast and cervical cancer screening practices and interventions among Chinese, Japanese and Vietnamese Americans. *Oncology Nursing Forum*, 32 (5), 995–1003

Linos A and Riza E (2000) Comparisons of cervical screening programmes in the European Union. *European Journal of Cancer*, 36, 2260–2265

Lowndes CM and Gill ON (2005) Cervical cancer, human papilloma virus and vaccination. *BMJ*, 331, 22 Oct

Lowy DR and Schiller JT (2006) Prophylactic human papillomavirus vaccines. *Journal of Clinical Investigation*, 116 (50), May, 1167–1173, http://www.jci.org

Mahdavi A, Bradley JM (2005) Vaccines against human papillomavirus and cervical cancer: promises and challenges. *Oncologist*, 10, 528–538

Marteau TM, Walker P, Giles J, Smail MP (1990) Anxieties in women undergoing colposcopy. *British Jnl Obstet Gynaecol*, 97, 859–861

McCaffrey K, Forrest F, Waller J, Desai M, Szarewski A and Wardle J (2003) Attitudes towards HPV testing: a qualitative study of beliefs among Indian, Pakistani, African Carribean and white British women in the UK. *British Journal of Cancer*, 88, 42–46

McCaffrey K and Irwig L (2005) Australian women's needs and preferences for information about HPV in cervical screening. *Journal of Medical Screening*, 12 (3), 134–141

Mitchell H (2006) The price of guidelines: revising the national guidelines for managing Australian women with abnormal Pap smears. *Sexual Health*, 3, 53–55

Moscicki AB, Burt VG, Kanowitz S, et al. (1999) The significance of squamous metaplasia in the development of low grade squamous intraepithelial lesions in young women. *Cancer*, 85, 1139–1144

Muir Gray JA (2001) The evolution of screening. *Pharmacoepidemiology and Drug Safety*, 10, 49–54

National Cervical Screening Program (2007): http://www.cancerscreening.gov.au/internet/screening/publishing.nsf/Content/cervical-1lp (accessed 1/3/07).

National Health and Medical Research Council (2004) *Principles of Practice, Standards and Guidelines for Providers of Cervical Screening Services for Indigenous Women*. NHMRC, Australia: http://www.cancerscreening.gov.au/internet/screening/publishing.nsf/Content/pubs2 (accessed 25/2/07)

National Health and Medical Research Council (2005) *Screening to Prevent Cervical Cancer: Guidelines for the Management of Asymptomatic Women with Screen Detected Abnormalities*. NHMRC, Australia: www.nhmrc.gov.au/publications (accessed 3/3/07)

NHS Cancer Screening Programmes (2006) *Taking Samples for Cervical Screening*. NHSCSP publication no 23. Department of Health, UK

Nuovo J, Melnikow J and Howell LP (2001) New tests for cervical cancer screening. *American Family Physician*, 64, 780–786

Owusu GA, Eve SB, Cready CM, et al. (2005) Race and ethnic disparities in cervical cancer screening in a safety-net system. *Maternal and Child Health Journal*, 9 (3), September, 285–295

Park S, Chang S and Chung C (2005) Effects of a cognition-emotion focused program to increase public participation in Papanicolaou smear screening. *Public Health Nursing*, 22 (4), 289–298

Parkin DM, Bray F, Ferlay J and Pisani P (2005) Global cancer statistics 2002. *CA Cancer J Clin*, 55, 74–108

Peto J, Gilham C, Fletcher O and Matthews FE (2004) The cervical cancer epidemic that screening has prevented in the UK. *Lancet*, 364, 249–256

Philips Z, Avis M and Whynes DK (2005) Knowledge of cervical cancer and screening in east-central England. *Int J Gynaecol Cancer*, 15, 639–645

Posner T and Vesney M (1988) *Prevention of Cervical Cancer: the Patient's View*. King's Fund, London

Rankow EJ and Tessaro I (1998) Cervical cancer risk and Papanicolaou screening in a sample of lesbian and bisexual women. *Journal of Family Practice*, 47 (2), 139–143

Ries LAG EM, Kosary CL, Hankey BF, et al. (2000) SEER Cancer Statistics Review, 1975–2000, National Cancer Institute, Bethesda, MD. http://seer.cancer.gov/csr/1975_2000 (accessed 2/3/07)

Rostad KE (2002) The psychological impact of abnormal cytology and colposcopy. *British Journal of Obstetrics and Gynaecology*, 109, April, 364–368

Sasieni P and Adams J (1999) Effect of screening on cervical cancer mortality in England and Wales: analysis of trends with an age period cohort model. *BMJ*, 318, 1244–1245

Sasieni P, Adams J and Cuzick J (2003) Benefits of cervical screening at different ages: evidence from the UK audit of screening histories. *British Journal of Cancer*, 89 (1), 88–93

Saslow D, Runowicz CD, Solomon D, et al. (2002) American Cancer Society. American Cancer Society guideline for the early detection of cervical neoplasia and cancer. *CA: a Cancer Journal for Clinicians*, 52 (6), Nov–Dec, 342–362

Schiffman M and Castle PE (2005) The promise of global cervical cancer prevention. *New England Journal of Medicine*, 353 (20), 17 November, 2101–2104

Smith M, French L and Barry HC (2003) Periodic abstinence from Pap (PAP) smear study: women's perceptions of Pap smear screening. *Ann Fam Med*, 1, 203–208

Slater DN (1998) False negative cervical smears: medico-legal fallacies and suggested remedies. *Cytopathology*, 9, 145–154

Somerset M and Peters T (1998) Intervening to reduce anxiety for women with mild dyskaryosis: do we know what works and why? *Journal of Advanced Nursing*, 28 (3), 563–570

Symonds P, Naftalin N and Shaw P (2003) A smear on audit. Implications of the Leicester cervical smear audit. *BJOG: An International Journal of Obstetrics & Gynaecology*, 110 (7), 646–648, July

Tiffen J and Mahon S (2006) Cervical cancer; what should we tell women about screening? *Clinical Journal of Oncology Nursing*, 10 (4), 527–531

Tseng D, Cox E, Plane MB and Hla KM (2001) Efficacy of patient letter reminders on cervical cancer screening; a meta-analysis. *Journal of General Internal Medicine*, 16 (18), August, 563–568

Waxman A (2005) Guidelines for cervical cancer screening: history and scientific rationale. *Clinical Obstetrics and Gynaecology*, 48 (1), 77–97

Wilson JMG and Jugner G (1968) *Principles and Practice of Screening for Disease*. WHO, Geneva

Wright TC, Cox JT, Massad LS, Carlson JD, Twiggs LB and Wilkinson EJ for 2001 ASCCP-sponsored consensus workshop (2003) 2001 consensus guidelines for the management of women with cervical intraepithelial neoplasia. *American Journal of Obstetrics and Gynaecology*, 189 (1), July, 295–304

Chapter 9

Cervical cancer in developing countries

'. . . it is a cancer that has disproportionately affected the world's most vulnerable women for generations. Why, then, was cervical cancer not an international health priority long ago?'

(Hunter 2006)

Introduction

Previous chapters have illustrated that cervical cancer is principally a problem of the socio-economically disadvantaged, who tend to have higher risk factors for the disease and are less active recipients of screening (see Chapter 8 and Chapter 10). The same is true on a global level. Of the 493,243 new cases of cervical cancer documented in GLOBCAN 2002, there were 273,505 cervical cancer deaths, of which approx 80% occurred in developing countries (Ferlay et al. 2004). The age standardised incidence of cervical cancer in the developing world is up to 61 per 100,000 compared with 11 per 100,000 in developed countries (Ferlay et al. 2004). Furthermore, because accurate incidence data is not available in most poorly-resourced countries, under-reporting is high (ACCP 2004). The actual figures may be much greater than these.

Cervical cancer is the most common cancer amongst women in developing nations (Denny 2005) with a lifetime risk of acquiring the disease of approximately 2–4% (Goldie et al. 2003). In the developed world it constitutes about 4% of all cancers, but in Latin America, sub-Saharan Africa and South and South-east Asia (where cervical cancer rates are highest) this figure rises to 15% (Parkin et al. 2002). Because cervical cancer tends to claim lives at a relatively young age, it has a terrible impact on the family. In developing countries the role of the mother is socially and economically pivotal. A motherless baby has a very poor chance of survival. In some developing countries such as Argentina, Chile, China, Peru, South Africa and Thailand cervical cancer kills more women than maternal mortality (Parkin et al. 2002).

It is an uncomfortable fact that much of the therapy described in this book is completely unattainable for the majority of patients suffering from cervical cancer. Despite having to manage an enormous caseload of oncology patients, developing nations have access to only 5% of the world's global cancer resources (Ferlay et al. 2001).

Comparisons have been made between the levels of cervical cancer found in the developing world today and those of the developed nations a few decades ago. The reduction in the incidence of cervical cancer in developed nations has been widely attributed to the success of cervical screening – more than 50% of women who develop cervical cancer have never been screened (Sung et al. 2000). Looking at data obtained in the mid-1980s, approximately 5% of women in developing countries had been screened in the preceding five years compared with 40% to 50% in the developed world (World Health Organisation 1986).

Whilst it is hoped that the implementation of screening in developing countries might improve cervical cancer statistics, in reality such programmes are beyond the resources of most. Disappointingly, even in those developing countries where screening has been intro-duced, it has not always successfully impacted on cervical cancer rates (Arrossi et al. 2003).

This chapter explores some of the issues associated with cervical cancer in low-resourced nations, beginning with a discussion of screening. Management of the cervical cancer patient is then examined using the country of Uganda to illustrate some of the many issues facing oncology health professionals in the developing world.

Cervical cancer screening in the developing countries

A literature search of 'cervical cancer' and 'developing countries' will principally yield information about the dynamics of setting up cervical cancer screening programmes. There is a large amount written on the subject in comparison to a small amount about the actual management of cervical cancer in a resource-poor setting.

In light of what we know about cervical cancer this is to be expected. It is a disease characterised by a distinct and detectable pre-invasive phase. Any management strategies are most efficiently and cost-effectively directed towards diagnosis and treatment at an early stage.

It is therefore disappointing that in spite of this extensive literature, little progress has been made in establishing screening in developing countries. In Africa, where cervical cancer rates are amongst the worst in the world, no country has managed to conduct sus-tainable, large, population-based screening programmes. Only a few countries in Asia have been able to make significant progress with cervical screening and Chile is the only country in South America with a successful mass screening programme (Cronje 2003). Cuba, Mexico and Costa Rica have achieved very limited changes in cervical cancer mortality following the introduction of cervical screening (Arrossi et al. 2003, Pan American Health Organisation 2004).

And yet is this really so surprising? Even within the developed world, where the infra-structure and resources are all available to promote success, cervical screening programmes have faced considerable teething problems (see Chapter 8). Some of the problems faced by developing nations are the same. For example, recent cervical screening programmes in Latin America and the Caribbean failed because of sub-optimal performance of cytol-ogy, lack of quality control and inefficiency of systems to follow up and treat women (Sankaranarayanan et al. 2005). These difficulties are not dissimilar to those described in Chapter 8 which had to be overcome in order to improve western cervical screening programmes. However, clearly most developing nations have much more to contend with. As well as these organisational issues, they face a whole plethora of other restrictive factors such as lack of health resources, competing health priorities, instability, war and, in some instances a culturally condoned lack of women's basic rights.

Nevertheless, the call for screening implementation in the developing world continues. The World Health Organisation's recommended goal for low income nations is to perform at least one cytologic test per woman, per lifetime, between the ages of 35 and 40. This has been estimated to have the potential to reduce the cervical cancer rate by 65% (WHO 1986).

The Alliance for Cervical Cancer Prevention has produced a useful document to guide the implementation of cervical screening in developing countries (ACCP 2004). They suggest that the instigation of a successful programme requires not only an appropriate infrastructure but also the necessary political commitment. In order to be of benefit it is important that two fundamental criteria are met:

(1) The incidence of cervical cancer must justify screening.
(2) Necessary resources must be available and committed for attaining wide screening coverage and ensuring that adequate systems are in place to manage screen positive women appropriately.

'Programmes should be planned strategically, be based on realistic assessment of needs and capacities, and utilize the most recent evidence on screening and treatment approaches. The poor performance of cervical cancer prevention programmes in some limited-resource settings has most often been the result of *poor planning and implementation and lack of systems for ongoing monitoring and evaluation*, irrespective of the screening test or treatment methods used. Establishing mechanisms and processes to support and sustain each component of a programme will go far to ensuring that services are effective, accessible and acceptable to women who need them.'

(ACCP, 2004, p. 21)

Difficulties with implementing screening in developing nations

Apart from the logistical and organisational problems with implementing a screening programme in a low resourced nation, there are two other basic hurdles to be overcome which are discussed in further detail below. These are:

(1) problems with the screening test
(2) problems with screening uptake

Problems with the screening test

It has been suggested that several factors should be present to constitute an 'ideal screening test' in the third world. Such a test should:

(1) have a high sensitivity, specificity and positive predictive value
(2) provide an immediate result
(3) be relatively easy to evaluate
(4) be inexpensive
(5) be acceptable to both clients and health care workers

(Cronje et al. 2003)

The foundation of modern cervical screening programmes in the developed world is the cervical smear test. Because of its gradual evolution and also possibly because of a lack of exploration into alternative techniques, the Pap smear has never been subjected to the type of testing which we have grown to associate with 'evidence-based medicine'. The extent to which the cervical smear test meets the above criteria is arguable.

The term 'sensitivity' as applied to cervical screening has already been discussed in Chapter 1 and Chapter 8. It has been difficult to come up with an exact figure for sensitivity because of methodological differences in trial design. However, it seems unlikely to greatly exceed 60%. Three recent reviews cited in Sankaranarayanan (2005) conclude that the sensitivity of the Pap test in detecting CIN 2–3 ranges from 47% to 62% (Fahey et al. 1995, Mitchell et al. 1998, Nanda et al. 2000). Whilst it might be expected that because of poorer equipment and working conditions this figure would be lower within developing nations, this is not necessarily the case. A sensitivity range of 44–78% has been put forward for low resourced nations, depending on the country involved and methodological factors in trial design (Sankaranarayanan et al. 2005).

To a degree, compensation for deficiencies in sensitivity can be made through increasing the frequency of screening. Two or three-yearly screening as found in developed nations provides something of a 'safety-net' for false negatives. Within the developing world, however, screening at this frequency is impossible. Resources are too limited to allow for regular re-testing and cultural and logistical factors mean that women are unlikely to attend with such regularity. To quote Carr (2004), 'Papanicolaou screening is at best an only moderately effective screening technique if it is done only once in a lifetime or infrequently.'

Turning to the second point – the immediacy of obtaining results – cervical cytology testing requires that samples are sent to a laboratory for examination and it may take days/weeks for a result to become available. The ramifications of this are that women need to make repeat visits for results and treatment. Return of patients within *developed* countries has been shown to be problematic (see Chapter 8). Within *developing* countries it is an even greater issue. There are a number of examples of this in the literature.

In one study by Cronje et al. (2003), 876 patients screened required a colposcopy, but only 468 women (56%) ever returned for the procedure. In another ACCP study conducted in Peru, only 23% of women with positive cytology had the diagnostic work-up and treatment that was required (Sankaranarayanan et al. 2005). A third study conducted in South Africa indicated that of the women who requested not to be treated at the screening visit, only 47% finally returned for treatment. In addition, only 25% of the women treated for CIN at the screening visit returned for their follow-up visit one year later (Denny 2005).

The third issue concerns the ease of evaluation. The cervical smear procedure requires a minimum of three groups of skilled people in order to produce an evaluable sample (Sankaranarayanan et al. 2005):

(1) doctors or nurses to collect the cells, prepare and fix the smear
(2) cytotechnicians to process, stain and read smears (cytotechnicians require 12–24 months training)
(3) cytopathologists to supervise and take responsibility for the final report

It also calls for an adequate infrastructure which includes a good laboratory, quality control measures and a system of communicating results to the women. Ideally, a positive cervical cytology test should be followed by colposcopy. Colposcopy is expensive both in terms of equipment and personnel. It requires a level of expertise generally found only in tertiary or urban health care facilities – if at all. It generates a need for histology testing, requiring further laboratory facilities and trained pathologists, all of which are in short supply in poor countries (Denny 2005).

Clearly, all of these factors carry an economic cost. Whilst cervical cytology is currently less expensive than some other types of testing (e.g. HPV DNA testing), there are also screening tests which are considerably less expensive still, such as visual techniques. Some of these alternative screening tests available are discussed later in this chapter.

Finally, there is the issue of acceptability. Any screening test which requires directly accessing cervical tissue is likely to be associated with acceptability problems. This is certainly the case for cervical smear testing. The cultural factors influencing cervical smear acceptability are also discussed in greater detail below.

In conclusion, because of the perceived shortcomings in cervical screening, the WHO proposal that developing nations aim to introduce at least one smear per lifetime for every woman has received a mixed response. There are some who doubt the efficacy of this approach. For example, to quote Cronje (2005): 'with a Pap smear sensitivity of 30–50%, a loss to follow-up of 33% and coverage of, say 60%, a maximum reduction [in cervical cancer] of 20% can be expected using this approach.'

Consequently, a number of research projects are currently being conducted in order to investigate other options for cervical screening. Some of these strategies are described below.

Cervicography

Cervicography is photography of the cervix following application of dilute acetic acid using a special camera known as a 'cerviscope'. A certified evaluator examines the slides. The sensitivity of the technique has been estimated to be 50% and its specificity 80%. It appears to be more sensitive for low grade rather than high grade lesions.

The potential problems associated with this approach are:

- requirement for advanced technology (camera, developing film, etc.)
- cost
- recall of patients

(Cronje 2005)

HPV DNA testing

As discussed in Chapter 2, the presence or absence of HPV, whilst not directly indicative of a cellular abnormality, certainly identifies a group of individuals that are at risk of developing one. It will be recalled that within the younger age groups a large proportion of women will be found to be positive for HPV but that these lesions are frequently transient and self-resolving. It is amongst women in their late thirties and forties that persistent, high risk HPV infection is cause for concern. Thus, HPV testing in this age range has been put forward as a possible screening strategy for developing nations. In some studies cervical HPV testing has been shown to perform better than cytology and visual inspection, but only amongst older women (ACCP 2004).

One of the advantages of the HPV test is that it is easy to collect – indeed, some studies have indicated self-collection by women is feasible. HPV detection in urine is another promising method which removes the need for a gynaecological examination altogether (Brinkman et al. 2002).

Negative factors associated with this technique are that it is highly expensive. Furthermore, whilst theoretically a simple test, it is also very sensitive and is subject to contamination (Walraven 2003). The fact that minute quantities of viral DNA can be detected in a specimen can be confusing. Whether a positive result for high risk HPV based on a tiny amount of DNA is as clinically significant as a positive result from a larger amount of DNA remains an unanswered question (Walraven 2003).

Visual inspection techniques

Visual inspection techniques involve assessment of the cervix with the naked eye following the simple insertion of a speculum. They can be conducted by nurses, midwives or other health professionals, do not require sophisticated equipment and are low in cost. Furthermore, they can be performed during the menses (Carr 2004).

Ideally, visual inspection techniques involve the application of a substance to the cervix to assist with the diagnosis. VIA (Visual Inspection with acetic acid) involves the application of dilute acetic acid (3–5%) resulting in a temporary whitening of pre-cancerous lesions. Visual inspection with Lugol's iodine (VILI) involves the application of iodine resulting in a brown colouration for normal cells and a yellow colour for pre-cancerous cells. It is possible that VILI may perform better than VIA, but to date the bulk of the research has been with VIA.

Visual inspection is considered to be at least as sensitive as cervical cytology with a somewhat lower specificity (Carr 2004). Two methodologically rigorous studies with a total of nearly 4000 women indicate the sensitivity and specificity of VIA for biopsy-proven, high grade lesions is approximately 70% (Carr 2004).

The low specificity of the test means that potentially a much greater number of positive results will be generated, requiring either further investigation (with colposcopy) or intervention ('screen and treat'). In one Nicaraguan study, the consequence of employing VIA was the detection of more than twice as many lesions as conventional cytology. This meant a quadruplicating of the number of patients referred for colposcopy and a doubling of the number of patients needing treatment for high grade lesions or invasive cancer (Claeys et al. 2003).

This lack of specificity has more serious implications in the 'screen and treat' setting. Clearly, visual techniques lend themselves to 'screen and treat' because there is no need to wait for results from a laboratory. However, a high number of false positives in this context would result in the unnecessary treatment of some women.

Nevertheless, there are still a number of proponents of the approach who argue that the benefits of visual screening tests outweigh the potential hazards of over-treating (Gaffikin et al. 2003b). Many centres employing 'screen and treat' use cryotherapy, a treatment which is associated with a low level of morbidity. Recently, the results of a large 'screen-and-treat' programme that combined visual inspection with immediate treatment of all screen-positive women was reported from Thailand. Although the study did not evaluate the efficacy of this approach, it did evaluate safety and acceptability. Not one single serious complication of cryotherapy was observed among 756 women who underwent cryotherapy. In addition, 95% of women who participated in the programme expressed satisfaction with their experience (Gaffikin et al. 2003a).

Another approach for cervical screening is combining VIA with one of the other screening techniques described. For example, one testing partnership, which has been examined in South Africa, is HPV DNA testing together with VIA (Denny et al. 2005). This trial indicated that the combination of these screening techniques in the context of 'screen and treat' could make a significant impact on the prevalence of CIN.

In conclusion, whilst VIA appears to show some promise as a screening tool in the developing world, there is a need for further research. There is currently only limited information about its performance in 'real-life' settings and a need for further, programme-based data (Gaffikin et al. 2003b, Sankaranarayanan et al. 2005). In one study by Cronjie et al. (2003) cytologic examination, cervicography, the direct acetic acid test, and speculoscopy were all assessed and the investigators concluded that no test was suitable for screening in developing countries. Either the sensitivity or specificity was too low (sensitivity in the case of cytologic examination, specificity in the case of the other tests). It was concluded that 'Two or more tests combined will increase the sensitivity, but the specificity remains low. Screening methods in developing countries remain an urgent problem.'

Box 9.1 Visual inspection with acetic acid

VIA (also referred to as direct visual inspection (DVI) cervicoscopy, the acetic acid test or the vinegar test) requires that a woman lie in the lithotomy or supine position. A speculum is passed to visualise the cervix which is then washed with a dilute solution (3–5%) of acetic acid for approximately 1–2 minutes. Thereafter, the cervix is examined with the naked eye or with a hand-held magnifying device (usually 4x magnification) and an adequate light source. The acetic acid causes 'whitening' (known as 'acetowhitening') of epithelial cells that contain a high nuclear-cytoplasmic ratio. A range of epithelial changes will appear acetowhite after the application of acetic acid and these include immature squamous metaplasia, infection of the cervix with HPV (both low and high risk types) and true cervical cancer precursors. Colposcopy examines the cervix in greater detail by using a significantly higher magnification. VIA simply determines the presence or absence of an acetowhite lesion in the region of the transformation zone of the cervix. (Denny 2005).

Generally there are three possible interpretations of a VIA test (Carr 2004):

(1) positive (acetowhite area present)
(2) negative (no acetowhite area present)
(3) suspicious for cervical cancer

Like cervical cytology, VIA is highly subjective and thus it is important to standardise definitions of what constitutes a positive and negative test and to ensure that quality control measures are in place (ACCP 2004).

Problems with the screening uptake

It has been suggested that unless the coverage of a cervical screening programme reaches 70% to 80% of women, the likely decrease in cervical cancer rate is insignificant (Cronje 2005). We have already examined some of the barriers to cervical screening in the developed world. Similarly, developing nations face significant problems with uptake of cervical screening practices. Some of the issues encountered are discussed below.

Cancer is associated with negative and frightening images in both developed and developing nations, as can be seen by the words used to describe it: 'devouring', 'eating', 'putridity' or 'plague' (Bingham et al. 2003). It is possible that these images are stronger in populations who have received less education and therefore have less capacity to dispel myths. Furthermore, the reality in many developing nations is that the majority of cancers are diagnosed at a later stage when treatment is less likely to be effective. Women in Mexico describe cervical cancer as the 'rotting or devouring of the womb' and say that treatment leaves them 'hueca' (sexually disabled). In Bolivia, cancer is described as a 'death sentence' that destines women to die slowly and painfully (Bingham et al. 2003). In South Africa, the general perception is also that cancer of the 'womb' is inevitably fatal (Wood et al. 1997).

Furthermore, cancer is stigmatising. In one Indian study a number of women stated that they would be shunned by family and friends if found to have a positive cervical smear because cancer is considered to be an infectious disease (Basu et al. 2006). A diagnosis of cervical cancer is commonly associated with an STD diagnosis. In South Africa and Kenya, many women believe a positive diagnosis means that they have AIDS ('HPV' and 'HIV' sound very similar).

Such beliefs have a powerful influence on health-associated behaviour – particularly regarding screening uptake. Non-attendance of screening is a major problem within developing nations. There are a number of reasons for this. Some are listed in Box 9.2. Others include:

(1) Lack of understanding of the concept of preventative medicine (Bingham et al. 2003, ACCP 2004)

Many women in developing nations would only consider seeking medical help if there was an obvious problem with their health. A good example of this can be seen in one South African study conducted by EngenderHealth in collaboration with the University of Cape Town. This qualitative trial involved more than 200 women in Khayelitsha, on the outskirts of Cape Town. Most of the women who attended screening did so because they perceived that they were ill and had heard they would receive respectful care. Their illness was usually unrelated to cervical cancer (EngenderHealth 2003).

(2) Economic reasons

Basu et al. (2006) questioned a cohort of women who declined uptake of screening facilities in India. The majority were housewives (75%), together with labourers, small traders and service-holders; 72% of the labourers were daily wage earners who would have to sacrifice pay to attend. Similar studies performed in Kenya show that many women must travel anywhere from two to eight hours for screening, at an average cost of a day's agricultural wage. Women will therefore come to clinics only when they are able to finance the trip, negotiate their home responsibilities and obtain support from their husbands. Furthermore when women do make the trip, they are not as likely to return if they are turned away or otherwise unable to be seen (Bingham et al. 2003).

(3) Lack of support from family/partner

A repeated theme associated with the screening behaviour of women in developing countries is that of lack of social empowerment. Women from lower socio-economic groups are frequently not allowed to make their own decisions and are required to request their partner's permission in order to seek medical care. Nearly half the Indian women questioned by Basu et al. (2006) whilst appreciating the potential benefit of screening could not participate because of other preoccupations or because of a lack of support within the family. In some countries the association between HPV and sexually-transmitted disease carries connotations of marital infidelity. This results in fear of having to explain positive results to a spouse and consequent avoidance of screening (Bingham et al. 2003). In South Africa, the pelvic examination is described as 'the hanging of the legs' and women refer to the experience as 'surrendering oneself'. A positive result is considered to suggest the woman is 'dirty' or 'promiscuous' and the whole procedure challenges the male's control over his wife (Buskens and Bradley 2002). The cooperation of the male partner is not only required for screening to take place but is also imperative for treatment to be effective and without complications. For example, women should not have sex for four weeks following therapy for high grade CIN. In one African study although most women were able to abstain from sex or use a condom, some reported that they were coerced into having sexual relations, or they were unable to obtain condoms. In some instances, men sought sexual partners elsewhere during this time period (PATH 2002 cited in Bingham et al. 2003).

(4) Fear, myths and misconceptions

Fear is a powerful disincentive for cervical screening – and that is not only fear of finding cancer but also of screening itself. Most women in developing countries have never seen a speculum and the sight of a tray containing one, together with a colposcope and other gynaecological examination equipment is extremely frightening. Approximately 20% (84/469) of non-attenders in the study by Basu et al. (2006) were scared of the tests, 62% thinking they would be painful. Misinformation regarding testing is also common in many communities; 13% of women in the above study thought a biopsy itself could cause cancer. 'Biopsy' in India is a word associated with a positive cancer diagnosis. It is also considered to cause spread of disease and hasten death.

(5) Quality of care and prior health experiences

Bingham et al. (2003) performed a large analysis of participation rates in cervical screening programmes in a number of developing countries (Bolivia, Peru, Kenya and South Africa). One of the major barriers to screening uptake was how women were treated at the clinic. Both the way in which they were spoken to by staff and the general appearance of the clinic were very important. Women appreciated being addressed by their names, and wanted providers to speak simply, softly and gently, and avoid brusque behaviour. The appearance and cleanliness of the clinic and provider were important, as were provisions to ensure privacy during examinations. Watkins et al. (2002) explored cervical screening uptake in a sample of women in rural Mexico and found the most frequent reason for not obtaining a Pap smear was anxiety regarding physical privacy (50%). A good standard of hygiene was also important. A common concern expressed by a number of women was that the specula were not properly cleaned before being used. It is helpful for women to see this process in order to increase their comfort with the screening process (Bingham et al. 2003).

Improving uptake of screening, treatment and follow-up

Simply making the services available, however, is insufficient to ensure that they are used. Services need to be accessible, acceptable, affordable and reliable.

(ACCP 2004, p. xvii)

It is important that a woman's screening experience is positive not only for her own wellbeing but also to promote the programme within a community – much information about cervical cancer screening spreads by word of mouth (ACCP 2004). Furthermore, a high standard of service will not only improve screening uptake but also promote better adherence to treatment and follow-up schedules.

Box 9.2 Reasons for non-attendance of cervical screening programme – India (Basu et al. 2006, reproduced with permission)	
I do not need any check up because I have no complaint	46%
I am scared of the tests	36%
My relative/neighbour had a problem when they had the test	28%
Let fate/god decide my destiny	19%
I feel shy to be examined even by female doctors	15%
I cannot have any gynaecological problem since my periods have stopped	13%
I feel shy to be examined by a male doctor	12%
I did not want to listen to anything about it	8%
I did not understand what it was all about	8%
I cannot afford treatment if cancer is detected	6%
I could not go because I had too many household works to attend to	40%
I could not go due to illness/other problems in the family	32%
My husband/relatives would not allow me to go	27%
I will lose my daily earning if I go	23%
I do not have anyone to accompany me and I cannot go alone	13.5%
My doctor told me the test would be useless	7%
If I have to stay away from the job for a few days I will lose it	2%
I will be asked to pay for the test	1%

As mentioned in the above section, one of the most powerful factors in making the service accessible is taking the time to talk with the women who attend and providing them with quality care (Bingham et al. 2003). On an organisational level engaging the support of traditional healers and influential community members in cervical screening programmes is also an important strategy in improving attendance rates. To quote Watkins et al. (2002): 'The responses of many women suggest that compliance with cervical cancer screening would be enhanced by addressing cultural beliefs, encouraging conversations about women's health issues, and increasing the number of female health care providers.'

Several outreach activities are described in the literature and are not dissimilar to approaches employed to improve screening attendance in developed nations (Chapter 8). They include (ACCP 2004):

- community health education
- home visits
- reaching out to social and family networks
- involving men
- tapping into cultural norms and traditions

Another way of addressing poor return rates is through linking screening with immediate treatment, ('screen and treat') (Denny 2005). Follow-up rates of 95% can be achieved if women are requested to return within two to six days of treatment. This rate falls to 85% if the result of the test is delayed by two weeks (Denny et al. 2000).

Treatment

Management of pre-invasive disease

'Improving an inexpensive kind of cryotherapy or finding an alternative for use in low-resource settings is a critical missing link that will translate improved screening into improved prevention.'

Schiffman and Castle (2005)

Box 9.3 Economic factors

The most important aspect of any screening programme is funding. Cervical neoplasia prevention programmes have to compete with other conditions and diseases (e.g. malnutrition, sanitation, housing, clean water supply, tuberculosis and HIV) for funding; subsequently, they often do not receive priority. Therefore, whatever method is used for the control of cervical cancer, it has to be affordable.

(Cronje 2005)

The average annual expenditure on health in most African countries is approximately US$3 per capita compared with US$5000 in the USA (http://cms.hhs.gov quoted in Denny 2005).

A number of studies have been performed to assess the cost of cervical screening strategies. These utilise computer models which have the capacity to estimate the costs using several different screening methods (Mandelblatt et al. 2002). Clearly it is important that such analyses are performed for each different screening project – what is cost effective in one country may not be in another (Goldhaber-Fiebert and Goldie 2006).

Legood et al. 2003 (cited in ACCP 2004) provide an indication of the costs of one screening project performed in Barshi, India. It was a large project with a population of 100,000 previously unscreened women. Mobile clinics were employed, utilising VIA, cytology and HPV testing. Women who tested positive were provided with transport to the rural hospital for diagnosis and treatment. On average the project screened 25,000 women pa.

About $1 million (US) was allocated to the project. The cost per eligible woman was calculated to be $4.30–12.40, depending on the screening test used; 21% of the total cost was attributable to programme-level costs including infrastructure changes, implementation and management. The overall recruitment and invitation costs were 6–17% of the total amount.

Unfortunately, many developing countries do not have the resources to perform relatively simple outpatient procedures such as LEEP and cryotherapy. Because of this, doctors will often resort to hysterectomy and cold knife cone biopsy (ACCP) for the management of pre-invasive disease. Such procedures carry a significant risk of complication and clearly have a negative impact on fertility.

Cryotherapy is probably the least expensive treatment and the easiest to apply, and therefore lends itself to the developing world setting. It is also very well tolerated with minimal side effects (Martin-Hirsch et al. 2004). The main negative experience reported by patients is pain during the procedure. Heavy bleeding is rare, although some women will experience profuse, watery vaginal discharge which may persist for a few weeks afterwards (Jacob et al. 2005). Because a large area is denuded from the cervix there is an increased potential for transmitting or acquiring HIV infection whilst healing is taking place. For this reason abstinence from sexual intercourse or use of condoms is advised for four weeks afterwards (Jacob et al. 2005).

The more problematic organisational aspect of the procedure is that it requires a continuous supply of nitrous oxide which is not always available. Although the technique can also be conducted using carbon dioxide, it is less dependable in terms of performance. Cryotherapy is not appropriate for very large lesions (Cronje 2005).

LEEP is more difficult to supply in the developing world because of a shortage of skilled providers, sophisticated equipment and also continuous power supply in some places. Furthermore, it calls for histology facilities which are costly and not commonly available (Jacob et al. 2005).

Management of invasive disease

The management of invasive cervical cancer continues to be a major challenge in many developing countries, particularly in sub-Saharan Africa, due to the lack of surgical facilities, skilled providers and radiotherapy services (Stewart and Kleihues 2003, cited ACCP 2004, p. 235).

As discussed in Chapter 1, the treatment of cervical cancer is stage dependent. Within any developed country the first step on diagnosing a patient with cervical cancer is to ensure that she is accurately staged. The FIGO staging of cervical cancer is clinical (see Chapter 1), although in many western countries additional medical imaging strategies are employed to improve its accuracy. Access to sophisticated medical imaging techniques in developing countries is very limited. In most areas the only feasible approach to staging is by speculum examination, vaginal and rectal examination and visualisation of the anal canal (proctoscopy).

Unfortunately, the majority of women will be diagnosed with cervical cancer only when their tumour has reached an advanced stage. Advanced cervical cancer is seen far more often in developing nations than it is in the developed world (ACCP 2004 p. 234). Between 1995–1997, 14.6% of cervical cancers in developing countries were diagnosed early, as opposed to 54% in USA (Sankaranarayanan et al. 1998). The remainder of cancers were only detected at a late stage.

Once again, the mainstay of therapy in many developing countries is surgery. Shortage of radiotherapy facilities is a major problem. Radiotherapy is available at only 16 of 50 countries in sub-Saharan Africa (Wabinga et al. 2003). To put this in perspective, the entire African continent has fewer radiotherapy machines than there are in Italy alone. Furthermore, even where radiotherapy resources are available, there is little data available concerning outcome of women treated with it (Wabinga et al. 2003).

One exception to this is a radiotherapy centre in Chandigarh, India, which has published some outcome data. Despite the fact that sophisticated radiotherapy techniques are not possible because of limited equipment, the results were surprisingly good, with overall and disease-free survivals of 44% and 52.2% respectively (Saibishkumar et al. 2006). Whether the same success rates can be claimed by other developing world centres is unknown. Certainly, in low resource countries chemoradiotherapy – the standard treatment in developing world countries – is a luxury which is beyond the reach of most patients. The addition of chemotherapy to radiotherapy regimens is reserved for high risk individuals (Saibishkumar et al. 2005).

Palliative care

'I saw one woman, and she said that she was in severe pain. She had pain when she urinated and when she defecated. She had blood, like haemorrhaging. She had bleeding every day, like menstruation. She had a lot of fever. And she had that bloody discharge that smelled bad.'

(quoted in Hunter 2006)

'I have the experience of one of my sisters. She died of cancer. I know many women who have died with cancer. They had bleeding. Day by day, they dried up. They get very, very skinny and yellow. That's how my sister died, very bony.'

(quoted in Hunter 2006)

The unfortunate reality of cervical cancer in poorly-resourced countries is that most women will only present to medical services when their disease is too advanced for any curative therapy.

Presenting features indicating advanced disease include:

- foul-smelling, bloody vaginal discharge
- blood in the urine
- bowel obstruction (vomiting, abdominal pain and distention)
- severe backache
- severe anaemia

• weight loss
• vesico-vaginal or vesico-rectal fistulas

As indicated in Chapter 10, the management of these types of problems is extremely difficult – even in countries with ample resources. Palliative care provision is even more problematic within the developing world, where even access to basic medications such as morphine can be blocked by political and administrative factors.

> Providing quality palliative care is challenging in most regions of the world, due to problems associated with the availability of medication, deficient health infrastructure, lack of training for providers, lack of counseling skills, discomfort in discussing the diagnosis and management with patients, and lack of community awareness of palliative care options.
>
> (ACCP 2004, p. 250)

In order to gain a fuller insight into some of the practical issues encountered by health professionals in under-resourced countries the following section focuses on just one developing nation: Uganda. This is one of many African countries which face an enormous health care burden as a result of cervical cancer. Box 9.4 provides accounts from palliative care nurses working in Uganda describing the reality of cervical cancer for many of their patients and the nursing challenges that it presents.

Box 9.4 Case studies

These accounts are from two nurses working in Hospice Uganda and describe nurses' experience of cervical cancer in this country.

Account 1

These patients come to Hospice with vaginal bleeding with foul smelling discharge and some times with leakage of urine when the tumour has infiltrated into the bladder. The patients' lives are in total chaos due to this type of cancer because it affects the whole patient. It affects the patient psychologically, socially, physically, emotionally and spiritually.

Socially: the patient with the leakage of urine is very smelly and does not want to be with people and the people also find it a problem because of the smell. The patient is always isolated and stays in bed all the time and she develops bed sores and all the other complications of being bedridden.

Physically: the patient has a lot of pain because of the tumour occupying the whole pelvis. They tend to complain of 'labour like pains'. This pain is like when the mother is in labour, you can imagine that pain being there for ever!

Emotionally: the patients feel angry and cry easily because they are sad about themselves and sometimes they become depressed completely. They are abandoned by their husbands because of the smell and unable to have penetrative sex.

Culturally: these patients are expected to fulfil their duty as women in bed which is a real problem for them and very painful. At the end of the day they are replaced.

Spiritually: there is a lot of questioning why me! Some patients would think that they are bewitched and a lot of money is spent in looking for the witch. Sometimes patients change from religion to religion looking for a cure. There have a feeling of guilt, thinking that they must have annoyed God that is why they are being punished like that.

Case study

Mary (not real name), 27 years old, Munyankole, married with no children, she was referred to Hospice with a history of inoperable cancer of the cervix. She was complaining of lower abdominal pain, vaginal foul discharge, pain in the vulva and pain in the sacral area. Mary was forced to get married to an old man because the husband of her choice had abandoned her because she was not having children and the parents needed cows to return them to the first husband.

Mary was in total pain.

She was welcomed made comfortable and helped to tell her story because she had visited so many health facilities with not much help.

After examination she was started on treatment for pain and the foul smell. A suggestion to go for palliative radiotherapy was given but she was financially incapacitated to afford the treatment.

Three days later Mary came back for review, her pain was less and the smell had vanished but she was complaining of excess watery discharge. She had even lost the feeling of a full bladder. Mary had developed vesicle vaginal fistula. She could not control her bladder any more.

Mary was counselled again and given a plastic pant to control the dribbling of urine and be able to walk a round and do her the washing. The old man had also abandoned her because he could not stand the wet bed and smell.

A return to her brother was organised who gave her room to live in. Mary's problems were too many but we continued to attend to them as they arose and continued to counsel her. We have managed to improve her quality of life and she is now a happy woman in spite of all the problems.

(Martha Rabwoni 2007)

Account 2
What problems do women with cancer of the cervix face?

Loss of roles, body image, abandonment, domestic violence, separation, neglect, etc.

Loss of roles
When a woman gets married, [she] is expected to produce children and make a big family. Many children bring prestige to the family and especially the man. Women also feel secure and protected when they have many children. She is also expected to play the caring role for the husband, children and husband's family. When cancer sets in, a woman loses that role and because she can no longer perform the expected roles/duties is either abandoned or sent back to her parents.

Women have no bargaining powers, they are forced to play sex and suffer excruciating pain.

Denying a man sex means domestic violence, harassment separation and abandonment and not only to wife but also the children. Therefore many women suffer unbearable pain to protect their children.

A woman said 'my husband demands sex despite the explanation that I experience pain whenever I have sex because the vagina has narrowed due to radiotherapy but he says he enjoys it because it is now tight.'

Some women are thrown out of the main house into a hut so that a man can bring another woman who will service him and play the expected roles.

One of the responses by cancer patients: 'I was bleeding and my husband stopped coming home, he stopped giving me any support not even school fees for my children. I can not support my children nor can I think of sex and yet he says no sex no support.'

Loss of body image
Because of cancer women lose the body image psychologically they feel they are no longer worth. The situation is made worse by husbands and husband's relatives (in-laws) affirming that they are no longer worth because they can not longer perform the expected roles.

The smelly vaginal discharge, VVF [vesico-vaginal fistulae], RVF [rectal-vaginal fistulae] cause a lot of distress in these women because they don't know how to manage the condition. Husbands and relatives avoid them because of the smell.

However, these conditions can be improved with good nursing care if they get a chance to reach a palliative care nurse. Simple easily available local materials can be used to improve the smell.

Issues faced by palliative care nurses

These patient[s] experience a lot of psychological pain.

Because they have lost their roles, body image, some of them are abandoned and yet they have no where to go either because the relatives died or are poor and not willing to receive them back home. There is no government or NGO support to care for these patients. It is difficult to see them go hungry, no where to sleep and without facilities to use. It is emotionally draining on nurses to face these situations especially when there is very little to offer in terms of material support. However if we do get a chance to talk to husbands who are usually the decision makers the situation in a home may change.

Therefore as nurse we play multiple roles, i.e. counseling the patient, husband and family. We play a role of a social worker, e.g. at times have to look for agencies that can pay school fees so that the children can study or advocate for the patients and the children's rights. Also we offer a spiritual guidance role, and offer to pray with the patient. These are the inclusive roles of a palliative care nurse in Africa.

The other challenge is nursing patients with little resources, i.e. no diapers for patients with VVF. We encourage hygiene, regular washing of local cottons used for diapers, and applying Vaseline to avoid excoriation by the padding themselves made with old cotton clothes that can soak the urine and held in place by a locally made plastic pant designed at Hospice.

Conclusion
Cancer of the cervix is one of the cancers that destroy the self esteem of women in Uganda. With little resources available a lot can be done, we need to sensitise husbands, family, community and work together to make these women lead a comfortable and meaningful life before they die.

(Rose Kiwanuka 2007)

Uganda – the problems of cervical cancer in a developing nation

Whilst in some developing nations the rate of cervical cancer has declined slightly or remained stable over the last two decades (south Asia and Latin America), in others it has increased. For example, incidence rates are increasing in sub-Saharan countries such as Uganda, Zimbabwe, Mali (Wabinga et al. 2000, Parkin et al. 2001). Today, Africa has one of the highest incidence rates of cervical cancer in the world. Five of the seven countries with the highest rates are in eastern or southern Africa (Walraven 2003).

Uganda is unusual amongst the African countries in that it has a cancer registry. The Kampala Cancer Registry was established 1951 and is one of the longest standing registries on the African continent. This is no mean feat. Data is very difficult to obtain – for example, death certificates are rarely completed for deaths occurring outside hospitals. Case finding is by active search from records obtained from path labs, hospitals and Hospice Uganda.

The registry indicates that in the 1990s the cancers with the highest incidence were Kaposi's sarcoma, prostate cancer and oesophageal cancer amongst men and cervical cancer, breast cancer and Kaposi's sarcoma amongst women. Gondos et al. (2005) used the Ugandan database to compare the five-year survival rates for cervical cancer in Uganda with those in America, as found in the SEER database. Overall the Ugandans had a significantly poorer outlook – indeed, their survival figures were even lower than those published for many other developing countries.

Uganda faces a number of health issues which serve to explain this disparity. Some of the factors – common to many other developing countries – are discussed below.

(1) Lack of resources
  Uganda is an extremely poor country. The annual per capita health expenditure is currently estimated at $36 ($8 by the government, the rest donor dependent and variable). Forty per cent of the population lives in absolute poverty (living on less than $1 a day and unable to afford enough food to consume 2000 to 3000 calories a day) (Kikule 2003).

  Uganda is typical of most developing world countries in that there is a lack of resources at every level of cancer care. In 1988 there were only two radiotherapy units and one chemotherapy unit in the country. Only an estimated 5% of patients had access to these facilities.

(2) Lack of screening

Currently there is no formal screening programme in Uganda, although visual screening has been introduced on a pilot basis. Otherwise, cervical smear screening is offered on an opportunistic basis, and is free in the gynaecological outpatient clinic and the post-natal/family planning clinics (Mutyaba 2006). Resources for screening are limited and it is common to find clinics that are without trained personnel and laboratories. They may also not have clean water, electricity, slides, spatulas and many of the other basics that are required (Walraven 2003).

The result of this is that many patients present for treatment when their tumour is far advanced and inoperable. Over 80% of women diagnosed with cervical cancer in Mulago (the biggest hospital in Uganda), have advanced disease (Mutyaba 2006). For most patients palliative care is the only treatment option.

Fortunately, Uganda has a palliative care facility – the same cannot be said of every developing nation. This hospice service was set up in 1993 in Kampala and provides mainly home-based care for cancer and AIDS patients. Hospice services are never refused if the patient is unable to pay and are probably one of the most highly utilised cancer services in Uganda.

(3) HIV/AIDS

It has already been established that HPV infection and cervical cancer progresses more rapidly in women with HIV (Carr 2004) (see Chapter 2). Treatment of HIV positive women has a much poorer outcome with a recurrence rate of CIN ranging from 20% to 60%, depending on the degree of immunosuppression (Cronje 2005).

Uganda has fortunately experienced a decline in HIV/AIDS in recent years. Since 1992, HIV prevalence in Uganda has dropped by more than 50%, and significant changes in HIV-related behaviours have been documented. Nevertheless, it is still a sizeable problem. The overall prevalence of HIV/AIDS is 7%: 10.7% in urban and 6.4% in rural populations. Transmission is mainly through heterosexual sex (75% to 80%). Mother-to-child-transmission accounts for 15–25% of new infections (CDC 2007).

(4) Political instability and war

The incidence of cervix cancer in Uganda increased substantially between the 1960s and the 1990s (Wabinga et al. 2003). It might be expected that this rise would be attributed to the AIDS epidemic, but in fact it is considered to be the result of the social disruption caused by the Amin dictatorship (Wabinga et al. 2003). This and the ensuing civil wars favoured the spread of HPV and other STDs (Wabinga et al. 2003). War appears to be a powerful promoter of sexually transmitted diseases. Another example can be seen in Vietnam. It has been suggested that the increase in incidence of cervical cancer there in recent decades is mainly attributable to the Vietnam war in the 1960s (Suba et al. 2006).

(5) Medical personnel

As with most developing countries, there is a shortage of doctors in Uganda; in Kampala there are only 50 per 100,000 people. Furthermore, the training of doctors and other health professionals appears not to identify cervical cancer as a priority. Mutyaba (2006) conducted a questionnaire study of 310 Ugandan medical workers including doctors, nurses and final year medical students in order to assess their level of understanding of cervical cancer. There was a 92% response rate. Less than 40% knew risk factors for cervical cancer. Of the female respondents, 65% didn't feel susceptible to cervical cancer and 81% had never been screened. Of the male respondents, 26% had partners who had never been screened. Only 14% of the final year medical students felt skilled enough to use a vaginal speculum and 87% had never performed a Pap smear.

(6) Female circumcision

Female circumcision is traditional practice in many African countries and involves the partial or total removal of the female external genitalia. It is an ancient tradition, performed among all ethnic and cultural groups including Christians, Muslims, Jews and followers of indigenous African religions. Whilst it is supposed to have a religious basis, there are no references to the practice in the Bible or Koran and it is not practised in Saudi, the centre of Islam (Manji 2006).

Female circumcision is associated with many complications, some of which may be life-threatening. Immediate complications include intense pain and haemorrhage which can lead to shock and death. Wound infection, tetanus, gangrene and other gynaecological problems are common long-term complications. Excessive scarring and the small vaginal opening resulting from the procedure lead to pain during intercourse and childbirth. Perineal tearing and prolonged labour can cause maternal and foetal death.

Management of cervical cancer is extremely difficult amongst women who have undergone female circumcision. Manji (2006) describes the problems associated with treating two Sudanese girls with cervical cancer needing brachytherapy. Surgical intervention was necessary for insertion of the radioactive sources.

It is estimated that over 120 million girls and women have undergone some form of genital mutilation and that mostly they live in the 28 African countries where this is common. Two million girls are considered to be at risk of the practice each year (Manji 2006).

The future

In conclusion, conventional screening for cervical cancer is not practical for the developing world. The most promising future control method of this cancer is immunization against HPV. In the meanwhile, new avenues of screening and treatments should be investigated.

(Cronje 2005)

The magnitude of the problem faced by under-resourced countries with regard to cervical cancer is enormous. Furthermore, it is easy to become disheartened about the future when faced with the practical difficulties of screening and cancer management.

However, some improvements are being made, such as the implementation of palliative care services. Another new source of hope is the HPV vaccine. The two pharmaceutical companies who are responsible for the development of HPV vaccines (Merck and Glaxo-Smith-Klein) have undertaken to provide their vaccines to developing countries at cost price.

Inevitably, the implementation of vaccination programmes would require overcoming some significant obstacles. The HPV types covered by current vaccines are different from those prevalent in African nations. Furthermore, vaccination campaigns will present new logistical challenges to health care agencies. Nevertheless, vaccination offers a very real hope for future generations in low resourced countries. In the meantime, it seems likely that we will continue to see many women suffering with advanced disease and many preventable deaths from cervical cancer in the countries which can least afford to manage them.

Conclusion

Cancer of the cervix is an enormous problem in the developing world. Here the disease is often only diagnosed at an advanced stage and as well as causing a tragic loss of life it also has significant social and economic sequelae. Some developing nations have instituted screening programmes but these are associated with logistical and cultural difficulties which limit their effectiveness. The development of cancer vaccines offers some hope in under-resourced nations although once again a number of hurdles will need to be overcome in order to successfully implement vaccination campaigns.

Resources

International Agency for Research on Cancer: http://screening.iarc.fr/cervicalindex.php?PHPSESSID=9520a58311a694e36cf4bf7f1b35a43c
Hospice Africa: http://www.hospiceafrica.or.ug/

References

Alliance for Cervical Cancer Prevention (ACCP) (2004) *Planning and Implementing Cervical Cancer Prevention and Control Programs: a Manual for Managers*. ACCP, Seattle

Arrossi S, Sankaranarayanan R and Parkin DM (2003) Incidence and mortality of cervical cancer in Latin America. *Salud Publica Mex*, 45, Suppl 3, 306–314

Basu P, Sarkar S, Mukherjee S, et al. (2006) Women's perceptions and social barriers determine compliance to cervical screening: results from a population based study in India. *Cancer Detection & Prevention*, 30 (4), 369–374

Bingham A, Bishop A, Coffey P, et al. (2003) Factors affecting utilization of cervical cancer prevention services in low-resource settings. *Salud pública Méx*, 45 (Suppl 3), 408–416

Brinkman JA, Jones WE, Gaffga AM, et al. (2002) Detection of human papillomavirus DNA in urine specimens from human immunodeficeincy virus-positive women. *J Clin Microbiol*, 40, 3155–3161

Buskens I and Bradley J (2002) *Women's Perspectives on Cervical Cancer Prevention Procedures*. EngenderHealth, New York

Carr KC (2004) Cervical cancer screening in low resource settings using visual inspection with acetic acid. *J Midwifery Women's Health*, 49, 329–337

Centres for Disease Control and Prevention (CDC) (2007) The emergency plan in Uganda (http://www.cdc.gov/nchstp/od/gap/countries/uganda.htm accessed 19/3/07)

Claeys P, De Vuyst H, Gonzalez C, Garcia A, Bello RE and Temmerman M (2003) Performance of the acetic acid test when used in field conditions as a screening test for cervical cancer. *Tropical Medicine and International Health*, 8, (8), 704–709

Cronje HS (2005) Screening for cervical cancer in the developing world. *Best Practice & Research in Clinical Obstetrics & Gynaecology*, 19 (4), 517–529

Cronje HS, Parham GP, Cooreman BF, de Beer A, Divall P and Bam RH (2003) A comparison of four screening methods for cervical neoplasia in a developing country. *American Journal of Obstetrics and Gynaecology*, 188 (2), 395–400

Denny L (2005) The prevention of cervical cancer in developing countries. *BJOG*, 112, September, 1204–1212

Denny L, Kuhn L, DeSouza M, Pollack A, Dupree W and Wright TC (2005) Screen-and-treat approaches for cervical cancer prevention in low-resource settings: a randomized, controlled trial. *JAMA*, 294 (17), 2173–2181

Denny L, Kuhn L, Pollack A, Wainright H and Wright Jr TC (2000) Evaluation of alternative methods of cervical cancer screening for resource-poor settings. *Cancer*, 89, 826–833

EngenderHealth (2003) *Women's Perspectives on Cervical Cancer Screening and Treatment: Participatory Action Research in Khayelitsha, South Africa* (report). EngenderHealth, New York

Fahey MT, Irwig L and Macaskill P (1995) Meta-analysis of Pap test accuracy. *American Journal of Epidemiology*, 141, 680–689

Ferlay J, Bray F, Pisawi P and Parkin DM (2001) *GLOBOCAN 2000. Cancer Incidence, Mortality and Prevalence Worldwide*. Version 1.0. IARC Cancer Base no. 5. IARC Press, Lyon

Ferlay J, Bray F, Pisani P and Parkin DM (2004) *GLOBOCAN 2002. Cancer Incidence, Mortality and Prevalence Worldwide*. Version 2.0. IARC Cancer Base no. 5. IARC Press, Lyon

Gaffikin L, Blumenthal P, Emerson M, et al. (2003a) Safety, acceptability and feasibility of a single visit approach to cervical cancer prevention in rural Thailand: a demonstration project. *Lancet*, 361, 814–820

Gaffikin L, Lauterbach M and Blumenthal PD (2003b) Performance of visual inspection with acetic acid for cervical cancer screening: a qualitative summary of evidence to date. *Obstetrical and Gynaecological Survey*, 58 (8), 543–550

Goldhaber-Fiebert JD and Goldie SJ (2006) Estimating the cost of cervical cancer screening in five developing countries. *Cost Effectiveness and Resource Allocation*, 4 (13) (www.resource-allocation.com/content/4/1/13)

Goldie SJ, Grima D, Kohli M, et al. (2003) A comprehensive natural history model of HPV infection and cervical cancer to estimate the clinical impact of a prophylactic HPV-16/18 vaccine. *Int J Cancer*, 106, 896–904

Gondos A, Brenner H, Wabinga H and Parkin DM (2005) Cancer survival in Kampala, Uganda. *British Journal of Cancer*, 92, 1808–1812

Hunter J (2006) Better late than never: reflections on the delayed prioritization of cervical cancer in international health. *Health Care for Women International*, 27, 2–17

Jacob M, Bradley J and Barone M (2005) Human papillomavirus vaccines: what does the future hold for preventing cervical cancer in resource-poor settings through immunization programmes? *Sexually Transmitted Diseases*, 32 (10), 635–640

Kikule E (2003) A good death in Uganda: survey of needs for palliative care for terminally ill people in urban areas. *BMJ*, 327, 192–194

Legood R, Gray AM, Mahe C, et al. (2003) Trial based cost effectiveness comparison of cervical cancer screening strategies in India. Presented at European Organisation for Research and Treatment of Cancer: Third European Conference on the Economies of Cancer, 7–9 Sept, Brussels, Belgium

Mandelblatt JS, Lawrence WF, Gaffikin L, et al. (2002) Costs and benefits of different strategies to screen for cervical cancer in less-developed countries. *Journal of the National Cancer Institute*, 94, (19), 1469–1483

Manji MF (2006) Female circumcision (female genital mutilation): a problem for brachytherapy in cervical cancer. *International Journal of Gynecological Cancer*, 16 (2), Mar–Apr, 675–680

Martin-Hirsch PL, Paraskevaidis E and Kitchener H (2004) Surgery for cervical intraepithelial neoplasia. *Cochrane Review*, Vol (2). Date most recent update: 10 Aug 2004

Mitchell MF, Schottenfeld D, Tortolera-Luna G, Cantor SB and Richards-Kortum R (1998) Colposcopy for the diagnosis of squamous intraepithelial lesions: a meta-analysis. *Obstet Gynaecol*, 91, 626–631

Mutyaba T, Mmiro FA and Weiderpass E (2006) Knowledge, attitudes and practices on cervical cancer screening among the medical workers of Mulago Hospital, Uganda. *BMC Medical Education*, 6, 13

Nanda K, McCrory DC, Myers ER, et al. (2000) Accuracy of the Papanicolaou test in screening for and follow-up of cervical cytologic abnormalities: a systematic review. *Ann Intern Med*, 132, 810–819

Pan American Health Organisation (2004) Scant progress on cervical cancer: www.paho.org/English/DD/PIN/ptoday04_nov04.htm (accessed 15/3/07)

Parkin DM, Bray FI and Devassa SS (2001) Cancer burden in the year 2000: the global picture. *European Journal of Cancer*, 37, (Suppl 8), S4–S66

Parkin DM, Whelan SL, Ferlay J, Teppo L and Thomas DB, (eds) (2002) *Cancer Incidence in Five Continents*. Vol VIII, IARC Scientific Publications, no. 143. IARC Press, Lyon

Program for Appropriate Technology in Health (PATH) (2002) Proceedings of the Western Kenya Cervical Cancer Prevention Project (WKCCPP) dissemination workshop. 7 March, Nairobi, Kenya. Copies of this report are available by contacting: accp@path.org or by writing to: Cervical Cancer Prevention Team, PATH, 1455 NW Leary Way, Seattle (WA) 98107 USA

Saibishkumar EP, Patel FD and Sharma SC (2005) Results of radiotherapy alone in the treatment of carcinoma of the uterine cervix: a retrospective analysis of 1069 patients. *Int J of Gynaecol Cancer*, 15 (5), 890–897

Saibishkumar EP, Patel FD, Sharma SC, et al. (2006) Prognostic value of response to external radiation in stage IIIB cancer cervix in predicting clinical outcomes: a retrospective analysis of 556 patients from India. *Radiother Oncol*, 79, 145–149

Sankaranarayanan R, Black RJ and Parkin DM (1998) *Cancer Survival in Developing Countries*. IARC Scientific Publications, no. 145. IARC Press, Lyon

Sankaranarayanan R, Gaffikin L, Jacob M, Sellors J and Robles S (2005) A critical assessment of screening methods for cervical neoplasia. *International Journal of Gynaecology and Obstetrics*, 89, S4–S12

Schiffman M and Castle PE (2005) The promise of global cervical cancer prevention. *New England Journal of Medicine*, 353 (20), 2101–2104

Stewart BW and Kleihues P (eds) (2005) *World Cancer Report*. IARC Press, Lyon

Suba EJ, Murphy SK, Donnelly ADD, Furia LM, Huynh M and Raab SS (2006) Systems analysis of real-world obstacles to successful cervical cancer prevention in developing countries. *American Journal of Public Health*, 96, 480–487

Sung HY, Kearney KA, Miller M, Kinney W, Sawaya GF and Hiatt RA (2000) Papanicolaou smear history and diagnosis of invasive cervical carcinoma among members of a large, prepaid health plan. *Cancer*, 88 (10), 2283–2289

Thomas G (2006) Cervical cancer; treatment challenges in the developing world. *Radiotherapy and Oncology*, 79, 139–141

Wabinga HR, Parkin DM, Wabwire-Mangen F and Nambooze S (2000) Trends in cancer incidence in Kyadondo County, Uganda, 1960–1997. *British Journal of Cancer*, 82 (9), 1585–1592

Wabinga H, Ramanakumar AV, Banura C, Luwaga A, Nambooze S and Parkin DM (2003) Survival of cervix cancer patients in Kampala, Uganda: 1995–1997. *British Journal of Cancer*, 89, 65–69

Walraven G (2003) Prevention of cervical cancer in South Africa: a daunting task? *African Journal of Reproductive Health*, 7 (2), 7–12

Watkins MM, Gabali C, Winklegy M, Gaona E and Lebaron S (2002) Barriers to cervical screening in rural Mexico. *International Journal of Gynaecologic Cancer*, 12 (5), 475–479

Wood K, Jewkes R and Abrahams N (1997) Cleaning the womb: constructions of cervical cancer and womb cancer among rural black women in South Africa. *Soc Sci Med*, 45, 283–294

World Health Organisation (WHO) (1986) Control of cancer of the cervix uteri. *Bulletin of the World Health Organisation*, 64, 607–618

Chapter 10

Survivorship, recurrence and symptom management in cervical cancer

'It ain't over when it's over.'

(from Alfano and Rowland 2006)

Introduction

As a result of cervical screening programmes, many women in developed nations will be diagnosed with pre-malignant cervical dysplasias or early stage cervical cancer which can be successfully managed with the strategies described in earlier chapters. The result of this is a population of cancer survivors. Whilst clearly the optimal treatment outcome, cancer survivorship is not without its challenges, some of which are discussed below.

For those women who do not respond to primary therapy a different set of challenges arises. Unfortunately, 10–25% of women with early invasive cervical cancer will experience a recurrence (Park et al. 2001). Some of these women will be successfully treated with second line therapy, but others will not and their disease will progress. Furthermore, a proportion of women only present when their cancer is already advanced: 5–15% of cervical cancer patients present with FIGO stage IVA or IVB disease (Pettersson 1995, Quinn et al. 2006).

The first part of this chapter looks at some of the issues faced by cervical cancer survivors as they try to come to terms with the disease and its sequelae, and continue with their lives. The second part examines disease recurrence and discusses the management of some of the symptoms of advanced cervical cancer.

To a certain extent the former could be regarded as a 'developed world' problem, whereas the latter is far more of a matter for the developing world. However, because most of the literature on advanced disease and symptom management is from studies conducted in developed countries, the issues are principally addressed from this perspective.

Survivorship

There is no cancer survivor that doesn't think about the cancer all of the time. It is an experience that changes you forever.

(Mahon and Casperson 1977)

Cervical cancer survivors face two significant challenges. One is the management of long-term, treatment-related toxicities, many of which have already been discussed in previous chapters. The second is the psychological adjustment to their diagnosis, and in particular the fear of recurrence.

In recent years there has been a growing body of literature in recognition of the expanding population of 'cancer survivors', the needs of whom have not necessarily been understood or met by existing health care provisions. Much of the literature relates to breast cancer or to 'cancer' in general, although there are a few studies which focus specifically on gynaecological or cervical cancer (Ashing-Giwa et al. 2004, Wenzel et al. 2005, Hodgkinson et al. 2006, Vistad et al. 2006).

The definition of 'survivorship' varies in this literature. On the whole, health professionals tend to interpret it as disease-free survival for five or more years. However, consumer groups may take it to include patients at any stage in the disease trajectory, including patients in remission or those with ongoing disease. The National Coalition for Cancer Survivorship's Charter states that: 'from the time of its discovery and for the balance of life, an individual diagnosed with cancer is a survivor' (National Coalition for Cancer Survivorship Databases in Hodgkinson et al. 2006).

The literature indicates that cancer survivorship brings with it a large range of challenges which have the potential to impact every aspect of the individual's life.

Common survivorship issues include:

- Ongoing fatigue.
- Cognitive changes: many cancer patients report cognitive changes and impaired thought processes. Anderson et al. (1989) found high levels of confusion amongst gynaecological cancer survivors. Some women reported that they no longer knew how to interpret body symptoms and had difficulty understanding how their bodies work.
- Body image concerns.
- Sexual response and functioning difficulties.
- Infertility: this has been identified as a particular problem for women with gynaecological malignancies who were of childbearing potential at the time of diagnosis and treatment (Anderson and Lutgendorf 1997, Wenzel et al. 2005).
- Post-traumatic stress disorder (PTSD).
- Family/caregiver distress.
- Personal distress, anxiety, depression.
- Fear of recurrence: fear of recurrence has been ranked as the single largest concern of breast cancer survivors and ovarian and other gynaecologic cancer survivors. In some patients these fears are further compounded by concerns about the risk of other family members being diagnosed with the disease (Spencer et al. 1999, Kattlove and Winn 2003, Alfano and Rowland 2006) and also by the fear of developing second malignancies (Anderson and Lutgendorf 1997).

Whilst some of the literature suggests that in general cervical cancer survivors do not suffer from lasting psychological morbidity (Hewitt et al. 2003, Wenzel et al 2005, Deimling et al. 2006), there are also a number of studies indicating that many women do have difficulty with long-term psychosocial adjustment (Vistad et al. 2006). Nightingale et al. (2006) in a systematic review of the literature found that the psychosocial impact of the disease was greatest in the two years following diagnosis, although some patients experienced substantial psychological morbidity more than five years after diagnosis.

This is confirmed by a recent Australian study by Hodgkinson et al. (2006) which examined the long-term impact of gynaecological malignancy on survivors. They found that from one to eight years after treatment most women reported normal levels of quality of life (QOL) and relationship adjustment. However, their overall level of functioning was at the lower end of the normal range and, more significantly, symptoms of anxiety were nearly three times higher than within the general community.

In this study, the number of years since diagnosis did not appear to affect levels of distress or perceived need, although longer-term survivors (more than three years post-diagnosis) were found to have significantly higher anxiety rates, poorer mental QOL and poorer physical QOL. Thus, perhaps counter-intuitively, longer survivorship periods are not necessarily associated with a reduction in levels of distress.

Of the survivors, 87% reported a need for supportive care services in the last month and a quarter felt they needed help in managing concerns about the cancer coming back. Wenzel et al. (2005) similarly found that at the time of interview (five to ten years post-cervical cancer diagnosis) 59% of survivors stated that they would probably participate in a counselling programme if it was available and 69% stated that they would have attended a support group programme during the initial treatment if it had been offered.

Notwithstanding all these challenges for cervical cancer survivors, some studies indicate that in retrospect, not every aspect of the diagnosis is perceived as negative. Two thirds of women in the study by Hodgkinson et al. (2006) reported some positive outcomes from the disease. For example, over half endorsed the comment, 'I have grown as a person' and just under half endorsed a number of other similarly positive statements such as: 'I realise how precious life is', 'I focus more on things that are important' and 'I have made a lot of positive changes in my life'.

In another study by Schultz et al. (2004), 47% of cervical cancer survivors felt that the cancer had improved their family life. A further 22% felt it had improved intimate relations, (although 23% reported damage to intimate relations). Interestingly, damaged relationships appeared to be more common with women who had received radiotherapy plus surgery rather than surgery alone (Schultz et al. 2004). Vistad et al. (2006) in a review of a large number of studies of QOL amongst cervical cancer survivors drew similar conclusions, suggesting that there would appear to be more psychosocial and sexual problems following radiotherapy compared with surgery.

Among cancer survivors in general, two factors have consistently been found to be associated with successful adaptation: perceived social support especially from the spouse/partner, and coping style (specifically, those with a positive, active coping style do well, while those who are negative, prone to distress, and feel helpless or hopeless have a harder time moving forward to reclaim their lives) (Spencer et al. 1998). Certain sub-groups of women have been found to experience marked survivorship issues, for example, the Latinas population in the USA (Ashing-Giwa et al. 2004).

Cervical cancer recurrence

Whilst fear of recurrence remains a significant survivorship issue for many women, it is fortunately something that most will never have to deal with. The recurrence rate with stage IB to IIA cervical cancer has been reported to be as low as 10% (Friedlander and Grogan 2002). Nevertheless, there are some sub-groups of women who remain at a high risk of recurrence – principally those with lymphatic involvement or bulky disease. Up to 70% of patients with nodal metastases or locally advanced tumours will relapse (Friedlander and Grogan 2002).

Psychosocial factors may also place some women at risk of developing advanced disease. Within first world nations, women who present with advanced cervical cancer are often amongst the disadvantaged and vulnerable of society (see Box 10.1).

The majority of cervical cancer recurrences occur within two years of primary remission (Goto et al. 2005). Recurrence later than five years is rare, occurring in less than 10% of cervical cancer patients (Takehara et al. 2001). Unfortunately, the prognosis in either situation is poor. Despite major advances in the management of early stage disease, recurrent and metastatic carcinoma of the uterine cervix remains for the most part incurable (Eralp et al. 2003). Between 50% to 60% of patients who recur have disease which has spread beyond the pelvis and is invariably intractable to treatment (Friedlander and Grogan 2002).

Box 10.1 Social factors and cervical cancer

A combination of factors is likely to contribute to an increased risk of developing advanced stage cervical cancer, including:

- poor cervical screening uptake
- high risk HPV acquisition behaviour
- poor access to health care facilities
- poor quality health care facilities

Thus, the profile of high risk individuals begins to emerge. Not surprisingly, these women tend to be amongst the vulnerable and disadvantaged in our society. They include:

- Women with physical disabilities: simply the physical problems associated with performing gynaecological examinations can result in these women missing out on cervical screening and the early detection of malignancy (Lane 2005). In Australia, almost 30% of women aged 70–75 with a physical disability have never had a cervical smear (Frohmader 2002).
- Women with intellectual/ mental disabilities: women with cognitive difficulties have been found to have poorer access to cervical cancer screening facilities and higher levels of dissatisfaction with the service they receive (Parish and Whisnant-Saville 2006). Intellectually disadvantaged women also have a high risk of sexual abuse which further impacts access to appropriate health care resources (Lane 2005).
- Minority group and non-English speaking women: reduced access to screening amongst ethnic minority groups has already been discussed in Chapter 8 and is likely to result in a higher incidence of poor prognosis cancer amongst this population.
- Refugee women: a combination of factors contributes to generally poorer health outcomes amongst refugee women, including lack of screening (Barnes and Harrison 2004). Furthermore, these women may have been exposed to physical violence, including rape and often face additional barriers related to culture and language (Lane 2005).
- Lesbian women: it should not be assumed that women who are lesbians have not had previous heterosexual relationships which place them at risk of acquiring cervical cancer (Rankow and Tessaro 1998). Celibate women or those who have had exclusively lesbian relationships have a negligible risk of acquiring cervical cancer, although there is a risk amongst lesbian women whose partners have been in heterosexual relationships.
- Lower socio-economic status: women living in socially deprived areas are at greater risk of acquiring advanced stage disease (Baker and Middleton 2003, Singh et al. 2004). Parikh et al. (2003) found an increased risk of invasive cancer of almost 100% between high and low social categories.
- Sexually abused women: women with a history of sexual abuse are less likely to present for cervical screening (Farley et al. 2002).
- Obese women: there is some data to suggest a lower uptake of cervical screening amongst obese women (Ferrante et al. 2006).

Advanced cervical cancer is also found amongst women who have none of these risk factors. However, primary health care workers who have access to women falling into any of these categories should be aware of their potential for developing advanced cervical cancer and of the resources which can be offered to them.

Detection of recurrence and prognostic factors

The schedule of follow-up after treatment for cervical cancer varies according to the stage of disease at diagnosis and the therapy received. Most centres follow patients for five to ten years. Patients will typically have a pelvic examination every three or four months for the first two years and six-monthly thereafter.

It is difficult to find data on the proportion of recurrences that are detected at routine follow-up and those which are picked up following the development of symptoms. In one

Table 10.1 Summary of outcomes for patients with recurrent cervical cancer (with permission from Friedlander and Grogan 2002)

Recurrence	Treatment options	Outcome
Central	Pelvic exenteration	30–60% five-year survival
Local recurrence following surgery	Chemotherapy and radiotherapy	6–77% five-year survival
Distant metastases	Cisplatin-based chemotherapy	17–50% response: 4–9 months median survival

study, 84% of patients were found to be symptomatic at time of recurrence (Gerdin et al. 1994). In another which looked specifically at late recurrence (after five years), two thirds of 27 patients had symptoms on diagnosis of recurrence. In this study although CT scanning was found to be useful in picking up recurrences, half were detected using simple clinical examinations and chest X-rays (Goto et al. 2005).

After recurrence, the five-year survival rate has been estimated to be 50% for patients with locally advanced disease and 16% for those with metastatic disease (Tambaro et al. 2004). Poor prognostic factors include large recurrences (Friedlander and Grogan 2002) and those involving the pelvic side wall rather than recurring centrally. A worrying triad of symptoms is unilateral leg oedema, sciatic pain and ureteral obstruction. This almost always indicates disease involving the pelvic side wall which is usually unresectable and requires palliative measures (Friedlander and Grogan 2002).

Other poor prognostic factors for post-recurrence therapy include advanced stage at presentation, short time to progression from initial diagnosis and poor performance status (Friedlander and Grogan 2002). Recurrence within a previously irradiated field and a poor response to chemotherapy are also likely to result in a less favourable outcome (Eralp et al. 2003).

Symptoms of recurrence include pain, anorexia, vaginal bleeding, cachexia and psychological problems (Freidlander and Grogan 2002). Some of these may be confused with treatment related toxicities, particularly from radiotherapy, which can make early detection of recurrence difficult.

Psychological factors

The psychological implications of being diagnosed with either advanced or recurrent cervical cancer are enormous and yet surprisingly have not been the subject of a great deal of literature.

Mahon and Casperson (1997) performed a qualitative study interviewing people with recurrent cancer and identified a number of themes. Many patients attempt to find some meaning for their recurrence asking themselves, 'Why me?' Death was also a common concern expressed by most interviewees. The treatment for recurrent cancer often appeared to be more arduous than primary therapy.

Treatment

Choice of therapy is determined by the extent of the disease and the therapy so far. In patients who have received primary radiotherapy, further radiotherapy is often not an option. In this situation surgery (for example pelvic exenteration) presents the only curative approach. Chemotherapy may also be considered, particularly for the management of distant metastases, but can only be regarded as palliative. Some of the issues surrounding use of radiotherapy, chemotherapy and surgery for extensive disease are discussed in Chapters 3, 4 and 5.

Where progressive disease cannot be controlled with conventional treatments the next option is palliation. At this time priorities shift from controlling the disease to achieving adequate pain control and the best quality of life possible. The following section aims to identify some palliative care problems which are specific to advanced stage cervical cancer and which present particularly difficult nursing management issues.

Symptom control in advanced cervical cancer

The range of symptoms associated with advanced cervical cancer is a direct reflection of the pattern of disease progression. In cervical cancer, local recurrence within the pelvis and to the regional lymphatics is much more common than distant spread. For this reason many of the symptoms are related to a large pelvic mass. This can cause pressure or infiltration effects on the bladder, rectum, pelvic blood vessels, ureters, lymphatics and pelvic nerve supply (Lickass 2002).

Where distant metastases are found, the most common sites are the lung (21%), para-aortic nodes (11%), abdominal cavity (8%) and supraclavicular nodes (7%). Bone metastases occur in approximately 16% of patients, predominantly in the lumbar and thoracic spine (Friedlander and Grogan 2002).

A whole range of symptoms can arise with advanced cervical cancer, many of which are common to a number of advanced malignancies. Some of these symptoms are listed in Box 10.2.

The following section will not discuss these symptoms because they are already adequately addressed in the literature. Instead, a small number of less common symptoms will be examined which are found specifically (although not exclusively) in advanced stage cervical cancer. These symptoms have been selected because they have not been widely discussed in the existing palliative care nursing literature and they present particularly difficult nursing problems.

The topics for discussion are:

- difficult pain syndromes in cervical cancer
- fistulas
- management of vaginal bleeding
- advanced lower limb lymphoedema
- ureteric obstruction

Box 10.2 Problems of advanced gynaecological cancer (McVey 2005)

- pain
- fatigue
- breathlessness
- anorexia
- nausea and vomiting
- constipation
- fungating wounds
- haemorrhage

Difficult pain syndromes

In the already substantial cancer pain literature one thing which is continuously re-iterated is that there are as many specific pain profiles as there are cervical cancer patients. This calls for thorough pain assessment, taking into account not only the extent of disease and other co-morbidities, but also psychological, personal and social factors.

Palliative care literature commonly refers to two types of pain: nocioceptive and neurological. The term 'nocioceptive pain' is applied to pain resulting from the stimulation of pain receptors. This may be through tissue injury, inflammation, cuts and burns. Conversely, 'neuropathic pain' is caused by abnormal nerve activity, for example from postherpetic neuralgia or direct damage to the nerve through tumour infiltration.

Advanced cervical cancer is associated with both nociceptive and neurological pain. However, it is the management of neurological pain which is particularly problematic. Neurological pain does not fit comfortably into the commonly used WHO pain ladder because it is not always responsive to increasing doses of opiates. The WHO model does have an 'adjuvant' category of analgesics containing medications for nerve pain but does not provide clear guidance on which agents are effective and the order in which they should be given (WHO 1986).

In advanced cervical cancer, tumour invasion into nervous and muscle tissue can result in two particularly troublesome pain complexes: lumbosacral plexopathy and the psoas syndrome. The aetiology of these complexes and their management is discussed below.

It is disappointing but perhaps not surprising that most of the literature on the subject describes medical pain management strategies. That is not to say that non-medical techniques such as guided imagery or therapeutic touch have no role, but just that there is a paucity of literature evaluating their efficacy in this context.

Lumbosacral plexopathy (LSP)

Lumbosacral plexopathy is a particularly troublesome pain syndrome observed in advanced cervical cancer. The lumbosacral plexus is composed of the lumbar, sacral and coccygeal nerves – that is the nerves supplying the lower limbs and perineum. Because of its location it is sometimes associated with localised tumour invasion in patients with pelvic tumours. Less commonly it may be the site of metastatic spread.

Lumbosacral plexopathy occurs in less than 1% of cancer patients (Jaeckle 1985, 2004). Over 90% of patients with the condition present with pain in the lower back, buttock, hip and thigh (Taylor et al. 1997). Yadav (2007a) identifies certain characteristics associated with this type of pain:

- It may be of unilateral onset but is confined to one side in 90% of cases.
- It is usually constant, dull, aching, or pressure-like, but rarely burning. Cramping may also be present.
- It may worsen at night-time or when the patient is supine, and patients generally have difficulty finding any comfortable position at all (Jaeckle 2004).
- It may radiate down the leg.
- Pain exacerbation may occur with prolonged ambulation or sitting.
- Up to one third of patients may have 'hot dry foot' syndrome as a result of sympathetic nerve involvement (Dalmau et al. 1989).

Other symptoms of LSP are muscle weakness and sensory abnormality. LSP may also be a long-term toxicity from radiotherapy; in which case it is generally associated with weakness and sensory loss rather than pain (Yadav 2007b).

Clinical diagnosis is often confirmed by medical imaging – usually MRI in preference to CT (Jaeckle 2004). Management may be through radiotherapy or chemotherapy, but where these are not feasible (for example, because of prior radiotherapy treatment) it will be pharmacological.

As already mentioned, the role of opiates in the management of nerve pain is the subject of some controversy. Whilst they would appear to have a function (Grond et al. 1999), unfortunately in a number of cases opiate toxicity will be reached without achieving adequate pain control. Oxycontin is possibly the most efficacious opiate in the management of nerve pain.

Additional medication options include:

- steroids or non-steroidal anti-inflammatory drugs
- antiepileptics (e.g. gabapentin 300–3600 mg/day (Caraceni et al. 1999), or the less costly sodium valproate and carbamazepine)
- tricyclic antidepressants (e.g. amitriptyline)
- a single dose (500 mg or 1 g) of intravenous magnesium sulfate has been used with success in a small sample of patients with neuropathic pain due to neoplastic plexopathy (Crosby et al. 2000)
- some anaesthetic agents (e.g. ketamine) have been used orally and in low doses with good effect (Kannan et al. 2002)
- lidocaine and clonidine have also been reported as having a role in neuropathic cancer pain, although not specifically in the management of LSP (Farrar et al. 2001)

In light of the paucity of evidence to guide which drug to use, the choice of agent is likely to be determined by physician preference, toxicity profile and cost.

Psoas syndrome

The psoas muscle is a long, spindle-shaped muscle whose function is to flex the thigh relative to the pelvis. On the whole, metastatic tumour involving skeletal muscles is an uncommon occurrence. It has been postulated that the frequent movement of muscles and/or the accumulation of lactic acid in them may prevent the establishment of metastatic deposits (Ampil et al. 2001). However, metastasis to the psoas has been reported with a number of primaries, including the gastrointestinal tract, bladder, kidney and cervix (Ampil et al. 2001).

Malignant psoas syndrome is associated with both nocioceptive and neuropathic pain and is characterised by:

- evidence of proximal lumbosacral plexopathy (neuropathic pain)
- painful, fixed flexion of the ipsilateral hip (nocioceptive pain)
- pain exacerbated by attempted extension of the hip ('positive psoas test')
- CT and/or pathological evidence of ipsilateral psoas major muscle malignant involvement, either from metastases or direct tumour involvement (Agar et al. 2004) (nocioceptive pain)

Pain may also be referred to the groin, thigh and anterior abdominal wall (Agar et al. 2004).

Symptom management requires a multimodal approach to address each of the specific processes which are occurring (Agar et al. 2004). Pharmacological management should include:

- opioids to control the muscle and nerve pain to a degree (Grond et al. 1999)
- agent/s to control the neuropathic pain (see LSP management above)
- muscle relaxants (e.g. diazepam) a very important component of therapy necessary to treat the muscle spasm

Once again, chemotherapy, radiotherapy, nerve blocks and surgery may all have a part to play. Surgical approaches involve removal of the psoas metastases.

Fistulas

'Probably the most distressing and demoralizing condition that a woman can experience. These unhappy women often become social outcasts.'

(Naru et al. 2004)

A fistula is an abnormal connection or passage between organs or vessels which do not usually communicate directly with one another. The close anatomical relationship of bladder, rectum, vagina and uterus render cervical cancer patients particularly susceptible to fistula formation (Naru et al 2004). There are a number of types of fistula:

- vesicovaginal (VVF) (bladder/vagina)
- urethrovaginal (UVF) (urethra/vagina)
- vesicouterine (VUF) (bladder/uterus)
- rectovaginal (RVF) (rectum/vagina)

Genital fistulas are a particular problem in developing countries, where 90% result from obstetric complications. Furthermore, because cervical cancer is generally only diagnosed at a late stage in these countries, fistula formation as a result of advanced pelvic disease is also seen relatively frequently. The resultant wetness, odour and discomfort can cause serious social problems (see Chapter 9).

In developed countries, the majority of genital fistulas are caused by gynaecological surgery, radiotherapy and malignancy (Thomas and Williams 2000, Romics et al. 2002, Naru et al. 2004). Here fistulas are much less common than in developing countries and are seen in approximately 1.8% of patients with cervical cancer (Emmert and Kohler 1996).

The main clinical symptoms depend on the type of fistula, but in one large series were found to be faecal or urinary leak through the vagina (44.7%), bleeding (31.5%) and local pain (5.3%) (Emmert and Kohler 1996). Recto-vagina fistulas are associated with the passage of flatus and stool from the vagina, foul-smelling vaginal discharge, recurrent or chronic vaginitis, excoriation of the perineal skin and dyspareunia (Burke 2005). Vesicovaginal fistulas are associated with continuous (day and night) incontinence. Symptoms are to a certain extent dependent on the fistula size. If a VVF is only small there may still be normal voiding in conjunction with watery discharge from the vagina (Romics et al. 2002).

Where there has been prior radiotherapy the risk of fistula is greatly increased and its management is more problematic. Because vascular damage progresses over several years some fistulas may only become apparent at a late stage and when there is little hope of successful closure. Emmert and Kohler (1996) looked at the interval from the last irradiation to presentation with fistula and found this to be a median of 11.6 months (RVF) or 8.7 months (VVF), although delays of up to 17 years have been reported (Ulhoi et al. 1994).

Other factors thought to contribute to fistula formation include anatomical distortion by fibroids or ovarian tumours, adhesions, sepsis, endometriosis, diabetes, cardiovascular disease, hypertension, advanced age and cigarette smoking (Thomas and Williams 2000, Burke 2005).

Management

A fistula which has been caused by trauma or treatment related toxicity may be amenable to surgical repair, but where caused by recurrent disease this is often not feasible. Whilst there may still be a role for surgical intervention, this may well involve the formation of an ileal conduit or colostomy.

Where the pelvic tissue quality has been substantially compromised by prior therapy conservative measures may be the only option. Emmert and Kohler (1996) found that slightly less than a quarter of patients with fistulas were treated surgically, the remainder being managed conservatively. For VVFs this will frequently necessitate catheterisation (often supra-pubic). RVF management involves the use of incontinence/sanitary pads and barrier cream to prevent skin excoriation. Malodorous discharge is a significant problem and one to which there appears to be no simple answer. It is discussed more fully in the following section about vaginal discharge.

Vaginal discharge, haemorrhage and odour

A common problem associated with pelvic recurrence is necrotic fungation of the tumour which erodes the top of the vagina. This can result in bleeding and malodourous discharge (Spencer and Fang 2005). Both of these present difficult nursing and management problems, as discussed below.

Bleeding

Bleeding in advanced cervical cancer generally results from tumour invasion of local blood vessels, sometimes in conjunction with cancer-induced coagulopathies. As with many terminal care topics, ethical and methodological difficulties mean that there are not many clinical trials in this area. Consequently, the approach to bleeding control is reliant on anecdotal reports or extrapolation of known therapies from the acute to the palliative setting. Box 10.3 lists some of the strategies that can be employed.

Radiotherapy may be helpful in intractable bleeding situations and is frequently administered as a single fraction (Onsrud et al. 2001). In some cases of advanced cervical cancer the maximum radiotherapy dose will already have been reached, leaving treatment options limited. Haemostasis may also be achieved surgically or through palliative embolisation which has been shown to have equivalent efficacy (Prommer 2005). Embolisation refers to diminishing blood flow through selected vessels by inserting haemostatic material and is generally performed under angiographic control (Broadley et al. 1995).

Where the above options are unsuccessful or not feasible, packing is commonly performed, often in combination with pharmacological agents. For example, packs can be soaked with acetone or formalin (Patsner 1993). Formalin is thought to 'fix' tissue, causing cross linkage of tissue proteins and may also be used topically in the prevention of radiation

---

Box 10.3 Options for palliation of bleeding (Prommer 2005, with permission)

Local measures:

- packing
- compression dressings
- topical haemostatics
- astringents/vasoconstrictors
- postural modifications
- radiation therapy
- palliative embolisation (inserting haemostatic material with radiography guidance)
- endoscopy

Systemic measures:

- plasma products
- platelet transfusions
- vitamin K
- DDAVP (vasopressin)
- recombinant FVIIa
- antifibrinolytic agents (e.g. tranexamic acid)

> **Box 10.4 Measures to be taken with the patient at risk of bleeding (Prommer 2005, with permission)**
>
> • Promote discussion with patient/family regarding the potential for haemorrhage.
> • Establish resuscitative status.
> • Teach family/caregivers management strategies (e.g. pressure).
> • Provide dark basins and dark towels.
> • Plan access to drugs and drug administration.
> • Make sedatives available (e.g. midazolam 2.5–5 mg IV or SC).
> • Provide phone numbers on hand for acute problems.
> • Plan in advance and chose options for respite care.

proctitis (Fletcher et al. 2002, Prommer 2005). The exact mechanism of haemostasis achieved by acetone is unknown but it is presumed to act as an astringent (Patsner 1993).

Where bleeding is caused or exacerbated by a coagulopathy this may be corrected through the use of systemic therapies including the administration of blood products (e.g. fresh frozen plasma) or antifibrinolytic agents (e.g. tranexamic acid).

'Massive bleeds' which are the result of large vessel erosion frequently carry a poor prognosis and therefore require the institution of measures of comfort as far as possible (see Box 10.4).

Malodourous discharge

Advanced cervical cancer may also be associated with malodorous vaginal discharge. Odour may arise from fistula formation, or from necrosis at the tumour site at the top of the vagina. Other contributory factors are thought to be the interaction of certain types of bacteria or an overgrowth of normal vaginal organisms (Von Greunigen et al. 2000). It is often the cause of considerable distress amongst both patients and their families and can be very difficult to manage. A number of therapies are suggested in the literature, although once again the evidence base for many is difficult to ascertain. Some suggested strategies are:

• Gentle douching using diluted peroxide, betadine, vinegar or normal saline (Spencer and Fang 2005). However, the role of douching in general is controversial and not well addressed in the literature.
• Metronidazole-topically using gel or liquid, or orally. There is controversy regarding appropriateness of systemic antibiotics for the management of local infections in terms of patient acceptability and bacterial resistance. Topical application of metronidazole gel has been found efficacious in cervical cancer (Von Greunigen et al. 2000)
• Charcoal dressings – a basket of charcoal in the patient's room may help reduce odour (Seaman 2006).
• Panty liners impregnated with deodoriser.

None of these strategies can claim to be wholly effective and the literature available to guide nursing practice in this area is extremely disappointing.

Lower limb lymphoedema (LLL) in palliative care

'It looks like a big club . . . It looks so dreadful, so it's just as well to bandage it so you don't have to see the wretched thing . . . my healthy leg is 46 [cm in circumference] and this one is 86 – the bad one.'

(Frid et al. 2006, Patient 2)

Lower limb lymphoedema as a post-operative/radiotherapy problem has already been discussed in Chapter 3. There is much less data concerning LLL amongst palliative care patients and in practice data from curative phase trials of lymphoedema are often, and probably incorrectly, applied to palliative situations (Frid et al. 2006).

In advanced cancer, lymphoedema may be compounded by a number of factors including:

- insufficiency of the kidney, liver or heart, any of which can lead to retention of fluid in tissue spaces
- local spread of disease in the pelvis and abdomen causing further blockage of lymphatic channels
- hypoproteinaemia from poor dietary intake, liver disease and renal failure, each of which may encourage fluid retention in the interstitium
- peritoneal seedings which can cause excess fluid production as a result of a local inflammatory response
- generalised debility and decreased mobility
- medications (e.g. taxotere or steroids in some cases as they lead to fluid retention)

(Sneddon 2005)

Oedema in palliative care patients is often gross, involving the root of the limb and adjacent body trunk. Skin condition may also be compromised, with symptoms such as lymphorrhoea (i.e. leakage of lymph through breaks in the skin) and hyperkeratosis (a warty, scaly change to the skin). In some patients, fungating lesions may develop on lymphoedematous skin making management even more problematic (Williams 2004).

Treatment goals in the palliative care setting are different from those in a curative situation and focus on comfort, maintaining mobility and preventing further complications secondary to the lymphoedema (Sitzia and Sobrido 1997).

Once again, evidence-based information regarding lymphoedema management in terminal disease is difficult to find. Measures like manual lymphatic drainage are often not effective at this stage – although some patients do experience symptomatic relief from the massage (Williams 2004). Alternative strategies include bandaging and utilisation of appropriate compression garments. This calls for skill and expertise. Incorrect bandaging or inappropriate use of compression pump may simply result in redistribution of fluid to other tissues – in particular the labia, perineum and internal vagina (Williams 2004).

It is in the palliative care setting that other measures of lymphoedema control may seem appropriate, for example pharmacological strategies like the use of potassium-sparing diuretics (Sneddon 2005).

Lymphorrhoea can present particular nursing management problems. It requires the application of absorbent dressings – although specifically which dressing to apply and how it should be attached to thin, friable skin is difficult to determine. Management of hyperkeratosis is similarly problematic. Board and Harlow (2002) suggest that it may be treated by the application of 50% white soft paraffin and 50% liquid paraffin, or, in severe cases, 5% salicylic acid, although the data supporting this recommendation is not specified.

Frid et al. (2006) performed a qualitative study in order to assess patients' experiences and perceptions of LLL, and how it was managed in the late stages of their disease. Thirteen patients were interviewed – nine women and four men. For some of them, LLL was distressing because of its association with disease recurrence and the impact it had on their lives at a time when every moment was precious. For others, LLL was not considered to be a major problem in the context of everything else they were going through.

Ureteric obstruction

Acute renal failure secondary to malignant ureteral obstruction is not uncommon for patients suffering from abdominopelvic malignancies (Kinn and Ohlsen 2003). Large pelvic masses may occlude both ureters leading to kidney failure. Left untreated, patients become progressively comatose and die, usually peacefully (Chang et al. 2006).

Conversely, ureteric obstruction can be relieved by either surgical or non-surgical techniques. Non-surgical techniques include the institution of anti-tumour measures such as chemotherapy or radiotherapy. The administration of corticosteroids may also be considered, presumably improving the patency of the ureters through reducing the level of tumour oedema. However, this approach is associated with a risk of sepsis and is not always effective (Chye and Lickiss 1994).

The two most commonly adopted surgical procedures are insertion of a percutaneous nephrostomy tube or insertion of retrograde ureteric stents. Sometimes a staged approach is used, beginning with nephrostomy tubes and then inserting stents at a later date (Chye and Lickiss 1994).

The decision to insert stents or nephrostomy tubes should not be undertaken lightly and in some cases is definitively contraindicated – particularly in developing countries. Patients with advanced cervical cancer can be expected to experience a greater level of post-procedural complications and it cannot be guaranteed that their overall quality of life will be improved (Tenaka et al. 2004). Post-procedural complications include haemorrhage, infection, stent breakage, blockage or migration (Chye and Lickiss 1994). Furthermore, whereas renal failure can result in a relatively peaceful death, stenting may simply allow the patient to survive for long enough for their tumour to progress. They may thus go on to develop additional, and possibly more discomforting, symptoms such as fistulas, tenesmus and uncontrollable pelvic pain.

Thus, a number of considerations need to be taken into account prior to intervening in situations of ureteric obstruction. Chang et al. (2006) suggest that the situations in which nephrostomy may be indicated are:

- renal obstruction due to a non-malignant complication such as previous surgery or radiotherapy
- renal obstruction due to untreated primary malignancy
- renal obstruction due to certain disease relapses in which there are viable treatment options

In other situations a thorough assessment of the individual patient is required, taking into account her age, premorbid health, quality-of-life and personal goals. The rate of disease progression is also an important factor to consider (Wilson et al. 2005).

Conclusion

This chapter has examined some of the long-term issues faced by women who have been treated for cervical cancer. Some of the challenges of survivorship have been discussed, as well as some of the problems associated with recurrent and advanced disease. In examining the care of patients with advanced disease, the focus has been on symptoms which present particularly difficult nursing problems. The chapter has been written from the perspective of the developed world, although it is recognised that many of the issues associated with advanced disease are much more pertinent to developing nations where resources are limited.

Resources

National Coalition for Cancer Survivorship: http://www.canceradvocacy.org/
Jo's Trust: www.jotrust.co.uk/
DIPEX: www.dipex.org
Palliative Care Australia: www.pallcare.org.au
National Council for Palliative Care: www.ncpc.org.uk/

References

Agar M, Broadbent A and Chye R (2004) The management of malignant psoas syndrome: case reports and literature review. *Journal of Pain and Symptom Management*, 28 (3), 282–293

Alfano CM and Rowland JH (2006) Recovery issues in cancer survivorship: a new challenge for supportive care. *The Cancer Journal*, 15 (5), 432–433

Ampil FL, Lall C and Datta R (2001) Palliative management of metastatic tumours involving the psoas muscle: case reports and review of the literature. *American Journal of Clinical Oncology*, 24 (3), 313–314

Andersen B and Lutgendorf S (1997) Quality of life in gynaecologic cancer survivors. *Ca Cancer J Clin*, 47, 218–225

Andersen BL, Andersen B and deProsse C (1989) Controlled, prospective longitudinal study of women with cancer: II Psychological outcomes. *J Consult Clin Psychol*, 57, 683–691

Ashing-Giwa KT, Kagawa-Singer M, Padilla GV, et al. (2004) The impact of cervical cancer and dysplasia: a qualitative, multiethnic study. *Psycho-oncology*, 13, 709–728

Baker D and Middleton E (2003) Cervical screening and health inequality in England in the 1990s. *J Epidemiol Community Health*, 57, 417–423

Barnes DM and Harrison CL (2004) Refugee women's reproductive health in early resettlement. *Journal of Obstetric, Gynecologic & Neonatal Nursing*, 33 (6), 723–728

Board J and Harlow W (2002) Lymphoedema 3: the available treatments for lymphoedema. *British Journal of Nursing*, 11 (7), 438–450

Broadley KE, Kurowska A, Dick R, Platts A and Tookman A (1995) The role of embolization in palliative care. *Palliative Medicine*, 9 (4), 331–335

Burke C (2005) Rectovaginal fistulas. *Clinical Journal of Oncology Nursing*, 9 (3), 295–297

Caraceni A, Zecca E, Martini C and De Conno F (1999) Gabapentin as an adjuvant to opioid analgesia for neuropathic cancer pain. *J Pain Symptom Management*, 17, 441–445

Chang HL, Lim HW, Su FH, Tsai ST and Wang YW (2006) Win or lose? Percutaneous nephrostomy for a terminal stage cervical-cancer patient featuring obstructive uropathy. *Journal of Palliative Care*, 22 (1), 57–60

Chye RWM and Lickiss JN (1994) Palliative care in malignant ureteric obstruction. *Annals of the Academy of Medicine*, 23 (2), 197–203

Crosby V, Wilcock A and Corcoran R (2000) The safety and efficacy of a single dose (500 mg or 1 g) of intravenous magnesium sulphate in neuropathic pain poorly responsive to strong opioid analgesics in patients with cancer. *Journal of Pain and Symptom Management*, 19 (1), 35–39

Dalmau J, Graus F and Marco M (1989) Hot and dry foot as initial manifestation of neoplastic lumbosacral plexopathy. *Neurology*, 39, 871–872

Deimling GT, Bowman KF, Sterns S, Wagner LJ and Kahana B (2006) Cancer-related health worries and psychological distress among older adult, long-term cancer survivors. *Psycho-oncology*, 15, 306–320

Emmert C and Kohler U (1996) Management of genital fistulas in patients with cervical cancer. *Archives of Gynecology & Obstetrics*, 259 (1),19–24

Eralp Y, Saip P, Sakar B, et al. (2003) Prognostic factors in patients with metastatic or recurrent carcinoma of the uterine cervix. *International Journal of Gynaecological Cancer*, 13 (4), 497–504

Farley M, Golding JM and Minkoff JR (2002) Is a history of trauma associated with a reduced likelihood of cervical cancer screening? *Journal of Family Practice*, 51 (10), 827–831

Farrar JT and Portenoy RK (2001) Neuropathic cancer pain: the role of adjuvant analgesics. *Oncology (Huntingdon)*, 15 (11), 1435–1442

Ferrante JM, Chen PH and Jacobs A (2006) Breast and cervical screening in obese minority women. *Journal of Women's Health*, 15 (5), 531–541

Fletcher H, Wharfe G, Mitchell S and Simon T (2002) Treatment of intractable vaginal bleeding with formaldehyde-soaked packs. *J Obstet Gynaecol*, 22, 570–571

Frid M, Strang P, Friedrichsen MJ and Johanssen K (2006) Lower limb lymphoedema: experiences and perceptions of cancer patients in the late palliative stage. *Journal of Palliative Care*, 22 (1), 5–11

Friedlander M and Grogan M (2002) Guidelines for the treatment of recurrent and metastatic cervical cancer. *The Oncologist*, 7, 342–347

Frohmader C (2002) *There is No Justice – Just Us! The Status of Women With Disabilities in Australia*. Women with Disabilities Australia (WWDA), Canberra

Gerdin E, Cnattingius S, Johnson P and Pettersson B (1994) Prognostic factors and relapse patterns in early-stage cervical carcinoma after brachytherapy and radical hysterectomy. *Gynecologic Oncology*, 53 (3), 314–319

Goto T, Kino N, Shirai T, Fujimura M, Takahashi M, Shiromizu K (2005) Late recurrence of invasive cervical cancer: twenty years experience in a single cancer institute. *The Journal of Obstetrics and Gynaecology Research*, 31 (6), 514–519

Grond S, Radbruch L, Meuser T, Sabatowski R, Loick G and Lehmann KA (1999) Assessment and treatment of neuropathic cancer pain following WHO guidelines. *Pain*, 79, 15–20

Hewitt M, Rowland JH and Yancik R (2003) Cancer survivors in the United States: age, health and disability. *J Gerentol A Biol Sci Med Sci*, 58 (1), 82–91

Hodgkinson K, Butow P, Fuchs A, et al. (2006) Long term survival from gynaecological cancer; psychosocial outcomes, supportive care needs and positive outcomes. *Gynaecologic Oncology*, 104, 381–389

Jaeckle KA, Young DF and Foley KM (1985) The natural history of lumbosacral plexopathy in cancer. *Neurology*, 35, 8–15

Jaeckle KA (2004) Neurological manifestations of neoplastic and radiation-induced plexopathies. *Seminars in Neurology*, 24 (4), 385–393

Kannan TR, Saxena A, Bhatnagar S and Barry A (2002) Oral ketamine as an adjuvant to oral morphine for neuropathic pain in cancer patients. *Journal of Pain & Symptom Management*, 23 (1), 60–65

Kattlove H and Winn RJ (2003) Ongoing care of patients after primary treatment for their cancer. *CA Cancer J Clin*, 53 (3), 172–196

Kinn AC and Ohlsen H (2003) Percutaneous nephrostomy – a retrospective study focussed on palliative indications. *APMIS Supplementum*, (109), 66–70

Lane L (2005) Social and cultural diversity, in Lancaster T and Nattress K (eds) *Gynaecological Cancer Care: a Guide to Practice*. Ausmed, Australia. pp. 303–311

Lickiss JN (2002) Palliative care and pain management, in Berek JS and Hacker NF (eds) *Practical Gynaecologic Oncology*, 2nd edn. Williams and Wilkins, Baltimore. pp. 687–705

Mahon SM and Casperson D (1997) Exploring the psychosocial meaning of recurrent cancer: a descriptive study. *Cancer Nursing*, 20 (3), 178–186

McVey P (2005) Advanced symptom management, in Lancaster T and Nattress K (eds) *Gynaecological Cancer Care: a Guide to Practice*. Ausmed, Australia. pp. 329–355

Mortimer PS (2000) Acute inflammatory episodes, in Twycross R, Jenns K and Todd J (eds) *Lymphoedema*. Radcliffe Medical Press, Oxford. pp.130–139

Naru T, Rizvi J and Talati J (2004) Surgical repair of genital fistulas. *The Journal of Gynaecology Research*, 30 (4), 293–296

National Coalition for Cancer Survivorship databases: http:www.canceradvocacy.org (accessed 9/6/07)

Nightingale A, Papacharalabous EN and Butler-Manuel SA (2006) Systematic literature review of the psychosocial impact of cervical cancer, Poster Presentation (no 0484). *International Journal of Gynaecological Cancer*, 6 (suppl 3), 736

Onsrud M, Hagen B and Strickert T (2001) 10 Gy single-fraction pelvic irradiation for palliation and life prolongation in patients with cancer of the cervix and corpus uteri. *Gynaecol Oncol*, 82, 234–239

Parikh S, Brennan P and Boffetta P (2003) Meta-analysis of social inequality and the risk of cervical cancer. *Int J of Cancer*, 105, 687–691

Parish SL and Whisnant Saville A (2006) Women with cognitive limitations living in the community: evidence of disability-based disparities in health care. *Mental Retardation*, 44, (4), 249–259

Park TK, Kim SN, Kwon JY and Mo HJ (2001) Postoperative adjuvant therapy in early invasive cervical cancer patients with histopathologic high-risk factors. *International Journal of Gynaecological Care*, 11 (6), 475–482

Patsner B (1993) Topical acetone for control of life-threatening vaginal haemorrhage from recurrent gynaecological cancer. *European Journal of Gynaecological Cancer*, 14, 33–35

Pettersson F (1995) *Annual Report of the Results of Treatment in Gynecologic Cancer*. Vol 22. International Federation of Gynaecology and Obstetrics, Stockholm, Sweden

Prommer E (2005) Management of bleeding in the terminally ill patient. *Haematology*, 10 (3), 167–175

Quinn MA, Benedet JL, Odicino F, et al. (2006) Carcinoma of the cervix uteri. FIGO Annual Report Vol 26. *International Journal of Gynaecology and Obstetrics*, 95 (Suppl 1), S43–S101

Rankow EJ and Tessaro I (1998) Cervical cancer risk and Papanicolaou screening in a sample of lesbian and bisexual women. *Journal of Family Practice*, 47 (2), Aug, 139–143

Romics I, Kelemen Zs and Fazakas Zs (2002) The diagnosis and management of vesicovaginal fistulas. *BJU International*, 89 (7), 764–766

Schultz P, Stava C, Beck ML and Vassilopoulou-Sellin (2004) Ethnic/racial differences on the physiologic health of cancer survivors. *Cancer*, 100, (1), 156–164

Seaman S (2006) Management of malignant, fungating wounds in advanced cancer. *Seminars in Oncology Nursing*, 22 (3), 185–193

Singh GK, Miller BA, Hankey BF and Edwards BK (2004) Persistent area socioeconomic disparities in US incidence of cervical cancer, mortality, stage and survival, 1975–2000. *Cancer*, 101 (5), 1051–1057

Sitzia J and Sobrido L (1997) Measurement of health-related quality of life of patients receiving conservative treatment for limb lymphoedema using the Nottingham Health Profile. *Quality of Life Research*, 6, 373–384

Sneddon M (2005) Lower limb lymphoedema, in Lancaster T and Nattress K (eds) *Gynaecological Cancer Care: a Guide to Practice*. Ausmed, Australia. pp. 213–234

Spencer C and Fang H (2005) Cervical cancer, in Lancaster T and Nattress K (eds) *Gynaecological cancer Care: a Guide to Practice*. Ausmed, Australia. pp. 63–77

Spencer SM, Carver CS and Price AA (1998) Psychological and social factors in adaptation, in Holland JC (ed.) *Psycho-oncology*. Oxford University Press, New York. pp. 211–222

Spencer SM, Lehman JM, Wynings C, et al. (1999) Concerns about breast cancer and relations to psychosocial well-being in a multiethnic sample of early-stage patients. *Health Psychol*, 18 (2), 159–168

Takehara K, Shigemasa K, Sawasaki T, Naito H and Fujii T (2001) Recurrence of invasive cervical carcinoma more than five years after initial therapy. *Obstet Gynecol*, 98, 680–684

Tambaro R, Scambia G, Di Maio M, et al. (2004) The role of chemotherapy in locally advanced, metastatic and recurrent cervical cancer. *Critical Reviews in Oncology-Hematology*, 52 (1), 33–44

Taylor BV, Kimmel DW, Krecke KN and Cascino TL (1997) Magnetic resonance imaging in cancer-related lumbosacral plexopathy. *Mayo Clin Proc*, 72, 823–829

Tenaka T, Yanase M and Takatsuka K (2004) Clinical course in patients with percutaneous nephrostomy for hydronephrosis associated with advanced cancer. *Acta Urologica Japonica*, 50 (7), 457–462

Thomas K and Williams G (2000) Medicolegal aspects of vesicovaginal fistulas. *BJU International*, 86 (3), 354–359

Ulhoi BP, Rosgaard A and Harling H (1994) Treatment of radiation-induced vesicovaginal fistula. *Ugeskr Laeger*, 156 (51), 7685–7687

Vistad I, Fossa SD and Dahl AA (2006) A critical review of patient-rated quality-of-life studies of long-term survivors of cervical cancer. *Gynaecologic Oncology*, 102, 563–572

Von Greunigen VE, Coleman RL, Li A, Heard MC, Miller DS and Hemsell DL (2000) Bacteriology and treatment of malodourous lower reproductive tract in gynecologic cancer patients. *Obstetrics and Gynecology*, 96 (1), 23–27

Wenzel L, DeAlba I, Habbal R, et al. (2005) Quality of life in long-term cervical cancer survivors. *Gynaecol Oncol*, 97, 310–317

Williams AE (2003) Lymphoedema, in Faithfull S and Wells M (eds) *Supportive Care in Radiotherapy*. Churchill Livingstone, Edinburgh. pp. 287–302

Williams AF (2004) Understanding and managing lymphoedema in people with advanced cancer. *Journal of Community Nursing*, 18, (11), 30–40

Wilson JR, Urwin GH and Stower MJ (2005) The role of percutaneous nephrostomy in malignant ureteric obstruction. *Annals of the Royal College of Surgeons of England*, 87 (1), 21–24

World Health Organisation (1986) *Cancer Pain Relief*. WHO, Geneva

Yadav RR (2007a) Neoplastic lumbosacral plexopathy. E-medicine: http://www.emedicine.com/pmr/topic90.htm (accessed 4/6/07)

Yadav RR (2007b) Radiation-induced lumbosacral plexopathy. eMedicine: http://www.emedicine.com/pmr/topic122.htm (accessed 4/6/07)

Chapter 11

Cervical cancer vaccines

'Before these vaccines are made available, it will be important to ensure that health-care providers are comfortable with, and skilled at, discussing the benefits of STI vaccines with parents and their young adolescent children.'

(Mays and Zimet 2004)

Introduction

The scientific developments of the last decade have resulted in therapies which stand to revolutionise the management of cervical cancer. Previous chapters have illustrated how 'traditional' medical strategies involving surgery, radiotherapy and chemotherapy each have a role in cervical cancer therapy. Similarly, screening campaigns can facilitate its early detection and therefore more effective intervention. However, none of these addresses the root cause of the disease and can actually prevent it from developing.

And yet this is the claim for cancer, or more accurately, HPV vaccines. Prophylactic vaccines, which were trialled in the early part of this century and are now commercially available, have the potential to virtually eradicate the disease if employed correctly. Therapeutic vaccines have a little way further to go in their development but it is hoped that one day they will play a role in the management of established disease. There is thus a very real possibility that cervical cancer could in forthcoming decades become a disease of the past – certainly within developed countries. Perhaps not surprisingly, the challenge will be to achieve similar results in developing nations where economic factors are so much more restrictive.

Below follows an analysis of the role of vaccines in cervical cancer, beginning with a review of some of the important clinical research which has been performed using preventative HPV vaccines and the issues surrounding the implementation of a vaccination programme. The chapter ends with a look at the current status of therapeutic vaccines for cancer and their possible role in the future management of cervical cancer.

The role of vaccines in cancer therapy

A vaccine can be defined as 'a foreign substance injected to stimulate the immune system to launch an immune response against the specific target or targets contained in the vaccine' (King 2004). In the case of cervical cancer it is HPV rather than actual cancer that provides the target for the vaccine. Indeed, the term 'cancer vaccine' is slightly misleading and would be more accurately replaced by 'HPV vaccine'. None of the clinical trials testing such vaccines use the development of cancer as an end point – this would clearly have been unethical in light of the knowledge we have about how cervical cancer progresses. Instead they looked at the development and persistence of HPV infection and CIN.

There are two categories of vaccine which are currently available or under investigation for the treatment of cervical cancer: prophylactic and therapeutic. Prophylactic (or preventative) vaccines have been around since the days of Jenner and his famous early clinical trials with smallpox. The principle of prophylactic vaccination is to stimulate the production of antibodies without actually causing the disease itself. Prophylactic vaccination has proved highly effective in reducing the incidence of infection with measles, diphtheria and rubella (by 99.9%), and has almost completely eradicated polio and smallpox (Frazer et al. 2006). Until now the closest we have come to a prophylactic vaccine for cancer is the hepatitis B vaccine, which has been effective in reducing the incidence of cirrhosis and primary hepatocellular cancer in Malaysia, Singapore and Taiwan (Chang et al. 1997, King 2004).

Therapeutic vaccines aim to treat the disease by boosting the immune system to fight it. They can be seen as a form of active immunotherapy inducing the host to make an immune response against his own tumour cells (King 2004). Clinical trials are underway looking at the role of therapeutic vaccines in a variety of cancers, including cancer of the cervix.

Both types of vaccine are discussed in greater detail below.

Prophylactic vaccines

A prophylactic vaccine prepares the host to recognise an invading antigen and induce a neutralising antibody response. A neutralising antibody response is a response in which an antibody is released which reacts with the infectious agent to destroy it or to inhibit its infectivity. One way in which neutralising antibodies are effective is by coating virions and preventing them from binding to cell surfaces. (A virion is another name for a virus particle.)

Prophylactic vaccines for cervical cancer use the HPV viral capsid as the antigen. This has been facilitated by the development of technology which can generate virus-like particles or VLPs. As discussed in Chapter 1, VLPs consist of viral capsids that resemble the whole virus but do not contain a DNA core. They can induce a neutralising antibody response but cannot replicate and are therefore without infectious or oncogenic risk (Kahn and Bernstein 2005).

The VLP approach has been used with great success in a number of vaccines, including hepatitis B and HPV vaccines (Ault 2006). HPV VLP vaccines have been found to be highly immunogenic even at relatively low antigen doses. They can induce antibody responses that are 40 times higher than those found after natural infection, and persist for at least 36 months (Kahn and Bernstein 2005). The antibodies that are made by the body in response to the vaccine are thought to move from the serum into the cervical mucus in order to have their virus neutralising effect (Kahn and Bernstein 2005).

Clinical trials of prophylactic vaccines

Several phase 1 trials of monovalent VLP vaccines have been completed, with each one reporting similar findings, indicating that VLP vaccines are safe, well tolerated and highly immunogenic. Most have used a three-dose regimen with injections given over a six-month period. Adverse events are generally mild and similar to those observed with other vaccines: injection site reactions such as pain, bruising, and erythema and systemic effects such as headache, fatigue and gastrointestinal complaints (Ault 2006).

In 2002, Koutsky et al. published an important proof of concept trial which was the first to show efficacy with a monovalent HPV 16 vaccine. Approximately 2400 college-age women received three injections of either the experimental vaccine or placebo. The authors reported 41 cases of persistent HPV 16 infection or cervical dysplasia in the placebo group versus no cases in the group of women receiving the vaccine. Thus, the vaccine was 100% efficacious in preventing persistent HPV 16 infection and 100% efficacious in preventing HPV 16-associated cervical dysplasia. Furthermore, there were no vaccine-related serious adverse events and nearly equal numbers of discontinuations resulting from vaccine-related adverse events in the vaccine and placebo arms (Koutsky et al. 2002).

However, as has already been discussed in Chapter 2, vaccination against one HPV strain is not going to be enough to prevent all the cases of cervical dysplasia. If immune responses to HPV are type-specific, to achieve maximum public health benefit prophylactic HPV vaccines need to protect against multiple HPV types.

For this reason, more complex vaccines against HPV have now been developed. Glaxo-SmithKline (Cervarix®) have developed a bivalent vaccine against HPV 16 and 18, which is currently available. Merck has also developed a quadrivalent vaccine against HPV 16, 18, 6 and 11 (Gardasil®). It is hoped that this will immunise against approximately 70% of cervical cancers in developed countries as well as conferring immunity against vulval and vaginal cancers. Furthermore, by including HPV 6 and 11 it should prevent 90% of genital warts (See Box 11.1).

Gardasil® is administered intramuscularly in a three-dose regimen requiring vaccination at months one, two and six. As with other VLP vaccines it was found to be well tolerated, with injection site reaction and fever the most commonly reported adverse events. Within Australia it is approved for use in females aged 9 to 26 years and males aged 9 to 15 years. Cervarix® has also now been licensed in Europe and Australia. It is to be used in the UK national vaccination programme which will begin in September 2008.

HPV vaccination – immunising the population

Although long-term data is still being collected from the early vaccine studies, there is now considered to be adequate clinical information to support the expansion of HPV vaccination nationally. Attempts have been made to examine the broader implications of general vaccination using computer models. One such study indicated that if 100% of adolescents were immunised with an HPV 16 and 18 vaccine which had 98% efficacy there is the potential to reduce cervical cancer by 50% (Goldie et al. 2003).

Similarly, pharmacoeconomic models have been used to assess the financial implications of a vaccination policy. For example, it has been calculated that within the USA the cost of treating cervical cancer exceeded $4.5 billion in 1994 – that is greater than the cost of any other single sexually transmitted infection with the exception of HIV (Lowndes 2006). Sanders and Taira (2003) estimated that vaccinating the entire US population of 12-year-old girls would prevent more than 200,000 HPV infections, 100,000 abnormal Pap tests and 3300 cases of cervical cancer. Life expectancy would be improved by 2.8 days or 4.0 quality-adjusted life days at a cost of $246 relative to current practices. This would include the cost of a booster vaccination every ten years. Similar life expectancy improvements have been reported for vaccination against measles, mumps and rubella, with each saving 2.7, 3.0 and 0.3 life-days, respectively (Frazer et al. 2006).

Kulasingham and Meyers (2003) also evaluated the economic impact of a vaccine for HPV and concluded that its cost-effectiveness would be significantly enhanced if it facilitated economies in cervical screening programmes. As discussed in Chapter 8, cervical screening is the least efficient in younger women because the detection of transient lesions is greatest. Furthermore, screening does not appear to be as effective against the relatively rare aggressive cancers that do occur in younger women. The findings in this study suggest that a vaccine which reduces the incidence of oncogenic HPV types during the peak ages of infection (generally the late teens and early twenties) could be economically attractive, particularly if it allowed for a delay in commencing cervical screening.

Box 11.1 Genital warts (Condyloma accuminata)

Each year 1 million new cases of genital warts are diagnosed (within the USA), two thirds of which are in women. The annual incidence of genital warts is 1–2% of the sexually active population (3–6 million people) (Scheinfeld and Lehman 2006). Although associated with HPV 6 and 11, patients with genital warts may be infected with numerous HPV sub-types. HPV sub-type has no bearing on treatment.

Genital warts are almost always spread by sexual contact. Approximately 70% of individuals who have sexual contact with an infected partner develop genital warts. The incubation period of HPV varies from three weeks to eight months, with a mean of 2–3 months after initial contact. The rate of sub-clinical infection is thought to be as high as 40%. Approximately 80% of individuals with genital warts are aged 17–33 years (Scheinfeld and Lehman 2006).

Genital warts can occur on the penis, groin, cervix, urethral meatus, vagina, anus, pubis, and oral cavity. Their contour can be flat, ceribriform, or verrucous and their colour white, skin coloured, pink, purple, red, or brown (Scheinfeld and Lehman 2006). Differential diagnosis could include neoplasm, molluscum contagiosum, condyloma lata, fibroepitheliomas and pearly penile papules (Kodner and Nasraty 2004). Although often asymptomatic, internal warts may cause discomfort, pain, bleeding or difficulty with intercourse, especially with larger, cauliflower-like lesions. Urethral lesions may impair urination (Kodner and Nasraty 2004).

Diagnosis of anal and genital warts is predominantly clinical. Biopsy, viral typing, acetowhite staining and other diagnostic measures are not routinely required. The goal of treatment is clearance of visible warts (Kodner and Nasraty 2004).

A number of treatment options are available and choice of therapy is based on the number, size, site and morphology of lesions as well as patient preference, cost, convenience, adverse effects and clinician experience (Kodner and Nasraty 2004). Unfortunately, after therapy recurrence is a problem, occurring within three months in 25–67% of cases. Recurrences are often at sites of previous genital warts and have been attributed to long-lived cells at the site of previous clearance that then reactivate (Scheinfeld and Lehman 2006).

Choice of treatment is reminiscent of therapy for CIN (Chapter 2) and can similarly be differentiated into destructive and excisional strategies. Destructive approaches involve the use of cytotoxic agents, laser or cryotherapy techniques.

Podophyllin and podophyllotoxin are topical cytotoxic agents, the former of which is applied in the doctor's office and the latter is applied by the patient. Trichloracetic acid (TCA) can also be used to treat genital warts. Imiquimod is a patient-applied immunomodulatory topical treatment. Treatment with 5FU cream (Efudex) is no longer recommended because of severe local side effects and teratogenicity (Kodner and Nasraty 2004).

Cryotherapy involves application of nitrous oxide or liquid nitrogen (–196°C) to genital warts, inducing dermal and vascular damage, and eventually causing cellular necrosis.

Excisional strategies involve either basic surgical removal or sometimes the employment of electrical techniques such as LEEP.

All treatment methods are associated with discomfort, erythema, epithelial erosion, ulceration at the treatment site, depigmentation and scarring (Kodner and Nasraty 2004). Local or even general anaesthesia may be required and treatment should be confined to the affected skin to minimise side effects. Clearly the therapy should not be worse than the disease (Ting and Dytoc 2004).

The cost per successful treatment course is US$200–300 for podofilox, cryotherapy, electrodessication, surgical excision, laser treatment and LEEP (Kodner and Nasraty 2004). The response rates for all treatments is 60% to 90% with a placebo effect of 0% to 50% (Kodner and Nasraty 2004).

Thus, within the scientific community the argument for immunising the population would appear to be compelling. However, in order for a vaccination programme to be successful, scientific approval alone is not enough. It is also necessary that it is perceived as useful and acceptable by the general public.

Unfortunately, there is widespread ignorance about HPV and its role in cervical cancer which renders much of the population ill informed about the utility of an HPV vaccine. In one study, 70% of adult women indicated that they had never heard of HPV. In this study even women who have been diagnosed with an abnormal Pap test or undergone a colposcopy do not necessarily understand the link between cervical dysplasia and HPV infection (Pitts and Clarke 2002).

In part this lack of understanding could be explained by poor media coverage of HPV and its links with cancer (Calloway et al. 2006). That said, one message which has been successfully conveyed to the public by the media is the association between cervical cancer and sexually transmitted disease. Indeed, it has been argued that this has probably been somewhat overplayed, resulting in unnecessary stigma being attached to a diagnosis of cervix cancer (Helmerhorst and Meijer 2002). This could ultimately compromise the acceptability of a vaccine – particularly because the optimal time at which to immunise with a preventative vaccine is prior to exposure to the virus. In the case of HPV, this means before commencing sexual activity, which effectively means vaccinating children.

The exact age at which sexual activity begins naturally varies between different individuals and in different cultures. This was illustrated by the Youth Risk Behaviour Survey (2006) which found that the proportion of high school students engaging in sexual intercourse was 41% amongst Caucasians, 68% amongst African Americans and 51% amongst Hispanics (Kimmel 2006). Whilst the overall average age of commencing sexual intercourse in the USA is thought to be around 16 years old (Family Health International 2003) it is also important to remember that many adolescents engage in other forms of potentially infective sexual activity long before this.

It has thus been suggested that in order to have the most protective effect, immunisation should be given to young adolescents at no later than 11 to 12 years of age (Mays and Zimet 2004). A school-based vaccination programme is likely to be the most efficient and cost-effective way to achieve this (Lowndes 2006).

In order to function effectively such an immunisation programme would require the co-operation and consent of a number of parties, including school governors, teachers, parents, health professionals and of course the adolescents themselves. Each of these groups is in turn influenced by a number of factors related to their knowledge about HPV, and their beliefs about vaccines. The literature to date has mainly concentrated on the role of three of the groups: the adolescent, the parent and the health professional.

HPV vaccination – the decision-making triangle

The adolescent

Although in legal terms still a minor, adolescents are clearly old enough to have their own view about vaccination – a view which will be largely influenced by peers, teachers, the media and their parents.

According to the health belief model (Hochbaum 1958), the individual's decision to accept vaccination involves balancing the risk of having the injection against the perceived benefit of preventing the disease. This involves a risk assessment on the part of the adolescent, who needs to determine their likelihood of contracting HPV or, more importantly, cervical cancer.

Just as knowledge of HPV and cervical cancer has been shown to be limited in adults, so it is amongst adolescents. Dell et al. (2000) questioned 523 high school students in

Canada about HPV and found only 13% had heard of it. Furthermore, only one in three of the students considered themselves to be at risk of acquiring an STD. For this reason the risk perception of acquiring the disease is likely to be low. To quote Kimmel (2006): 'Adolescents seldom consider the future consequences of their actions, and it is unlikely that the fear of HPV and cervical cancer would change their sexual behavior, especially when cervical cancer may take years to develop.'

It is therefore a little surprising that there are also a number of studies indicating a high level of acceptability of vaccination amongst adolescents (Rosenthal 2005). It is possible that this could be an indication of the development of a more open attitude to discussing sexual health with young people – possibly in response to the high media profile of HPV vaccines. In the past, studies have indicated that a disappointingly low proportion of adolescents discuss sexual health matters with their doctor. Although Dell et al. (2000) found 82% of students had seen a doctor in the previous year, only 58% of the sample had time to talk with them alone and only 21% discussed sexual issues. Among sexually experienced students only 44% had talked with a doctor or a nurse about sexual health.

Introduction of HPV immunisation into schools would require discussion of sexual matters at an early age and it has been argued that this may have significant health benefits for adolescents (Sturm et al. 2005). Young people could be better assisted in the development of decision-making skills concerning other aspects of sexual health. For example, health professionals could provide guidance in adolescents' evaluation of health-related information encountered in the media and on the Internet, help them to assess the pros and cons of a health behaviour, and teach them to ask relevant questions.

Parental endorsement is also likely to be a key factor in vaccine uptake amongst adolescents. Conversely, some adolescents will not wish their parents to be aware of their level of sexual activity, and this in turn could prevent them from accepting vaccination. Parental attitudes towards vaccination are similarly influenced by a number of factors, some of which are discussed below.

The parent

Some adults find the very concept of offering HPV vaccination to adolescents distasteful. They consider HPV-related education to be inappropriate, feeling that it promotes under-age sexual activity, condones sexual promiscuity and reflects a general decline in morality (Frazer et al. 2006). People with such a view are likely to be resistant on all levels to the implementation of an HPV vaccination programme.

Fortunately these individuals appear to be in the minority. Davis et al. (2004) surveyed almost 600 parents or guardians of adolescents regarding HPV vaccination. Initially, 55% responded favourably to an HPV vaccine for their child – a number which increased to approximately 75% after a brief educational intervention. Rosenthal (2005), in a recent review of the literature, concludes that HPV vaccination is highly acceptable to parents because the protection it affords against cancer and related HPV diseases outweigh the potential risks.

Parental attitudes towards vaccination are obviously coloured by a number of important influences, with the media once again playing an important part (see Box 11.2). Social factors would also appear to be highly relevant. Streefland et al. (1999) looked at immunisation in a number of different countries and found that societal norms were very persuasive behavioural prompts. They identified a phenomenon which they described as 'bandwagoning' whereby parents choose to vaccinate their child simply because everyone else does: 'people have their children vaccinated because everybody does so and it seems the normal thing to do . . . because it is what good mothers seem to do.' (Streefland et al. 1999, quoted in Sturm et al. 2005)

In the same way that adolescents are influenced by parental attitudes to vaccination, so parents are influenced by their health providers. In one study of infant vaccination more than 50% of parents cited the fact that their doctor was participating in the study as a

---

Box 11.2 Vaccine education and the role of the media

Although 93% of parents in the USA regard vaccination as safe, there remains an active minority who are anti-vaccination. These people express views suggesting that children receive more vaccinations than are good for them or that vaccinations weaken the immune system (Kimmel 2006). Indeed, for many years vaccinations have been blamed for a number of medical conditions that elude clear causal explanations. For example, in the late nineteenth century the smallpox vaccine was falsely linked to syphilis and leprosy. More recently, vaccinations have been put forth as possible causes of sudden infant death syndrome and autism (Sturm et al. 2005).

Such health messages have traditionally been fuelled by the media and not necessarily well supported by evidence. For example, in the 1970s negative press surrounding the pertussis vaccination in the UK led to a fall in coverage from 81% in 1974 to 31% in 1976. This was followed by a spike in pertussis rates (Gangarosa et al. 1998). Similarly, in Sweden, following reports that pertussis was no longer a serious illness, vaccine coverage fell from 90% in 1974 to 12% in 1979. Disease rates subsequently multiplied thirty-fold (Gangarosa et al. 1998). The media has a significant influence on the public and health professionals alike.

In their analysis of anti-vaccination print coverage in the 1990s, Leask and Chapman (1998) identified eight recurrent subtexts or themes, including 'cover-up' (a conspiracy to withhold information from the public), 'totalitarianism' (vaccination as a threat to individual civil liberties and an excessive exertion of governmental control) and 'poisons' (vaccines as toxic agents composed of dangerous chemicals). White Caucasian women with orientation towards alternative medicine are the most likely group to refuse vaccination (Sturm et al. 2005).

The role of the media is likely to be very significant in the success of an HPV vaccination campaign. It has the potential to disseminate HPV-associated information which might increase the perceived utility of a vaccine and reduce the emotiveness associated with the 'sexually transmitted disease' aspect of HPV. Unfortunately, to date it has failed to meet this challenge. Generally, media coverage has been neither comprehensive nor accurate (Calloway et al. 2006). In their analysis of the media coverage of HPV vaccination Calloway et al. made the following assessment: 'If only relying on newspapers for information, readers could get an incomplete picture or fail to understand the complexity of the association between HPV infection and cervical cancer. This, in turn, could influence the public's willingness to accept a vaccine.'

---

reason for their involvement (Langley et al. 1998). Another study of hepatitis B vaccination in adolescence found that the best predictor of parental acceptance was the belief that vaccination was regarded as important by the provider (Rosenthal et al. 1999)

These findings suggest that the success of immunisation programmes will to a large extent rest with health care providers, who must be willing and able to discuss STD vaccination. Unfortunately, a number of studies indicate that primary health care providers are reluctant to discuss sexuality-related issues with adolescents and their parents (Mays and Zimet 2004). The role of health professionals in HPV vaccination is discussed below.

The health professional

The attitudes of health professionals to STD vaccination has been the subject of much recent research and, encouragingly, many studies report a high degree of acceptability (Ault 2006). Raley et al. (2004) found that 79% of fellows of the American College of Obstetricians and Gynecologists would accept an HPV preventative vaccine as part of their practice – particularly if endorsed by a professional organisation such as ACOG, the American Academy of Pediatrics, the Committee on Immunization Practices, or the American Academy of Family Physicians.

Box 11.3 Some questions before starting an HPV vaccination programme (after Lowndes and Gill 2005, with permission)

(1) Does the vaccine cover the HPV type in that country?
(2) Will the vaccine help confer immunity against other HPV types?
(3) Will a vaccination programme be acceptable to adolescents and their parents?
(4) Will a vaccination programme involve boys too?
(5) When will boosters be given, if ever?
(6) How will the programme impact existing screening programmes?
(7) Will the vaccine have any effect on pre-existing HPV infections and should it involve older, sexually active adults?
(8) Are there any population sub-groups who should be particularly targeted?
(9) What will the cost and cost-effectiveness be?

Mays and Zimet (2004) also found AAP endorsement to be an important factor in health professional promotion of vaccination. Another important factor was the age of the adolescent patient. Health professionals appear to find it easier to endorse vaccination amongst older individuals. Also, those health professionals who had greater clinical involvement with adolescents tended to be more willing to recommend vaccination to the parents of those adolescents.

Prophylactic vaccines – where do we go from here?

Any large-scale vaccine programme is clearly linked with significant logistical and practical problems. Furthermore, in the absence of mature data from the vaccine studies a number of important clinical questions remain unanswered. Some of these unanswered questions are listed in Box 11.3 and discussed in greater detail below.

Who should be vaccinated?

It has already been established that the primary target group is young adolescent females. However, is there any benefit vaccinating subjects after they have been exposed to the virus? For example, is it helpful to vaccinate sexually active women who have an existing HPV infection? These are questions which have not been fully answered by the research. Nevertheless, in women who are already infected it is at least feasible that the vaccine could reduce the spread of infection from one genital site to others, and possibly even have a therapeutic effect against established lesions (Lowy and Schiller 2006). If there is any benefit in vaccinating women who have had sexual activity this is likely to be inversely proportional to the degree of sexual activity they have had (Lowy and Schiller 2006).

The next question is: should males be vaccinated as well as females? We know that some males carry oncogenic strains of HPV. We also know that they can carry other strains of the virus which can result in debilitating and unpleasant genital warts (see Box 11.1). Finally, it would also appear that the immunogenicity of the HPV vaccines is the same in men as it is in women (Asif et al. 2006).

Mathematical models have been used to estimate the reduction in HPV prevalence that would be achieved by vaccinating males as well as females (Lowndes 2006). They have varied in their findings but some have predicted it to be more effective at reducing HPV infection than vaccinating women alone. One study concluded that by vaccinating both men and women there would be a 44% decrease in the prevalence of the vaccine-HPV types, as opposed to a 30% decrease from vaccinating just women (Hughes et al. 2002).

Box 11.4 Anal cancer and HPV

It has been known for some time that men who have sex with men (MSM) appear to have a significantly higher incidence of anal cancer than the general population. The incidence of anal cancer amongst women is 1.3 per 100,000 and men 1.2 per 100,000 (Workman 2003). However, amongst homosexuals this number rises to 25–37 per 100,000. This rate is comparable with the rate of cervical cancer amongst women prior to the implementation of screening programmes (Klenke and Palefsky 2003)

There are a number of similarities between anal and cervical cancer. Both diseases are HPV related and both are associated with an identifiable 'pre-malignant' phase. In cervical cancer this is cervical intra-epithelial neoplasia (CIN) and in anal cancer it is anal intra-epithelial neoplasia (AIN). AIN generally arises at the proximal part of the anal canal, known as the dentate line. This is a transitional zone where the glandular mucosa of the rectum meets the squamous mucosa of the anus. Also, as with cervical carcinoma, anal carcinomas are mainly associated with squamous histology.

Similarly, presenting symptoms are subtle with both cancers, meaning that in many instances anal cancer is not diagnosed until it is at a relatively advanced stage. Although half the patients presenting with anal cancer will have a mass, only 30% will have the sensation of a mass. The larger the size of the mass, the poorer the prognosis. Other early symptoms are pain (30%), bleeding (45%) and a history of warts (50% of homosexuals) (Ryan et al. 2000).

Since the 1970s, the treatment of choice for cancer of the anus has changed from surgery with abdominoperineal resection to chemoradiotherapy. The prognosis and quality of life of patients has consequently improved considerably. The five-year survival rate for people with anal cancer is 53%. The cancer specific survival rate is estimated to be 84% (Maggard and Beanes 2003).

The presence of HIV significantly increases the risk of contracting anal cancer. Indeed, all HIV-infected individuals, are at risk for developing anal cancer – not just men who have sex with men. Amongst persons living with HIV/AIDS, the relative risk of developing squamous cell anal cancer is thought to be approximately thirty-fold higher than for uninfected persons (Frisch et al. 2001). Homosexual males with AIDS have an even higher risk – 84 times higher than that of the general population (Melbye et al.1994). For this reason it has been argued that screening programmes for anal cancer should be implemented among men who have sex with men, or at least amongst HIV-positive individuals (Goldie 1999).

If vaccines are effective in both sexes, it was the consensus of a recent worldwide panel of experts that *any* sexually active individual should be given the opportunity to become vaccinated (Frazer et al. 2006).

Ultimately, the decision of whether or not to include males in vaccination campaigns is likely to be made on a financial basis and the financial benefit of vaccinating boys is questionable. One study estimated the reduction in cervical cancer cases to be 95.4% if just women are vaccinated compared with 98.8% if boys are vaccinated, but at a substantially greater cost (Taira 2004 in Frazer et al.). Another option could be just to vaccinate 'high risk' groups such as men who have sex with men. It is more likely that this would be financially viable in view of the much higher risk of this group acquiring HPV-related disease (see Box 11.4).

How often should vaccinations be given?

To be of maximum benefit a vaccine should confer long-term immunity – this is particularly important within third world countries, where cost and logistical factors make administering boosters problematic. However, gathering the necessary long-term data about the duration of immunity takes time. For example, hepatitis B vaccines have been available for nearly two decades and yet the need for boosters has been debated as recently as 2000 (Jacob et al. 2005).

Although it has been established that vaccination brings about immune responses which are substantially higher than HPV infection alone, whether this leads to an increased duration of immunity is not known. Some studies have shown that antibody responses can be detected nearly four years after vaccination, but there is not long enough follow-up data to know whether they endure for longer than this. Furthermore, the level of antibody which is necessary to give protection against future infection is also unknown (Frazer et al. 2006). These are issues which can only be answered as further follow-up analyses are performed and the existing data matures.

Will vaccines be effective for other HPV types which are not included in the vaccine?

Because the currently available HPV vaccines are only effective against limited oncogenic HPV types (16 and 18) there are still a large number of other HPV sub-groups which are not covered. Work is currently under way to modify vaccines to include more HPV types. Once again, this is of particular relevance in developing countries where different strains of HPV are more prevalent. Although HPV 16 and 18 are the predominant oncogenic HPV strains in Europe, Asia and North America, in other countries this is not the case. For example, in Africa HPV 45 is more common and in South America HPV 31. A vaccine containing 16, 18, 45, 31, 33, 52 would theoretically prevent 87% of types worldwide but the cost of this would need to be balanced against the benefit it would bring (Lowndes 2006).

Assuming that programmes are instigated with only existing vaccines (to HPV 16 and 18) there could be two possible sequeles:

(1) Instead of developing cancer as a result of HPV 16 or 18 infection, women will be susceptible to development of 'replacement' cervical cancer. This means that the other, strains of HPV would replace 16 and 18 in causing infection and dysplasia. It would possibly take longer to acquire infection with these other subtypes because HPV 16 and 18 are known to be the most oncogenic strains.
(2) There may be cross-immunity between vaccines. It would appear that certain HPV vaccines are capable of inducing immune responses against other HPV types (Kadish and Einstein 2005). This has been noted specifically between strains of HPV which are similar (e.g. types 16, 31 and 33 or type 18 and 45) (Lowndes 2006). Boursarghin et al. (2002) demonstrated that as many as 40% of VLP vaccine recipients developed low titre neutralising antibodies against HPV types other than those included in the vaccine.

Will the HPV mutate so that it is no longer susceptible to a preventative vaccine?

Because of the way HPV uses the replication machinery of the host cell to propagate its genome it has low 'error' rates, with the result that it appears to be a very stable virus over time. It is thus thought to be unlikely that mutant strains of the virus will make the vaccine redundant.

How will vaccination programmes affect current screening programmes?

It is important that vaccination programmes are set up in parallel with existing screening programmes and are complementary to then. Currently, 50% of cervical cancer cases arise in women who do not attend screening (Nuovo et al. 2001, Lowndes 2006). It is to be hoped that vaccination of such non-attenders would significantly impact cervical cancer incidence.

An effective vaccination campaign could affect both the frequency and the type of screening available.

(1) Frequency of screening
    It is to be hoped that vaccination will ultimately reduce the requirement to screen women as regularly as today, although this may not occur for quite some time. In view of the existence of other HPV strains which are not covered by current vaccines, and until further data is forthcoming regarding the ongoing levels of immunity that vaccination confers, the general recommendation is that women should be encouraged to adhere to the general screening recommendations for their country (Frazer et al. 2006).

(2) Method of screening
    If, as anticipated, vaccination does significantly reduce the population prevalence of HPV 16 and 18 it could be that HPV testing rather than cervical cytology will become the primary screening tool. This has the potential to decrease screening costs and possibly also improve the performance of screening programmes (Lowndes 2006)

Who will fund the vaccination programmes in the developed world?

This will vary according to national policy. Gardasil® has been licensed by the European Commission and FDA. In the USA it has been included in the US vaccines for Children Program that provides free immunisation to those who need them and the US Department of Health is also considering government funding. The Australian Government is currently providing the new vaccine free to all women and girls aged between 12 and 26 through the National HPV Vaccination Program. In the UK the Joint Committee on Vaccination and Immunisation (JCVI) has recommended the use of HPV vaccines and vaccination of 12–13-year-old girls is scheduled to begin in September 2008.

Implications for the developing world

As illustrated in Chapter 8, cervical cancer is a huge problem within the developing world and the problems of immunising the population are equally enormous. Whilst implementation of a vaccination programme in third world countries encompasses many of the considerations already discussed, there are also a number of additional factors related to logistical, political, cultural and climatic considerations.

Most successful vaccination campaigns have been realised in countries in which there is already a functioning immunisation programme which has good supplies and information systems, well-trained providers, good quality control mechanisms, strong public education programmes, free or low-cost services, effective supervision and regular audits (Frazer et al. 2006). Many developing countries lack the resources, infrastructure and supplies to sustain such a vaccine programme. Cooperation between government and international organisations such as the World Health Organisation (WHO) and Global Alliance for Vaccines and Immunization (GAVI) will be crucial to the success of vaccination programmes within third world countries (Roden and Wu 2006).

Uptake of immunisation within the developing world is often extremely poor. For example, after years of setting up and substantial international financial backing, coverage of the six childhood vaccinations is reported to be as low as 30% in some developing countries (Jacob et al. 2005); 40% of children are though not to have been vaccinated against measles and more than 50% of the children in sub-Saharan Africa in 1999 had not received the DPT3 vaccination (Jacob et al. 2005). The addition of a new vaccine will challenge already stretched third world health resources even further.

Targeting adolescents for vaccination is also likely to be problematic. Although a school-based programme makes sense in the developed nations, large proportions of children in developing nations do not attend school. For example, in India (where the cervical cancer rate is 35 per 100,000), less than 50% of school-aged girls attend school in some states (IIPS 2000). Furthermore, in developing countries girls often leave school early because of marriage or a need to earn an income.

Possibilities for cheaper vaccination strategies are being explored for use in the developing world. For example, 'needle-free' vaccines are likely to be easier to implement than widespread injections. Recent studies have shown that both HPV 16 and 18 VLPs are immunogenic when administered orally (Gerber et al. 2001). It is also possible that vaccines could be developed within E. coli cells rather than the more costly insect or yeast cells which are currently used (Roden and Wu 2006). The development of vaccines which are stable at ambient temperatures would be enormously useful in resource poor areas and is currently under investigation (Roden and Wu 2006).

Will vaccines be effective amongst immunocompromised people?

It has already been mentioned that HPV-associated disease is a particular problem for the immunosuppressed, such as people with HIV/AIDS or transplant recipients on immunosuppressive drugs (see Chapter 1). HPV prophylaxis could potentially be very important for these patients. At this time it is unclear how they would respond to a vaccine, and whether additional boosters would be necessary. The issue is not so much the safety of the vaccine, (the vaccine is assumed to be safe because it does not contain the oncogenic parts of the virus), but rather its efficacy.

Most HIV positive patients do appear to seroconvert following vaccination, although response strongly correlates with CD4 counts (Roden and Wu 2006). Possibly higher vaccine doses and more frequent boosters would be required for this population. Furthermore, immunodeficient patients often suffer from cancers arising from the less common HPV types which are not covered by the currently available vaccines. Finally, many HIV positive patients will have pre-existing HPV infections, reducing the likelihood of success with a prophylactic vaccine (Roden and Wu 2006).

Therapeutic vaccines

A therapeutic vaccine is one which is used to *treat* a disease by somehow 'alerting' the immune system to an established pathogen or malignancy. Prophylactic vaccines are in some ways simpler than therapeutic ones because they need only raise an immune response sufficient to limit infection and prevent clinical disease. A therapeutic vaccine must elicit an immune response that can clear an already established infection, necessitating making the immune system do something which it has failed to do in the primary infection. In other words, the therapeutic vaccine has to 'do better than nature' (Jansen and Shaw 2004).

Although HPV vaccines have been developed which are capable of inducing humoural and cell-mediated immunity in cervical cancer, none has yet demonstrated efficacy in eliminating cervical dysplasia, cancer or genital warts. In some ways the vaccines have not yet adequately mimicked critical aspects of a curative immune response (Lowy and Schiller 2006).

Therapeutic vaccines may be manufactured from a whole tumour cell, a protein from a tumour associated antigen, protein fragments (i.e. peptides) or lysates (broken membranes of a tumour cell) (King 2004). There are two types – autologous and allogeneic.

Autologous vaccines are patient specific. They are made using the patient's own tumour cells. Allogeneic vaccines can be regarded as 'off the shelf' and can be used for any patient (King 2004).

Most therapeutic vaccines consist of a vaccine target (the antigen against which an immune response is sought) combined with a carrier protein and possibly an 'adjuvant'. This is an agent which is added to the vaccine as a further 'boost' to the immune system.

Because a therapeutic vaccine must attack every infected cell regardless of its stage in the life cycle, in the context of cervical cancer, targeting the gene products of E6 and E7 has been found to be effective. These gene products are present in most HPV-infected cells because they are 'early' proteins, expressed soon after the virus has invaded the host (Jansen and Shaw 2004).

Therapeutic vaccines remain experimental in the treatment of cervical cancer – and indeed for all cancers. Whilst the concept is an attractive one, the fact that no therapeutic vaccines have yet been approved by the FDA suggests that it is a more complex approach than it appears. Although the Canadian authorities have approved one therapeutic vaccine (Melacine®) for the treatment of stage IV melanoma, it had a response rate of less than 10% when compared with conventional melanoma chemotherapy (King 2004). The reason for its approval, however, was its low level of toxicity. It is this aspect of vaccine therapy which motivates the continued search for its clinical application.

Conclusion

The development of preventative vaccines for cervical cancer is likely to impact enormously on the prevalence of the disease within developed countries and it is to be hoped that in the future it will eradicate it completely. In the interim, logistical problems regarding the implementation of vaccination schemes have to be addressed. The potential benefit of vaccination within the developing world is enormous, but so are the organisational and cultural issues associated with vaccination campaigns. Therapeutic vaccines are still largely experimental and their role in the management of the disease is yet to be seen.

Frequently asked questions

(1) Should I have the vaccine?
    The vaccine is most likely to be effective if given before sexual activity has begun and therefore is currently being offered to young women (i.e. in their teens and early twenties). It may also have benefit after sexual activity has commenced.
(2) Am I at high risk?
    Certain factors do put women at high risk of acquiring HPV infection, such as multiple sexual partners. Other factors seem to increase the likelihood of the infection progressing to cancer (e.g. smoking, immunosuppression). Vaccination will be offered to all women of relevant age regardless of risk factors when implemented as part of a national campaign.
(3) My mother/grandmother had cervical cancer – does that increase my risk?
    No, there does not appear to be any familial link with cervix cancer.
(4) What are the side effects of the vaccine?
    VLP vaccines are associated with mild to negligible toxicities. The patient product information with Gardasil® states that its toxicities are: injection site reactions; fever; hypersensitivity including bronchospasm; dizziness, syncope; GI upset: http://www.merck.com/product/usa/pi_circulars/g/gardasil/gardasil_ppi.pdf (accessed 25/6/07)
(5) How long does the vaccine last for?
    This is not yet known. The current recommendation for Gardasil® is a three-injection course (second injection at three months and third at six months). There is no current recommendation for a booster.

(6) What does it cost?
This will vary between countries. In some it will be given free as part of an immuni-sation programme. In others there will be a charge.

(7) Where do I go for it?
Your primary health care doctor will be able to guide you.

(8) Will I still need regular cervical smears?
Yes, the vaccine will not offer 100% guarantee of preventing an HPV infection because it only contains two high risk HPV subtypes.

(9) I am pregnant. Can I still receive the vaccine?
Vaccination with Gardasil® is not recommended during pregnancy, although if immunisation occurs accidentally during this time it is not considered unsafe. Vacci-nation whilst lactating is considered acceptable (Wain 2007).

(10) If I get the vaccine, should my husband have it too?
Vaccination for males is not currently recommended. Once you have immunity, 'reinfection' by an HPV-carrying partner should not occur (provided it is the same strain of HPV).

Resources

Australian Government Dept Health and Aging: http://www.health.gov.au/cervicalcancer
Merck: www.gardasil.com
GlaxoSmithKlein: http://www.gsk.com.au/products_vaccines_detail.aspx?view=122

References

Asif M, Siddiqui A and Perry CM (2006) Human papillomavirus quadrivalent (types 6, 11, 16, 18) Recombinant Vaccine (Gardasil®). *Drugs*, 66 (9), 1263–1271

Ault K (2006) Vaccines for the prevention of human papillomavirus and associated gynaecologic diseases: a review. *Obstetrical and Gynecological Survey*, 61 (6) Supplement 1, June, S26–S31

Boursarghin L, Combita A and Touze A (2002) Immunization with HPV L1 VLPs induced cross-neutralizing antibodies. In: Twentieth International Papillomavirus Conference, Paris

Calloway C, Jorgensen CM, Saraiya M and Tsui J (2006) A content analysis of news coverage of the HPV vaccine by US newspapers, January 2002–June 2005. *Journal of Women's Health*, 15 (7), 803–809

Center for Diseases Control (2006) Youth Risk Behavior Surveillance – United States, 2005. *Morbidity and Mortality Weekly Report*. Surveillance Summaries 9 June, 55 (SS5): http://www.cdc.gov/mmwr/PDF/SS/SS5505.pdf (accessed 24/1/07)

Chang MH, Chen CJ, Lai MS, et al. (1997) Universal hepatitis B vaccinations in Taiwan and the incidence of hepatocellular carcinoma in children. *New England Journal of Medicine*, 336, 1855–1859

Davis K, Dickman ED, Ferris D, et al. (2004) Human papillomavirus vaccine acceptability among parents of 10- to 15-year-old adolescents. *J Low Genit Tract Dis*, 8, 188–194

Dell DL, Chen H, Ahmad F and Stewart DE (2000) Knowledge about human papillomavirus among adolescents. Obstet Gynecol, 96, 653–656

Family Health International (2003) Reproductive health of young adults: http://www.fhi.org/training/en/modules/ADOL/s1pg15.htm (accessed 24/1/07)

Frazer IH, Cox JT, Mayeaux EJ, et al. (2006) Advances in prevention of cervical cancer and other human papillomavirus-related diseases. *Paediatric Infectious disease Journal*, 25 (2), Supplement, February, S65–S81

Frisch M, Biggar RJ, Engels EA and Goedert JJ (2001) Association of cancer with AIDS-related immunosuppression in adults. *JAMA*, 285,1736–1745

Gangarosa EJ, Galazka AM, Wolfe CR, et al. (1998) Impact of anti-vaccine movements on pertussis control: the untold story. *Lancet*, 351 (9099), 31 Jan, 356–361

Gerber S, Lane C, Brown DM, et al. (2001) Human papillomavirus-like particles are efficient oral immunogens when coadministered with Escherichia coli heat-labile enterotoxin mutant R192G or CpG DNA. *J Virol*, 75, 4752–4760

Goldie SJ, Grima D, Kohli M, Wright TC, Weinstein M and Franco E (2003) A comprehensive natural history model of HPV infection and cervical cancer to estimate the clinical impact of a prophylactic HPV 16/18 vaccine. *Int J Cancer*, 106, 896–904

Goldie SJ, Kuntz KM, Weinstein MC, Freedberg KA, Welton ML and Palefsky JM (1999) The clinical effectiveness and cost-effectiveness of screening for anal squamous intraepithelial lesions in homosexual and bisexual HIV-positive men. *JAMA*, 281, 1822–1829

Helmerhorst TJ and Meijer CJ (2002) Cervical cancer should be considered as a rare complication of oncogenic HPV infection rather than a STD. *International Journal of Gynecological Cancer*, 12 (3), 235–236, May–June

Hochbaum GM (1958) *Public Participation in Medical Screening Programmes: a Sociopsychological Study*. PHS publication number 572, US Government Printing Office, Washington, DC

Hughes JP, Garnett GP and Koutsky L (2002) The theoretical population-level impact of a prophylactic human papilloma virus vaccine. *Epidemiology*, 13, 631–639

International Institute for Population Sciences (IIPS) and ORC MACRO (2000) *National Family Health Survey* (NFHS-2) (1998–1999). IIPS, Mumbai, India

Jacob M, Bradley J and Barone M (2005) Human papillomavirus vaccines: what does the future hold for preventing cervical cancer in resource-poor settings through immunization programs? *Sexually Transmitted Diseases*, 32 (10), 635–640

Jansen KU and Shaw AR (2004) Human papillomavirus vaccines and prevention of cervical cancer. *Annual Review of Medicine*, 55, 319–331

Kadish AS and Einstein MH (2005) Vaccine strategies for human papillomavirus associated cancers. *Current Opinion in Oncology*, 17 (5), 456–461

Kahn JA and Bernstein DI (2005) Human papillomavirus vaccines and adolescents. *Current Opinion on Obstetrics and Gynaecology*, 17, 476–482

Kimmel SS (2006) Practical implementation of HPV vaccines in clinical practice. *Journal of Family Practice*, 55 (Suppl), November, 18–22

King SE (2004) Therapeutic cancer vaccines: an emerging treatment option. *Clinical Journal of Oncology Nursing*, 8 (3), 271–278

Klenke BJ and Palefsky JM (2003) Anal cancer: an HIV-associated cancer. *Haematology/Oncology Clinics of North America*, 17, 859–872

Kodner CM and Nasraty S (2004) Management of genital warts. *American Family Physician*, 70 (12), 15 December, 2335–2342

Koutsky LA, Ault KA, Wheeler CM, et al. (2002) A controlled trial of human papillomavirus type 16 vaccine. *New England Journal of Medicine*, 347, 1645–1651

Kulasingham SL and Myers ER (2003) Potential health and economic impact of adding a human papillomavirus vaccine to screening programs. *JAMA*, 290 (6), 13 August, 781–789

Langley JM, Halperin SA, Mills EL, et al. (1998) Parental willingness to enter a child in a controlled vaccine trial. *Clin Invest Med*, 21, 12–16

Leask J and Chapman S (1998) An attempt to swindle nature: press anti-immunisation reportage 1993–1997. *Aust N Z J Public Health*, 22, 17–26

Lowndes CM (2006) Vaccines for cervical cancer. *Epidemiol Infect*, 134, 1–12

Lowndes CM and Gill ON (2005) Cervical cancer, human papilloma virus and vaccination. *BMJ*, 331, 915–916

Lowy DR and Schiller JT (2006) Prophylactic human papillomavirus vaccines. *Journal of Clinical Investigation* (http://www.jci.org), 116 (5), 1167–1173

Maggard MA and Beanes SR (2003) Anal canal cancer; a population-based reappraisal. *Diseases of the Colon and Rectum*, 17, 354–356

Mahdavi A and Bradley JM (2005) Vaccines against human papillomavirus and cervical cancer; promises and challenges. *Oncologist*, 10, 528–538

Mays R and Zimet G (2004) Recommending STI vaccination to parents of adolescents: the attitudes of nurse practitioners. *Journal of the American Sexually Transmitted Diseases Association*, 31 (7), 428–432

Melbye M, Cote T, Kessler L, et al. (1994) A high incidence of anal cancer among AIDs patients. The AIDS/Cancer Working Group. *Lancet*, 343, 636–639

Nuovo J, Melnikow J and Howell LP (2001) New tests for cervical cancer screening. *American Family Physician*, 64, 780–786

Parkin DM, Bray F, Ferlay J and Pisani P (2005) Global cancer statistics 2002. *CA Cancer J Clin*, 55, 74–108

Pitts M and Clarke T (2002) Human papillomavirus infections and risks of cervical cancer: what do women know? *Health Education Research*, 17 (6), 706–714

Raley JC, Followwill KA, Zimet GD, et al. (2004) Gynecologists' attitudes regarding human papilloma virus vaccination: a survey of Fellows of the American College of Obstetricians and Gynecologists. *Infect Dis Obstet Gynecol*, 12, 127–133

Roden R and Wu TC (2006) How will HPV vaccine affect cervical cancer? *Nature Reviews/Cancer*, 6, Oct, 753–763

Rosenthal SL, Lewis LM, Succop PA, et al. (1999) College students' attitudes regarding vaccination to prevent genital herpes. *Sex Transm Dis*, 26, 438–443

Rosenthal SL (2005) Protecting their adolescents from harm: parental views on STI vaccination. *J Adolesc Health*, 37, 177–178

Ryan DP, Compton CC and Mayer RJ (2000) Medical progress: carcinoma of the anal canal. *New England Journal of Medicine*, 342 (11), 792–800

Sanders GD and Taira AV (2003) Cost-effectiveness of a potential vaccine for human papillomavirus. *Emerg Infect Dis*, 9, 37–48

Scheinfeld JD and Lehman DS (2006) An evidence-based review of medical and surgical treatment of genital warts. *Dermatology Online Journal*, 12 (3): http://dermatology.cdlib.org/123/reviews/warts/scheinfeld.html (accessed 2/7/07)

Schiffman M and Castle PE (2005) The promise of global cervical cancer prevention. *New England Journal of Medicine*, 353 (20), 2101–2104

Streefland P, Chowdhury AMR and Ramos-Jimenez P (1999) Patterns of vaccination acceptance. *Soc Sci Med*, 49, 1705–1716

Sturm L, Mays R and Zimet G (2005) Parental beliefs and decision-making about child and adolescent immunization: from polio to sexually transmitted infections. *Journal of Developmental and Behavioral Pediatrics*, 26 (6), 441–452

Taira AV (2004) Evaluating human papillomavirus vaccination programs. *Emerg Infect Dis*, 10, 1915–1923

Ting PT and Dytoc MT (2004) Therapy of external anogenital warts and molluscum contagiosum: a literature review. *Dermatologic Therapy*, 17 (1), March, 68–101

Wain G (2007) Gardasil® in the prevention of cervical cancer. *Medicine Today*, 7 (12), 55–57

Workman C (2003) Anal cancer, in Hoy J and Lewin S (eds) *HIV Management in Australasia: a Guide for Clinical Care*. Australian Society for HIV Medicine, Sydney

Youth Risk Behaviour Survey (2006) http://www.cdc.gov/MMWR/PDF/ss/ss5505.pdf accessed 1/7/08

Zimet GD, Perkins SM, Sturm LA, Blair RM, Juliar BE and Mays RM (2005) Predictors of STI vaccine acceptability among parents and their adolescent children. *Journal of Adolescent Health*, 37, 179–186

Index

Note: page numbers in *italics* refer to figures, those in **bold** refer to tables and boxes.

3.